Human Milk *in the* NICU

Policy into Practice

Lois D. W. Arnold, PhD, MPH
Faculty
Healthy Children Project

Adjunct Faculty
Union Institute and University

Program Coordinator
National Commission on Donor Milk Banking
American Breastfeeding Institute
East Sandwich, Massachusetts

JONES AND BARTLETT PUBLISHERS
Sudbury, Massachusetts
BOSTON TORONTO LONDON SINGAPORE

World Headquarters
Jones and Bartlett Publishers
40 Tall Pine Drive
Sudbury, MA 01776
978-443-5000
info@jbpub.com
www.jbpub.com

Jones and Bartlett Publishers
Canada
6339 Ormindale Way
Mississauga, Ontario L5V 1J2
Canada

Jones and Bartlett Publishers
International
Barb House, Barb Mews
London W6 7PA
United Kingdom

Jones and Bartlett's books and products are available through most bookstores and online booksellers. To contact Jones and Bartlett Publishers directly, call 800-832-0034, fax 978-443-8000, or visit our website, www.jbpub.com.

Substantial discounts on bulk quantities of Jones and Bartlett's publications are available to corporations, professional associations, and other qualified organizations. For details and specific discount information, contact the special sales department at Jones and Bartlett via the above contact information or send an email to specialsales@jbpub.com.

The author, editor, and publisher have made every effort to provide accurate information. However, they are not responsible for errors, omissions, or for any outcomes related to the use of the contents of this book and take no responsibility for the use of the products and procedures described. Treatments and side effects described in this book may not be applicable to all people; likewise, some people may require a dose or experience a side effect that is not described herein. Drugs and medical devices are discussed that may have limited availability controlled by the Food and Drug Administration (FDA) for use only in a research study or clinical trial. Research, clinical practice, and government regulations often change the accepted standard in this field. When consideration is being given to use of any drug in the clinical setting, the health care provider or reader is responsible for determining FDA status of the drug, reading the package insert, and reviewing prescribing information for the most up-to-date recommendations on dose, precautions, and contraindications, and determining the appropriate usage for the product. This is especially important in the case of drugs that are new or seldom used.

Production Credits
Publisher: Kevin Sullivan
Acquisitions Editor: Emily Ekle
Acquisitions Editor: Amy Sibley
Associate Editor: Patricia Donnelly
Editorial Assistant: Rachel Shuster
Associate Production Editor: Katie Spiegel
Marketing Manager: Rebecca Wasley
V.P., Manufacturing and Inventory Control: Therese Connell
Composition: Paw Print Media
Cover Design: Kate Ternullo
Cover Image: © Dejan Novakov/Dreamstime.com
Printing and Binding: Malloy, Inc.
Cover Printing: Malloy, Inc.

Library of Congress Cataloging-in-Publication Data
Arnold, Lois D. W.
Human milk in the NICU : policy into practice / Lois D.W. Arnold.
p. ; cm.
Includes bibliographical references and index.
ISBN-13: 978-0-7637-6133-2
ISBN-10: 0-7637-6133-8
1. Neonatal intensive care. 2. Breast milk. 3. Newborn infants—Nutrition. 4. Breastfeeding. I. Title.
[DNLM: 1. Breast Feeding. 2. Intensive Care, Neonatal—organization & administration. 3. Infant Nutritional Physiological Phenomena. 4. Milk Banks—organization & administration. 5. Milk, Human. 6. Mothers—education. WS 125 A755h 2010]
RJ253.5.A76 2010
618.92'01—dc22

2009024156

6048
Printed in the United States of America
13 12 11 10 09 10 9 8 7 6 5 4 3 2 1

Dedication

This book is for all the mothers of preterm and critically ill infants who have shared their NICU journeys with me. May the experiences of future mothers and their preterm and sick infants be more positive as a result of sharing your stories of pain and frustration.

Contents

Preface

Learning I was pregnant on Valentine's Day, 1978, was an unexpected gift and started my journey in the field of maternal and child health. Breastfeeding went swimmingly for Katy and me—we were awash in milk! My sister, a pediatric nurse practitioner, found me a donor milk bank in Honolulu, and I became a donor to the Hawaii Mothers' Milk Bank. Eventually I gave up my other career as a marine biologist, becoming the assistant administrator for the milk bank and earning a master's in public health. Along the way I helped to found the Human Milk Banking Association of North America and later became its executive director for nearly 9 years in the organization's infancy. A move to New England and a private practice as an IBCLC specializing in mothers of premature infants and women returning to work eventually led to my working for Healthy Children Project and becoming part of its faculty. That, in turn, led to a PhD in public health policy from the Union Institute and University.

Throughout my life, I have enjoyed solving puzzles, from crosswords to jigsaws to Sudoku. This book has been similar to the completion of a puzzle because it is a fitting of all the pieces of my professional life over the last 30 years or so into one big picture. It is a distillation of ingredients from research in different but interconnected fields.

Acknowledgments

This project would not have been possible without the support of the American Breastfeeding Institute. The model policies for both NICUs and donor human milk banks originally were created as part of a much larger project. My fellow Healthy Children Project faculty member, Elyse Blair, RN, IBCLC, was the lead in developing the NICU policies, and I was the lead in developing the donor milk banking policies. Each policy went through several reviews and periods for comment. Both sets of policies have been heavily modified for publication in this book.

I am indebted to my doctoral committee at the Union Institute and University, which included UI&U faculty Bethe Hagens, PhD (core) and Marianne Matzo, PhD, RN (second reader); consulting faculty Mary Joyce, PhD, and Kathleen Kendall-Tackett, PhD, IBCLC; peers Kajsa Brimdyr, PhD, and Kate Barnes, PhD; and independent consultant Karin Cadwell, PhD, RN, FAAN, IBCLC. Much of the material on donor human milk banking in this book had its origins in my doctoral dissertation, *Donor Human Milk Banking: Creating Public Heath Policy in the 21st Century.* The strategic plan for donor human milk banking was the centerpiece of the dissertation.

I am also indebted to Kathleen Marinelli, MD, FAAP, FABM, IBCLC, for ongoing consultations during the writing of this book, which provided me with information about the fine points of medical care of preterm infants. I am also grateful to my fellow faculty members from Healthy Children Project, Barbara O'Connor and Cindy Turner-Maffei, who have contributed thoughts and materials throughout the writing process and who have provided support and encouragement. They are enormously appreciated.

I would like to thank my colleague and mentor, Karin Cadwell, Healthy Children Project's director, without whose encouragement, support, and editorial expertise this book would never have come to fruition. She has read every word, occasionally putting chapters of this book higher on her agenda than her own projects. Throughout the process, beginning with my doctoral work, she has been there for me as a true friend and movie buddy and has helped me maintain my sense of humor.

Finally, my daughter, Katy, and my sister, Hannah, have each contributed in their own special ways to this book. They have my undying love and affection.

Part I

Setting the Stage

chapter one

Introduction

Thirty years ago I was fortunate enough to have a healthy baby girl who breastfed on the delivery table. Her skills at breastfeeding greatly exceeded my own, and she established and maintained a milk supply that was in excess of her needs, so I became a donor to a human milk bank that supplied processed, donated milk to premature infants. Over the weeks and months of donating and then becoming paid staff at the milk bank, I learned from the mothers and the babies who were being helped by my milk about the difficulties of having an infant in the neonatal intensive care unit (NICU).

At that time, little emphasis was placed on having the mother supply her own milk; either formula or donor milk from the milk bank was used. Since then the emphasis has shifted to include more mothers in the care and feeding of their babies, and protocols and procedures have been written about the storage and handling of a mother's milk in the NICU. My role has evolved, from the periphery of the NICU as milk bank staff, to a lactation consultant in the community helping mothers of NICU babies maintain their milk supply, to educator and trainer of healthcare providers, including NICU staff, in lactation management including how to help mothers succeed at breastfeeding or supply their own milk for a hospitalized infant.

As I travel around the country teaching, I encounter a wide variation in practice from NICU to NICU. A few have developed protocols and policies for feeding premature infants and caring for them based on the research literature. The majority, I have found, are not developing *evidence-based* policies or protocols. Practice reflects staff competency in implementing protocols and policies. Without policies that reflect best practices and research evidence, NICUs practice in outdated ways, to the detriment of the very infants they are trying to help grow into healthy individuals and to the frustration and discouragement of mothers.

What follows is a case study that will be referred to frequently as the chapters progress. It is a single actual case but is representative of many cases I have heard over the years. Mother after mother, hospital after hospital, the experiences to which I have been privy have been very similar. This book is dedicated to these mothers in the hope that the things that can and should change in the NICU will do so and future mothers like Bonnie will have a very different experience.

On December 23, 2007, at noon, Bonnie, a 28-year-old pregnant woman entered the emergency room (ER) of a community hospital with symptoms of cramping and bleeding. The physician in the ER performed a pelvic exam to determine the status of the cervix and then ordered an ultrasound to visualize the placenta. The technician had difficulty visualizing the head of the fetus with the external ultrasound and decided to perform an internal ultrasound, a procedure that increased the amount and severity of the cramping and bleeding. Bonnie reported this to the physician and nurse in the ER and they assured her that everything was fine; that the placenta was intact and her cervix was not dilated. The physician ordered the nurse to start an IV, informing the mother that she would be given pain medication and sent home. No arrangements were made to move the mother to the hospital's obstetric unit. However, the on-call obstetrician briefly visited Bonnie in the ER, warning her that she should report any illicit drug use right now because both she and the baby would be tested for drugs and the staff would find out if she were using drugs. Bonnie informed the obstetrician that she was not using any illicit drugs. The obstetrician's response was that drug use was associated with many premature births.

Bonnie started having intense pain in her back and began to perspire. She asked the nurse if she could go to the bathroom. Unassisted, in the bathroom, she realized something was not right. She returned to the ER bed and called the nurse, saying that she very concerned about how she was feeling. The nurse reassured her that everything was fine. Bonnie said she felt as though she had to push, and the nurse replied, "Oh, honey, you don't have to push. You're not that far along." With Bonnie's repeated insistence, the nurse examined the mother only to discover that the baby's head was crowning. The nurse called for the doctor, but before the doctor arrived, Bonnie delivered the male fetus with the amniotic sac intact. The time was approximately 3:30 p.m., more than 3 hours after Bonnie had arrived at the ER.

The baby lay on the ER bed for minutes until the doctor returned. Bonnie asked what was happening and the doctor told her that she had had a miscarriage. Then Bonnie heard her baby cry. Although staff from the respiratory therapy department were then called, they were unequipped to intubate the newborn, who was transported to the hospital's newborn nursery. There, the staff was again unprepared to care for this very critical baby. It was estimated that he was born at approximately 24 weeks' gestation, weighing 865 grams. A transport team was called from another facility in the area with a level 3 NICU. Due to bad weather, it took the transport team over 2 hours to arrive and get the infant stable enough for ambulance transport.

Bonnie was admitted to the maternity unit, where she told the staff that she wanted to provide breastmilk for her son. She also told the nurses that she knew that she would need to start pumping before 6 hours postpartum to ensure an optimal milk supply. The nursing staff promised to bring Bonnie an electric breast pump. However, by 6.5 hours postpartum, she was still without a pump. One of Bonnie's family members arrived to visit and began advocating for the pump delivery. Finally the pump arrived with assurance from the nurse that when Bonnie called to say that she was ready to begin using the pump, a nurse would come to instruct her. However, after multiple unanswered calls to the nurses' station, the family member helped Bonnie initiate pumping her breasts.

Bonnie was not ever encouraged by the maternity staff regarding frequent pumping. Instead, she was told by the nurses that rest was more important than pumping her breasts. When Bonnie was discharged the next morning, the discharge nurses present told her that she would probably not be able to locate an electric pump in the community for several days because of the holidays and the hospital had no pump to lend her. Bonnie's discharge education regarding lactation consisted of one sentence, "Be sure to wear a good supportive bra 24 hours a day so that you don't get engorged."

Following her hospital discharge, Bonnie drove 2 hours to be with her baby. She was determined to provide breastmilk for him but the NICU nurses gave scant education regarding how to do so. During her son's 110-day stay in the NICU, no support or positive reinforcement was ever given by the nurses regarding the expression of her milk.

On December 24, Bonnie was visited by the lactation consultant (LC) in the NICU where her baby had been admitted and explained to the LC that while pumping, her nipples were filling the tunnel of the pump flange and the nipple skin was being rubbed and was becoming sore. Bonnie requested larger flanges for her pump kit but was told by the LC that this was not necessary. She instructed Bonnie to pump for 15 minutes per session and that she should pump 8 to 10 times per day. The LC also instructed the mother how to store and label her pumped milk. On December 25, Bonnie's baby boy suffered from a level 4 cerebral hemorrhage that resulted in seizures and temporary respiratory failure. The LC came to see Bonnie, but she was too distressed to talk about her milk. Bonnie did not see the LC or anyone else from the lactation staff for months.

Over the days and weeks, Bonnie came to sometimes feel that the staff preferred to give her baby formula. On several occasions, the nurses actually referred to Bonnie's milk as formula. After one pumping session where she pumped only an ounce of milk, the nurse said to Bonnie, "Is that all you got?" Bonnie felt devastated. By this time Bonnie had returned to work in the city where she lived, was driving every evening to see her son and setting her alarm faithfully to pump every 2 hours day and night. One of the NICU's nurse practitioners misinformed Bonnie that if she drank too much milk while she was pumping, she would make her son lactose intolerant.

Because of a family history of diabetes and the connection between cow's milk proteins and diabetes, Bonnie had requested that fortification of her milk with cow's-milk-based fortifiers be discussed with her prior to administration. After her son had been in the NICU for 29 days, Bonnie discovered a box of fortifier sitting next to her son's crib. She learned from the nurse that fortifier had been added to her milk without her permission. On another occasion, Bonnie was watching her son's nurse mix the breastmilk with cow's milk based fortifier, pouring the extra breastmilk down the sink drain. Bonnie was hurt and angered by the waste of her milk. Now Bonnie began to question everything that was done to her son. She requested that the neonatologists on staff research another way to fortify her milk. In the meantime, Bonnie was requesting information from neonatologists around the country. Following research and discussion, she came to the conclusion that at this facility, fortifier would be the safest way to ensure her infant was receiving necessary nutrients.

Bonnie was unable to visit her son every day because winter driving conditions were often hazardous, but she asked to be told if her milk reserve was getting low so that she could bring additional milk to the NICU. She was told that although the nurse would pass this message on, "in report, many things get lost in translation" and if Bonnie wanted to make sure there was milk for her baby she would have to monitor that herself. When Bonnie began monitoring her milk, she discovered that after several weeks of feedings, her colostrum was still in the freezer.

Bonnie asked her son's nurses repeatedly about putting her baby to breast and was told that it was much more stressful for her son to breastfeed, and so bottle-feeding was much easier for him to tolerate. The nurses said he had to learn to bottle-feed before he could breastfeed and that his discharge would be held up until he could take all of his feedings by bottle. When Bonnie asked for help to put her baby to breast, it was clear that most of the staff had no idea how to help her, although the nurses would stand and watch her attempt to put the baby to breast, never offering help. She was also told to wait until the LC was on duty to get help with breastfeeding. One LC left a breastfeeding pillow for Bonnie as the full extent of her help. Another LC encouraged Bonnie to use a nipple shield because nipple shields had been researched and were found to be 90% effective in transitioning premature infants to the breast. Proper placement of the shield was not taught. Discouraged by the lactation support, Bonnie decided to just bottle-feed her milk in order to get her son discharged sooner. She thought she would have more success trying to breastfeed in her own home.

Skin-to-skin care is vital to the growth and development of premature infants and to breastfeeding success, yet this was another competency lacking in the nursing staff. Bonnie was never encouraged to hold her baby skin to skin. When after a week in the NICU, she began to ask repeatedly when she could hold her baby, she was told he was too critical to be held. By January 9, Bonnie was allowed to hold her clothed and wrapped baby on her lap on a pillow. Her persistence resulted in holding her son skin to skin for the first time on January 15, but the neonatologist told her, "Just this once. Don't expect this every time you are here." When the LC on the unit was asked about the NICU policy regarding skin-to-skin care, the LC replied that there was no policy because the doctors and the nurses could not agree on issues pertaining to skin-to skin-care. But Bonnie continued to be insistent about more skin-to-skin care. On February 21 she was told that she could begin holding her baby skin to skin for 1 hour only, once per week, 30 minutes after he had been fed. Once again, Bonnie was told by the nursing staff that skin-to-skin contact was too stressful, that he would get cold and that he was too little for more skin-to-skin contact. After a month of this discouragement, Bonnie again requested to hold her baby and she was told that he was then over 4 pounds and was too big for skin-to-skin care. Bonnie was extremely distraught at the contradiction and asked a friend, Maryanne, who worked elsewhere in the hospital, to advocate for her and her son. Maryanne spoke with the neonatologist who wrote an order allowing Bonnie to hold her baby skin to skin whenever she requested. The nursing staff told Bonnie that the neonatologist's order meant that skin-to-skin contact would only be allowed at the discretion of the nurses. One nurse said that babies need to stay in the crib because their bones hurt if they are held too much. Other nurses continued to tell Bonnie that her son would get too cold if held skin to skin.

One morning Bonnie walked into the NICU and found her baby lying in the isolette wearing only a T-shirt and diaper. The warmer had been shut off to transition the infant to room air. Bonnie thought her son felt cold so she took his temperature and discovered that it was 36°C. Bonnie swaddled him in blankets. Forty-five minutes later, the attending nurse came into the room and told Bonnie that the baby was cold. When Bonnie asked why the infant had not been swaddled, the nurse told Bonnie that she had been checking the infant's monitor leads. Bonnie said that she wanted to hold the baby skin to skin. The nurse did not respond. A new nurse then took charge of the infant's care after a shift change. She came into the room where Bonnie and her baby were skin to skin, pulled the blanket off them and told Bonnie she was going to place the infant back in the isolette because he was too cold. Bonnie told her that the point of doing skin-to-skin was to warm the infant. The nurse replied that she was in charge of the infant's well-being regardless of the mother's wishes. The neonatologist then came in to see Bonnie, and the nurse left the room. Bonnie asked again if it was harmful to hold her baby skin to skin. The neonatologist said it was fine. The nurse came back into the room and said that she was going to place the baby back in the isolette because the neonatologist had ordered it. When the mother refused to give up her son, the nurse asked her if she wanted to talk to the doctor or the supervisor. The mother said she wanted the doctor, who confirmed that it was fine for the baby to be held skin to skin. The nurse responded by taking the baby's temperature, threatening that if it was not warm enough, she was going to place the baby back in the isolette. The baby's temperature was already rising in the skin-to-skin position, and the nurse expressed surprise.

Bonnie reported this incident to the manager of the NICU in a private conversation in the manager's office. During that conversation the NICU manager joked and invalidated Bonnie's many concerns and complaints regarding the care of her infant. The manager promised that she would investigate why the baby had been left unswaddled. Two days later, the manager reported to Bonnie that the nurse said that she had left the baby swaddled and that the baby had been swaddled when Bonnie came in. The manager told Bonnie that perhaps a doctor had examined the baby and that was why the baby was not covered. The nurse manager told Bonnie that she was obviously having difficulty growing as a mother and had made arrangements for a counselor to interview her. Bonnie was grief stricken and frightened, feeling that the manager had accused her of being an unfit mother. Bonnie's mother called the hospital in order to connect her daughter with the hospital's patient advocate, only to discover that the patient advocate for the NICU was the nurse manager! Bonnie was promised that a nurse from the NICU would be assigned to serve as her advocate and the lack of a primary care nurse and the numerous nurses caring for her infant would be resolved so that fewer nurses would take care of him and get to know him better. None of these promises was fulfilled.

Near the end of his stay in the NICU, Bonnie's son had LASIK eye surgery in order to stop the progression of retinopathy of prematurity. The attending neonatologist promised Bonnie that her son would be aggressively weaned from the ventilator following surgery. However, when Bonnie came to visit her son the next morning, the baby's nurse reported that morphine had been administered for pain and that he had also been given the morphine during the night. When Bonnie questioned this intervention, reminding the nurse that the neonatologist had promised aggressive weaning from the ventilator, the nurse said that the doctor to whom she had spoken had approved an order to give the infant morphine. Bonnie asked to talk to the neonatologist herself. The nurse left, and 5 minutes later a nurse practitioner came to tell Bonnie that the plan was to administer naloxone (Narcan) and begin weaning the baby from the ventilator as quickly as possible. The nurse who had administered the morphine was sent home and another nurse was assigned to the baby.

Later, Bonnie's son had a cerebral reservoir surgically implanted to regulate the increase in cerebrospinal fluid in the brain. The neurosurgeon was trying to avoid placing a shunt as he was showing signs of regulating the fluid on his own. Head circumference became a critical measurement as it dictated when the neonatologist might tap the reservoir. One day the baby's head had grown a centimeter overnight. This is what had been reported during shift change and then relayed to the neonatologist. Bonnie, who had been spending a great amount of time with her baby, questioned that finding. The neonatologist said he would go back and check the information before tapping the reservoir. When he returned he told Bonnie that the information had been miscommunicated by the nurses and that her baby's head had *not* increased to that degree overnight. His reservoir was not tapped.

When I analyze this case, it is clear that there was little continuity of care or lactation management in the care of Bonnie and her baby. Staff was not consistent about addressing skin-to-skin issues and the other care issues concerning Bonnie and her son. Although Bonnie experienced kindness occasionally during her 110-day interaction with the staff, the majority of the time Bonnie felt as if she were an outsider looking in and observing the care of her baby. No effort was made to include Bonnie in the life and care of her son. Her wishes were consistently excluded from the plan of care.

Bonnie had access to community resources, and friends and family members who were versed in the research literature related to the benefits of human milk for premature infants and the benefits of skin-to-skin contact. Her resources also had experience with counseling mothers in the NICU as well as national access to neonatologists who volunteered to provide Bonnie with the pros and cons of practices such as fortifying the mother's milk and whether or not to vaccinate the premature infant prior to discharge. Supportive individuals were also familiar with the principles of biomedical ethics and could apply those principles to her case and help her to make decisions based on *informed* consent. However, in terms of resources within the NICU, Bonnie's experience mirrors that of many other mothers around the United States who have been disenfranchised regarding the care of their infants.

Providing expressed milk and skin-to-skin care may be among the only ways mothers have of being involved in the care of their premature infants. Frequent enough expression in order to maintain a milk supply is time consuming and may be exhausting. It is accompanied by the stress and worry of having a premature and sick baby. Negotiations with NICU staff in order to participate in their babies' care and to parent their infants is an additional stress. There may be the spoken or unspoken threat that if the mother puts up too many arguments for the care she wants, then she could have the baby removed entirely from her care and placed in foster care. Barriers actively prevent the mother from participating in these functions or she is deterred by lack of appropriate support or misinformation from staff. This denies her of her fundamental rights as a mother. The baby is denied his human right to achieve optimal health and sometimes even to survive.

Bonnie's case demonstrates the lack of a number of policies and practices that every mother should expect as a routine part of her and her prematurely born baby's care, including the following:

- Respect from obstetric care providers that includes a belief in the mother's sense of what her own body is telling her.
- Value and support of a mother's choice to breastfeed or provide milk for her premature infant throughout the maternity care system, even if she is not part of the team caring for the baby.
- Lactation support that is evidence-based, daily, and appropriate for the age and stage of the baby. Lactation care providers should be capable of critical thinking and not use the same intervention (such as dropping off pillows) for every mother as a solution.
- Adequate and accurate basic lactation care that can be provided by any member of the baby's and mother's healthcare team.
- Care providers who are supportive and encouraging of the mother's efforts to provide her milk, without disparaging remarks about either the quality or quantity of her milk and who do not waste expressed milk.
- Policies in the NICU that reflect the enormous amount of research on the benefits of skin-to-skin or kangaroo care for *all* babies. Practice from *all*

staff that reflects these policies and is reflected in consistent information and support for the mother from all care providers.
- Clear and accurate communications between members of the healthcare team, resulting in continuity of care.
- An independent patient advocate who will arbitrate ethical issues under the oversight of the hospital ethics committee.

Another disturbing element of Bonnie's case is that the NICU was housed in a teaching hospital for both physicians and nurses. The lack of continuity, policy, procedure, and staff competency was being modeled for future neonatologists and nurses whose practice will reflect both what they are taught in classroom learning and clinical observation and practice observation.

Dr. Adik Levin served as head of the Neonatal and Infants' Department at the Tallinn Children's Hospital in Estonia. With Dr. Beverly Chalmers, he wrote a book entitled *Humane Perinatal Care* (2001). In it he describes a model of NICU care that results in better weight gain in preterm infants, shortened duration of infections (by 3–5 days), reduced need for antibiotic treatment, lower rates of respiratory infection in the first year, and other immunological benefits. This model transfers the majority of care of preterm infants to their mothers who room with their babies 24 hours a day and provide their routine care from the first days of life. The hospital staff provides technical and medical care and trains the mother in the skills she needs in order to care for her fragile infant. The mother's milk is valued and she feeds her baby, either through a tube or directly at the breast. Skin-to-skin care is initiated as soon as possible after the birth and as continuously as possible. The amount of contact between staff and the baby is minimized to reduce the potential for infection and to optimize the biological and psychological ties between the mother and baby.

According to Levin:

> Traditionally the experience of having a baby in a NICU or special care baby unit (SCBU) is a traumatic one for parents and probably also for babies. It is characterized by separation of mother and baby, with minimal contact between them, and especially little skin-to-skin contact, as well as feeding with breastmilk substitutes either totally or in addition to breastmilk. In most of the industrialized world these practices (with minimal variations) are accepted as essential means of

> providing optimal care for the sick or preterm newborn. (Chalmers & Levin, 2001, p. 14)
>
> The evidence suggests that it is not ethical to continue using the traditional approach. We cannot in all honesty continue using that painful, less effective and costly treatment when more effective, less painful, and less costly alternatives are available. Nor can we continue to deprive newborns and their mothers of contact with each other. We can no longer ignore the insensitive aspects of our current models of care. (Chalmers & Levin, 2001, p. 16)

I have written this book to provide parents as well as healthcare providers with the rationales for removing barriers to human milk feeding and skin-to-skin care in the NICU and model protocols and procedures to reduce barriers to these important components of premature infant care. What should the ideal NICU look like in terms of supporting breastfeeding and skin-to-skin care of the mother/infant couplet? For parents who do not experience the standard of practice envisioned in this book, they can use this information to better advocate for themselves and their infants and to apply consumer pressure to NICUs to change the way they practice. For healthcare providers, this book provides a thought process and models for achieving the standard of practice that has already been established in the research literature.

REFERENCES

Chalmers, B., & Levin, A. (2001). *Humane perinatal care*. Tallinn, Estonia: TEA Publishers.

Part II

The Rationale for Using Human Milk in the NICU for Preterm and Sick Infants

chapter two

Establishing the Need: Why Human Milk Is Important to a Nation's Public Health

NUTRITIONAL PROGRAMMING: A MODEL

Many people believe, erroneously, that formula is at least as good as human milk, if not better. Many of us were fed manufactured formula or homemade milk mixtures as infants and we appear to be healthy adults. If we are not healthy, then the message from our culture is that it is our personal responsibility to make our own good health. It's our lifestyle choices, our environment, or even our genes that are to blame for whatever disease or condition we develop after infancy. We are told that exercising more, drinking less, and losing weight will cure our ills. We are told that if our mother had breast cancer we will probably get it unless we cut out fats from our diet and stop drinking alcohol. We are told that living near the Love Canal or working with asbestos or eating too much sugar is the reason for our ill health. While parts of these assumptions are well accepted, another consideration is that we are what we were fed.

Lucas (1994) has defined nutritional programming clearly as an event that can influence long-term outcomes in an individual in one of two ways by (1) causing "induction, deletion, or impaired development of a somatic structure resulting from a stimulus or insult at a critical period" (p. 288); or (2) "physiological 'setting' by an early stimulus or insult at a critical period, with long-term consequences for function" (p. 288). Fetal development itself is a highly programmed event and can be impacted by a number of things. For example, in the 1950s, thalidomide was prescribed for pregnant women to control nausea and morning sickness. The drug interrupted the development of limb buds in the fetus, and babies were born without arms or with very poorly developed arms that were greatly shortened. In this case, the teratogen caused the insult and the limbs did not develop. The current campaign by the March of Dimes to prevent spinal cord defects in developing fetuses by increasing the amount of folic acid in the mother's diet both preconception and postconception is an example of a campaign based on the documented impact of maternal nutrition on the proper programming of embryological development of the spinal column—without enough folic acid, the spinal cord is left exposed, without vertebral or connective tissue protection, allowing damage to the nerves that can cause paralysis and loss of body functions. In this case, low levels of a nutrient required during a critical period causes impaired development of a somatic structure.

Humans are born at a much more immature state than most other mammals. Once a baby is born, development of organs, organ systems, and physiological function continues to occur. Functional development can also be impacted by the interruption of the programmed sequence of events that must occur. This is the second type of insult that Lucas discusses. If a message is not given or the wrong message is sent during the critical period, programming will be different. Nutrition in early infancy is a prime candidate as a programmer. In animal studies cited by Lucas (1994), inadequate nutrition (undernutrition) in rats permanently affected brain size, brain cell number, and later learning behavior and memory. Undernourished fetal rats also showed later abnormalities in pancreatic function, with a reduction in the number of pancreatic cells and reduced insulin secretion.

If a baby is born prematurely, programmed development is enormously interrupted. Instead of receiving oxygen from its mother's bloodstream, the baby must expand its lungs, breathe, and exchange oxygen across a membrane. Instead of obtaining nutrients through the mother's bloodstream via the placenta, the baby must learn how to extract them from an IV made up of synthetic nutrients or rapidly develop its gastrointestinal tract for gastric feeding. To be the least interruptive of development, nutrients need to be delivered in as natural, complete, and nonsynthetic a form as possible, so that development can occur as normally as possible. This means that species-specific human milk will have advantages to the infant's development over formula that is manufactured out of things babies would never be exposed to if the natural progression of development were to occur. Lucas's seminal study of the impact of randomized diets in a preterm population is being conducted prospectively to look at long-term outcomes (Lucas, Morley, Cole, & Gore, 1994). This study supports his contention that the type of nutrition an infant receives programs short-term and long-term outcomes in humans and is extremely important to the health and well-being of individuals over their life span.

What Are the Short-Term Outcome Differences?

One of the most important short-term outcomes in the preterm population that has been studied by Lucas and Cole (1990; see also Morley & Lucas, 1994) as part of a long-term prospective study is the lower incidence of necrotizing enterocolitis (NEC) in preterm infants (see **Box 2-1**). In infants who were fed formula exclusively, the disease was 6–10 times more common than in those infants fed human milk exclusively. Pasteurized donor milk (see Part IV of this book) was as protective as raw maternal milk. NEC was three times more common in those who received both human milk and formula. Lucas and Cole estimated that in the United Kingdom, 500 cases of NEC each year and 100 deaths from NEC per year could be prevented by human milk feeding.

The financial costs of prematurity are high. Russell et al. (2007) analyzed the cost to the United States of hospitalization for preterm and low-birth-weight infants born in 2001. Eight percent of all infant hospital stays were for prematurity or low birth weight and cost the country approximately $5.8 billion (confidence interval $4.9–$6.7 billion). This represents 47% of costs for all infant hospitalizations. In other words, a very small proportion of infants accounts for a very large percentage of hospital costs during infancy. The financial costs of a single case of NEC are also extremely high and are additive to a family's bill. Bisquera, Cooper, and Berseth (2002) estimate that the average length of stay in the NICU was 60 days longer than that of control subjects (premature infants without NEC) and cost approximately $186,200 in excess of what the length of stay for control subjects cost for each case of surgical NEC. Infants with medical NEC cases (nonsurgical) stayed an average of 22 days longer in the hospital and incur costs of approximately $73,700 more than those of control subjects. In Bisquera and colleagues' (2002) multicenter study, "the yearly additional hospital charges for NEC were $6.5 million or $216,666 per survivor" (p. 423). If adjusted for inflation and increase in healthcare costs between 2001 and the present, these figures would be even more astounding. The demographics of prematurity tell us that

Box 2-1 What Is NEC?

NEC is the leading cause of infant mortality in the United States and is a disease of prematurity (Kosloske, 2001). The more premature the infant is, the higher the risk of developing NEC. The etiology of NEC is poorly understood, but human milk is the single agent that has proven over and over again to be the most effective means of preventing NEC. Symptoms of NEC include abdominal distention, gastrointestinal bleeding, and air in the bowel wall that can be seen on X-ray. Feeding intolerance, vomiting, and signs of sepsis (infection) are also seen. When NEC is suspected or diagnosed, feedings are stopped and intensive medical therapy is begun. Therapy includes antibiotics, IV fluids, gastric suctioning, and frequently ventilator and oxygen support (Bisquera et al. 2002; Kosloske, 2001). If allowed to progress, portions of the intestine become ischemic (anemic because of lack of blood flow to the area) and gangrenous and may perforate, sending infection into the rest of the body. The end of the small intestine where it attaches to the large intestine (the ileum) is the area most likely to be affected, with the colon next and then the rest of the small intestine (the jejunum) (Kosloske, 2001). Since the small intestine is the location of nearly all nutrient absorption, any disruption of its integrity can compromise nutritional status of an infant. During cases of NEC, oral feedings are stopped, slowing the infant's rate of growth. In about 35% of cases, surgery is required to remove the gangrenous or infected portions of the gut (Bisquera, Cooper, & Berseth, 2000). Healthy portions of the gut are then resected, leaving the infant with a lifelong condition called short-gut syndrome. With less mucosal surface area available, nutrients are poorly absorbed, special diets are frequently required, and growth faltering may occur. According to Kosloske (2001) approximately one third of infants with surgical cases of NEC do not survive, with others dying later of complications such as short-gut syndrome. In cases of NEC that respond to medical treatment and do not require surgery, the mortality rate approximates 20%.

the groups at highest risk for delivering prematurely are poorly educated low-income women who do not have access to adequate prenatal care or good nutrition, are substance abusers, etc. This population is Medicaid eligible, so state Medicaid programs cover the costs of hospitalization for preterm infants. Tax dollars, both state and federal, fund Medicaid. According to Russell et al. (2007), 42% of the hospital stays were eligible for Medicaid coverage. Prematurity and NEC are a crisis in public health.

Beyond the short-term costs of NEC, there may be long-term costs as well. Survivors of surgery for NEC may have lifelong issues with malabsorption and require costly special nutritional support. In a meta-analysis, Rees, Pierro, and Eaton (2007) report that 45% of children who had NEC were neurodevelopmentally impaired, including a higher risk of cerebral palsy and visual, cognitive, and psychomotor impairment, requiring more medical interventions, a greater need for social services, and long-term special education services.

How Was the Study Done?

The methodology of Lucas's study is important to consider. All babies in the study were born prematurely, were low birth weight, and tube fed the assigned diet. Mothers who wished to provide their own milk were allowed to do so. If the mothers chose not to provide their own milk, the babies were randomly assigned to either preterm or term formulas or banked donor breastmilk as feedings. If the mother chose to provide her own milk but supplementation was required, supplements were randomized to one of the same three types of feedings. This methodology is important as it allows comparison of outcomes by the type of feeding as opposed to the manner in which it was fed. The act of feeding at the breast per se may provide benefits to the infant separate from the milk. In Lucas's studies, breastfeeding did not occur, although some babies were fed their mother's milk. The study therefore looks at the effects of the milk itself vs. the formula itself[1] (Lucas et al., 1994; Morley & Lucas, 1994). All of the babies who participated in this study were born between January 1982 and March 1985. Individual infants who survived are now adults and are still being studied for physiological outcomes. Previous studies on the impact of nutrition on development have not been as long term.

Does It Make a Difference? Long-Term Outcomes

One of the first questions explored in this prospective study—developmental status—was when the cohort was 18 months old (Lucas et al., 1994). At 18 months of postterm age, infants who were fed banked breastmilk had higher scores on the Bayley psychomotor and mental development indices than infants fed a standard term formula, despite the term formula having a higher nutrient content. No differences were seen when the banked breastmilk-fed children were compared to those fed the preterm formula, despite

[1] In this study, the banked human milk was collected passively from the breast in a milk cup (breast shield) while the donor fed her infant on the other breast. This so-called drip milk is lower in fat content than expressed milk, and it could be a significant reason for the lack of infant growth observed in many studies of banked human milk that utilized this type of collection method. Milk that is actively pumped from the breast contains much higher fat content because of the negative pressure exerted by the pump (see Arnold, 1997).

the much lower nutrient content of the preterm formula compared to TF. The same children were again assessed developmentally between the ages of 7.5 and 8 years and results reported for the group assigned to receive their own mother's expressed milk vs. preterm formula. An abbreviated Anglicized Wechsler Intelligence Scale was used to assess IQ. When compared with the formula-fed group, the expressed milk group had an overall IQ advantage of 8.3 points (Lucas, Morley, Cole, Lister, & Leeson-Payne, 1992). Consistent with the rat studies mentioned earlier showing memory and learning deficits with undernutrition, it would appear that Lucas has demonstrated a programming link between early nutrition in the preterm population and later neurological development.

While no individual can be guaranteed an *increase* in IQ from being breastfed, what is striking is the *loss* of potential. For an infant born with an anomaly or genetic defect that impacts the nervous system and later intelligence, such as Down syndrome, the loss of even two or three points of IQ could mean the difference between that person being institutionalized or being able to live in a group home and hold a job. Human milk feeding from birth therefore becomes an extremely important programming tool to help individuals achieve their optimal potential. More recent studies in preterm populations have found a dose-dependent relationship between developmental scores and the amount of human milk that is fed. Looking at neurodevelopmental outcomes of 1035 extremely low-birth-weight infants at 18–22 months corrected age, Vohr et al. (2006) found that

> . . . for every additional 10 ml/kg per day increase in breast milk ingestion, the [Bayley] Mental Development Index increased by 0.53 points, the Psychomotor Development Index increased by 0.63 points, the Behavior Rating Scale percentile score increased by 0.82 points, and the likelihood of rehospitalization decreased by 6%. (p. e116)

The authors point out that these improvements in scores may have significant impact on the need for special education services among this high-risk population. "The potential long-term benefit of receiving breast milk may be to optimize cognitive potential and reduce the need for early intervention and special education services" (p. e116).

Another example of probable nutritional programming may be found in two of the models for the development of diabetes. Epidemiological studies have noted a link between insulin-dependent diabetes mellitus (IDDM) and lack of breastfeeding (for a review of several different models of formula-induced diabetes see Cadwell & Turner-Maffei, 2002). In one model, infants fed a cow's-milk-based formula from birth are exposed to a protein (bovine serum albumin) that looks very similar to a protein produced by the beta cells of the pancreas. In this model, susceptible individuals (i.e., those with a genetic history of diabetes) may mount an immune response to the cow's milk protein. Eventually they may also mount an immune response to their own body's beta cells. With this autoimmune response, there is a cessation of insulin production and a progression to IDDM (Martin, Trink, Daneman, Dosch, & Robinson, 1991; Karjalainen et al., 1992). This model is strengthened by the comparison of two populations that are genetically very close. Thorsdottir et al. (2000) analyzed the two variants of β-casein in milk from Icelandic cows and found that β-casein was significantly lower in them than in the milk from Scandinavian cows. They postulate that this may be the reason why Iceland has a lower incidence of IDDM than Sweden.

In a second model, the link may be that the formula-fed infant cannot move glucose into cells for use as a source of energy because the insulin receptors on the cell are blocked by something inappropriate in the formula, possibly saturated fats that are used in formula because they have a long shelf life. A condition called "hyperinsulinemia" (overproduction of insulin) occurs as the body makes further demands for more insulin that cannot function properly. Eventually the beta cells of the pancreas simply wear out from this overproduction and cease to function, and the individual becomes an insulin-dependent diabetic (Lucas et al. 1980; Pettitt, Forman, Hanson, Knowler, & Bennett, 1997; Wallensteen, Lindblad, Zetterstrom, & Persson, 1991). In these two examples, the body's ability to produce insulin is impaired by an inappropriate type of feeding that misprograms the pancreas. The insult of cow's milk components during a critical period of development (see Lucas's definition of nutritional programming earlier in this section), even in its modified form in formula, sets up a chain of reactions and events that are physiologically different from the chain of events that would occur if the infant had been fed only human milk. Though it may take some time for the outcome of IDDM to be expressed, the critical period is early in extrauterine life. Disruption of this period results in chronic lifelong disease that has been programmed in the first weeks of life by the parents' choice of feeding.

THE HAZARDS OF FORMULA

The Centers for Disease Control and Prevention (CDC) and the U.S. Public Health Service have put forward a focus on chronic disease prevention because chronic disease costs the nation substantial amounts of money in healthcare costs each year. An example of this may be found in recent reports and recommendations that have emerged focusing on what parents can do to prevent childhood obesity, which, in turn, could lead to diseases such as diabetes, heart disease, hypertension, etc. As the evidence becomes stronger and stronger for the relationship between early programming for these diseases through nutrition, the U.S. government has decided to devote financial and creative resources on promoting breastfeeding. Unfortunately, promotion is only part of the story. The World Health Organization recognizes that besides promotion efforts, mothers need individualized support to help them succeed at breastfeeding, and they need to be protected from cultural roadblocks that make breastfeeding difficult. For example, most U.S. states have enacted legislation to protect a woman's right to breastfeed in public. A majority of states have also enacted legislation that protects a breastfeeding mother's right to be supported in the workplace. The supportive employer provides a safe and clean place (not a toilet stall!) to express milk and to store her milk so that her infant can continue to be fed human milk even after she returns to work (see Baldwin and Vance 2009; USBC, 2005).

Table 2-1 summarizes by condition or organ system studies that demonstrate the long-term programmed negative consequences of formula feeding. These studies are primarily epidemiological in nature, correlating the association of a certain disease or physiological outcome with feeding. Where possible, the results of each study are expressed in terms of elevated risk or hazard created by formula feeding. In the past, these studies often expressed their findings in terms of the benefits of breastfeeding rather than the hazards of formula feeding. Studies indicate, however, that when one is trying to convince parents to breastfeed, the benefits of breastfeeding are not compelling enough; delineating the hazards of formula feeding works better, because parents are not aware of the elevated risks (Haynes, 2003).[2] Simi-

---

[2] This has proven true again recently as the federal government created a national breastfeeding campaign trying to inform parents of the benefits of breastfeeding. When conducting social marketing focus group research to determine the extent of knowledge about breastfeeding/formula feeding among individuals who had never been pregnant, many individuals stated that they were really shocked to learn about the hazards and increased risks of formula feeding and had trouble believing it. When shown the research, they were angered that they had not heard this information before from healthcare providers (Haynes, personal communication, August 2003). Based on what these individuals and prospective parents said in focus groups, the government campaign featured ads created by the Ad Council that hit hard at the risks and deleterious outcomes of formula feeding. The campaign was delayed by protests from and heavy lobbying by formula companies and finally released in June 2004 in a much watered-down version.

Table 2-1 The Epidemiological Evidence Against Formula Feeding: Hazards to Infants and Children

Acute illness, chronic disease, or deficit	*Reference*
Allergies	
Longer duration of breastfeeding (less formula) was protective against asthma and wheeze in young children.	Dell & To, 2001
The increased exposure to allergens in formula increased the rates of asthma in young children. Increased breastfeeding (less exposure to formula) combined with the protective factors of breastfeeding reduced the rates of asthma in young children.	Gdalevich, Mimouni, & Mimouni, 2001
A meta-analysis concluded that exclusive breastfeeding for the first 3 months of life protects against allergic rhinitis in infants and children.	Mimouni Bloch, Mimouni, Mimouni, & Gdalevich, 2002
The risk of asthma increased if exclusive breastfeeding was stopped before 4 months. There was a substantial reduction in risk of asthma at 6 years of age if exclusive breastfeeding occurred for at least 4 months.	Oddy, 2000; Oddy, Peat, & de Klerk, 2002
Cancers	
Breast cancer	
Having been formula fed as an infant increased the risk of developing breast cancer as an adult.	Freudenheim et al., 1994
Childhood cancers	
Infants who were artificially fed or breastfed for less than 6 months had an increased risk of developing lymphoma (5.6 times, 8.2 times respectively) before age 15 than those infants breastfed for longer than 6 months.	Davis, Savitz, & Graubard, 1988
Risk of all childhood cancers was increased 1.8 times for artificially fed infants and increased 1.9 times when compared with infants who were breastfed longer than 6 months.	Davis et al., 1988
Shorter duration of breastfeeding (< 6 months) was associated with an increased risk of childhood lymphomas.	Shu et al., 1995
Cardiovascular conditions	
Formula-fed children had higher LDL cholesterol (bad cholesterol) concentrations, lower HDL cholesterol concentrations, and a higher LDL:HDL ratio, which are risk factors for later cardiovascular disease.	Ravelli, van der Meulen, Osmond, Barker, & Bleker, 2000
Preterm formula consumption in a cohort of preterm infants was associated with higher blood pressures 13–16 years later. Results were true when comparisons were made between formula-fed groups and donor milk-fed groups.	Singhal, Cole, & Lucas, 2001

(*continues*)

Table 2-1 (*Continued*)

Acute illness, chronic disease, or deficit	*Reference*
Higher LDL levels, higher LDL:HDL ratios and higher concentration of C-reactive protein were found in formula-fed preterm infants at age 13–16 years.	Singhal, Cole, Fewtrell, & Lucas, 2004
Accelerated growth in the neonatal period from formula feeding may have an association with later cardiovascular problems.	Singhal, Cole, Fewtrell, Deanfield, & Lucas, 2004
Gastrointestinal conditions	
Celiac disease	
Children breastfed for less than 30 days were four times more likely to develop celiac disease than children breastfed for longer.	Auricchio et al., 1983
Crohn's disease	
Children with Crohn's disease were less likely to have been breastfed, more likely to have received formula from birth, and more likely to have had diarrheal illnesses during infancy.	Koletzko, Sherman, Corey, Griffiths, & Smith, 1989
Breastfeeding had a dose-dependent inverse relationship with development of Crohn's disease.	Rigas et al., 1993
Diarrhea	
Increasing breastfeeding duration decreased episodes of gastroenteritis. Exclusive breastfeeding for 4 months reduced the risk of early first episodes of gastroenteritis.	Forman et al., 1984
Short/no breastfeeding (< 6 months) increased the incidence of diarrhea in the first year of age. Increased formula feeding also increased the severity of diarrhea in infants age 7–12 months.	Ruuska, 1992
Infants who were mixed fed were 4.2 times more likely to die of diarrhea than exclusively breastfed infants. Infants who were artificially fed were 14.2 times more likely to die from diarrhea.	Victora et al., 1989
General GI problems	
Formula feeding was started earlier and was more frequent in infants with severe esophageal and gastric lesions.	Benhamou et al., 1998
Hernias	
Inguinal hernias were 51% more likely to occur in formula-fed infants than in breastfed infants. A dose-response relationship was noted in this case-control study.	Pisacane et al., 1995

Table 2-1 *(Continued)*

Acute illness, chronic disease, or deficit	*Reference*
Necrotizing enterocolitis	
A disease of prematurity, 400 cases and 100 deaths a year from NEC could be prevented in the United Kingdom if infants were fed human milk.	Lucas & Cole, 1990
Pyloric stenosis	
Mixed-fed and artificially fed infants were 2 and 2.7 times more likely to develop hypertrophic pyloric stenosis than exclusively breastfed infants.	Pisacane, et al., 1996
Ulcerative colitis	
Formula feeding increased the risk of ulcerative colitis.	Rigas, et al., 1993
Immune system problems	
Arthritis	
Formula feeding was associated with a 60% increased risk of developing juvenile rheumatoid arthritis.	Mason, et al., 1995
Formula feeding increased the risk of rheumatoid arthritis by 26% compared to breastfeeding for 1 to 12 months and 54 percent compared to being breastfed for 13 months or longer.	Pikwer, et al., 2008
Diabetes—Type I and Type II	
Early cow's milk exposure increased the risk of Type I diabetes approximately 1.5 times.	Gerstein, 1994
Formula feeding increased the risk of childhood Type I (insulin-dependent) diabetes.	McKinney et al., 1999
Formula feeding by mothers who were diabetic during pregnancy increased the risk of their children becoming diabetic.	Pettitt & Knowler, 1998
Exclusive formula feeding was associated with higher weights and higher rates of Type II diabetes (noninsulin dependent) in three age groups when compared with those breastfed exclusively for 2 months.	Pettitt et al., 1997
Adults who were formula fed as infants had higher mean blood glucose levels after a standard glucose tolerance test than those who were exclusively breastfed infants.	Ravelli et al., 2000
Longer exclusive and total breastfeeding is an independent protective factor against Type I diabetes.	Sadauskaite-Kuehne, Ludvigsson, Padaiga, Jasinskiene, & Samuelsson, 2004

(continues)

Table 2-1 (*Continued*)

Acute illness, chronic disease, or deficit	*Reference*
A nutrient-enriched diet (preterm formula) in a preterm population was associated with greater insulin resistance in adolescents aged 13–16.	Singhal, Fewtrell, Cole, & Lucas, 2003
Early introduction of cow's-milk products is independently associated with an increased risk of Type I diabetes.	Virtanen et al., 1993
Breastfeeding reduces the risk of Type II diabetes in native Canadian children by about 75%.	Young et al., 2002
Glandular development	
The thymus gland, an important gland in the development of the immune system, is significantly smaller in formula-fed infants.	Hasselbalch, Jeppesen, Engelmann, Michaelsen, & Nielsen, 1996
Infectious diseases and resulting conditions	
The risk of neonatal sepsis in a formula-fed high-risk population was 18 times greater than in a similar breastfed population.	Ashraf et al., 1991
Incidence of diarrhea in the first year of life was two times higher in the formula-fed group than in the breastfed group.	Dewey, Heinig, & Nommsen-Rivers, 1995
The percentage of any otitis media in the formula-fed group was 19% higher.	
Middle ear infections were much more common in formula-fed infants. There was a dose-response relationship, with exclusive breastfeeding being the most protective against otitis media.	Duncan, Holberg, Wright, Martinez, & Taussig, 1993
Fully bottle-fed infants were 10 times more likely to be hospitalized for infectious diseases than their breastfed counterparts. They spent 10 times more days in the hospital in the first year of life than exclusively breastfed infants.	Ellestad-Sayed, Coodin, Dilling, & Haworth, 1979
Infants with cleft palates who were bottle fed expressed human milk had much lower rates of ear infection than when bottle fed formula.	Paradise, Elster, & Tan, 1994
Neurological outcomes	
Formula-fed preterm infants had slower brainstem maturation than their breastfed counterparts.	Amin, Merle, Orlando, Dalzell, & Guillet, 2000
At ages 8–18 years, children fed formula as infants had consistent and statistically significantly lower IQ scores, lower reading comprehension and math scores, lower teacher ratings of reading and math skills, and lower exam scores.	Horwood & Fergusson, 1998
Exclusively formula-fed infants had a 60% higher rate of retinopathy of prematurity than those fed human milk.	Hylander, Strobino, Pezzullo, & Dhanireddy, 2001

Table 2-1 *(Continued)*

Acute illness, chronic disease, or deficit	*Reference*
Preterm infants who consumed formula only during the first month of life compared to their mother's own milk had an average IQ deficit of 8.3 points.	Lucas et al., 1992
Babies who were formula fed had lower scores on the Bayley Mental Development Index at 2 years of age. Longer durations of breastfeeding made larger differences.	Rogan & Gladen, 1993
Long term stereoscopic development was significantly lower in infants fed formulas with and without added DHA than in breastfed infants.	Singhal et al., 2007
Obesity	
The prevalence of obesity in artificially fed infants was twice the prevalence of obesity in breastfed children. A dose-response relationship between increasing duration of breastfeeding and decreasing prevalence of obesity was seen.	von Kries et al., 1999
High leptin levels associated with obesity were found in 13- to 16-year-old adolescents who were fed preterm formula compared to banked donor milk.	Singhal et al., 2002
Respiratory diseases	
Formula feeding elevates the risk of acute lower respiratory infection.	Pisacane et al.,1994
The rate of hospitalization for respiratory infections during the first 18 months of life was 18% for formula fed infants vs. 11.2% for breastfed infants.	Chen, Yu, & Li, 1988
Urogenital tract conditions	
Formula-fed infants had an increased risk of developing urinary tract infections compared to breastfed infants.	Pisacane et al., 1992

Source: Adapted from Arnold, 2005. Used with permission.

larly, when one is trying to convince healthcare providers of the importance of breastfeeding or the use of human milk, enumerating the benefits is not enough. Many healthcare providers are also unaware of the risks associated with formula feeding, and have given little thought to the concept of nutritional programming in infancy and its relation to later health/illness.

Even in studies where the associations of formula feeding with adverse outcomes later in life are weak, it may be that the definition of feeding method is not clear. Research has shown repeatedly that the biggest differences in health outcomes among populations come when the quantity of human milk consumed is the greatest. In other words, exclusive (full) breastfeeding (no formula, supplements, or solids at all) carries the biggest advantage (Cadwell, 2002; Raisler, Alexander, & O'Campo, 1999).

The increased risks of illness from formula feeding bring with them increased costs to the healthcare system. In its issue paper entitled *Economic Benefits of Breastfeeding*, the United States Breastfeeding Committee (USBC, 2002) delineates the additional medical and nonmedical costs of artificial feeding (formula feeding). It should be noted that this document is based on costs in the first years of the 21st century. As the century progresses, these figures will need to be adjusted upward.

FEEDING CONTROVERSIES EMERGING FROM A FORMULA-FEEDING MODEL

Growth

The reference fetus model is used to measure growth of a preterm baby. The rate at which a fetus gains weight over each trimester has been calculated. Neonatologists use this intrauterine accretion rate as a comparison for how well the premature baby is growing. Infants who do not meet this daily rate of increase are of concern. However, the circumstances of the preterm infant are very different from the fetus. In the latter, the mother's metabolism is doing all the work for the fetus, but the extrauterine preterm infant must spend energy to do his own breathing, digesting, thermoregulating, and excreting. Therefore, growth could be expected to be slower. The reference fetus model is not an ideal model, but currently it is the only one being applied. Intrauterine accretion rates are desirable because the brain cannot develop optimally if it is nutritionally compromised (see Wight & Morton, 2008, p. 220 for a discussion of growth standards for the preterm infant).

Preterm infants do not grow as rapidly when they are fed human milk, either maternal or donor, compared with preterm infants fed formula substitutes. This is a concern when the reference fetus model is being used as a standard. It is accepted that human milk is inadequate in terms of the minerals, vitamins, protein, and energy needs of the preterm infant (see Wight & Morton, 2008, for a review of feeding the preterm infant). Preterm infants have high needs for these nutrients because they are trying to grow in adverse circumstances. We must consider, however, that this slower rate of growth in preterm infants may not be only due to the composition of human milk but also the scheduling of feedings and the restrictions on the amount of human milk given to these infants. There is also the remaining question of whether rapid growth in the preterm infant is really desirable (see **Box 2-2**).

Volume Restriction—Are We Starving Them?

Term infants allowed to feed at the breast on cue will feed 10–12 times (sometimes more frequently) in a 24-hour period for a feeding interval of ≤ 2 hours, because human milk is so digestible and gastric emptying times are short. Yet preterm infants are rarely fed on demand, or cue, and volumes are restricted. Historically, before using a mother's own milk in the NICU became popular and before the creation of preterm formulas that had higher caloric content and modified proteins for easier digestion, preterm infants were fed standard term formulas. These formulas created metabolic stress for infants, so neonatologists began diluting formula and feeding smaller amounts of it at 3 to 4 hour intervals to cause fewer feeding-related complications for these critically ill infants. As human milk was introduced into the NICU on a regular basis, it was fed on the established schedule and was also diluted.

In the early 1980s as an employee of a milk bank, I received daily feeding logs for the NICU so I could determine how much banked donor milk to deliver to the NICU freezers. Orders would read "2 cc MOM or DM (banked donor human milk) 1/4 strength q 4," meaning that every 4 hours the infant would be fed 2 cc of his own mother's milk or banked donor milk that had been diluted one part milk to three parts sterile water. Considering that human milk is approximately 87% water, it is small wonder that preterm infants didn't grow; they were really being starved! This feeding regimen has carried over into today's practices; human milk is still treated somewhat like formula. Although rarely diluted today, it is still fed in restricted amounts on schedules that usually are every 2–3 hours.

Hamosh (1994) recommends avoiding use of restricted volumes when feeding preterm infants (see also Arnold, 2002). Sharpe (2002) suggests that many preterm infants could be fed more frequently and larger volumes per kilogram per day. Thureen and Hay (2001) propose that earlier and larger quantities be fed to preterm infants. Ziegler, Thureen, and Carlson (2002) also note that preterm infants frequently grow at a slower rate than they did in utero because their nutrient intakes are deficient when compared to nutrient uptakes of the fetus. They advocate aggressive practice or practice that exceeds standard practice.

Box 2-2 A Digression on Growth—When Too Much of a Good Thing Becomes Problematic

Childhood obesity is a major public health problem in many countries, not just the United States. It has been show in numerous epidemiological studies that the duration of breastfeeding is inversely related to the prevalence of obesity in school-age children and younger; i.e., the longer the duration of breastfeeding, the lower the prevalence of obesity (see Toschke, Grote, Koletzko, & von Kries, 2004; von Kries et al., 1999).

It is also now known that exclusively breastfed term infants have a very different pattern of weight gain from formula-fed infants. Breastfed babies gain weight more rapidly in the first 3 months of life and then their rate of gain slows compared to formula-fed infants. The formula-fed infants continue to grow at a much faster rate. If breastfed babies' weight gain patterns are the norm and are the standard of growth against which all other types of feeding-related weight gain should be measured, then the faster rate of growth exhibited by formula-fed babies after 3 months of age should be considered abnormal. Does this continued faster rate of weight gain contribute to obesity in childhood? Are these infants being programmed to be obese?

In this regard, the proceedings of a 2004 conference supported by the European Commission are revealing reading. Funded by the European Union, the Infant Nutrition Cluster is a group of three research projects looking at the programming effects of early nutrition on later health. One study looks at the issue of childhood obesity and whether it is the result of programming by infant nutrition; another looks at the effects of maternal fatty acid consumption on fetal and neonatal development; and the third looks at nutritional interventions to prevent Type I diabetes, which is a major and increasing health problem for children in Europe (see Koletzko, Dodds, Akerblom, & Ashwell, 2005).

While most of the book addresses the term infant, what about the preterm infant, who may be more vulnerable to external programming influences simply because he is less developed and mature? Several studies cited by Rolland-Cachera (2005) report that "rapid weight gain after low birth weight is associated with large subsequent weight gain and a central body fat pattern" (p. 36) (see Cameron, Pettifor, De Wet, & Norris, 2003; Eid, 1970; Monteiro, Victora, Barros, & Monteiro, 2003; Ong, Ahmed, Emmet, Preece, & Dunger, 2000). One might ask, therefore, what else is being sacrificed on the altar of rapid weight gain for preterm infants? Are we sacrificing future health by focusing on weight gain rather than other measures such as increase in head circumference and measures of increase in lean body mass? Are we programming preterm infants to have higher risks of obesity and insulin-dependent diabetes because we are focusing almost solely on rapid weight gain rather than the quality of the weight gain?

Wight & Morton (2008) report that about 90% of U.S.-born extremely low-birth-weight infants are discharged from the NICU "weighing less than the tenth percentile for corrected gestational age" (p. 221). Turning a preterm infant who is appropriate for gestational age at birth into a small-for-gestational-age infant at discharge is called "extrauterine growth restriction" and appears to be relatively common (Wight & Morton, 2008). Wight and Morton cite an intake of 150 cc/kg/day as the historic target but comment that this may be inadequate to meet optimal growth. Wight and Morton also cite a study by Hay et al. (1999) in which 180 cc/kg/day of *fortified* human milk is the recommended intake to achieve adequate growth. In the United States, this volume seems to be the upper limit in many NICUs. But this is not the case in Scandinavian NICUs and those in other parts of the world where it is common practice to see babies being fed 220–250 cc/kg/day.

Gastric Residuals—Testing . . . Testing . . .

With increased volumes, neonatologists also become concerned about undigested material left in the gut and frequently check to see if any residual is left in the gut. Gastric residuals should not be allowed to interfere with feeding according to Ziegler et al. (2002). Sharpe points out that the mucins inherent in human milk generate a mucus-like substance in the gut that is slow to break down. This substance is often mistaken for feeding residual when it is actually a protective coating. Frequent checking for residuals can injure the mucosa of the gut and interrupt a baby's progress (Sharpe, 2002). Human milk-fed preterm infants have faster gastric emptying times than preterm formula-fed infants and fewer residuals as a result. They are more likely to achieve full enteral feedings faster as well, which translates into shorter hospital stays (Wight & Morton, 2008).

Minimal Enteral Nutrition and Timing of Introduction of Feeds

According to Ziegler et al. (2002), aggressive nutrition means starting parenteral nutrition (feeding through an IV line) on the first day of life rather than delaying, as is common, and also starting minimal enteral feedings early. Also known as *trophic feedings* and *GI priming*, minimal enteral nutrition is beneficial to the infant. In utero, he has been swallowing amniotic fluid, helping prepare the GI tract for extrauterine nutrition. It is therefore physiologically abnormal for the gut to be empty, and lack of something in the premature baby's gut will cause it to atrophy. For the premature infant, early enteral nutrition (trophic feedings) with human milk should be started on the day of birth to stimulate gut maturation. According to Yu (2005), "early initiation of enteral feeding in sub-nutritional trophic quantity is vital for promoting gut motility and bile secretion, inducing lactase activity, and reducing sepsis and cholestatic jaundice . . . Preterm breastmilk expressed from the infant's own mother is the milk of choice" (p. 737).

Lucas and Cole (1990) found that delay in starting enteral feedings was associated with a significant reduction in the incidence of NEC among formula-fed infants. This was not the case with infants fed human milk. These infants could start enteral feedings much earlier without serious consequences. Neonatologists at the University of Leipzig attributed their low rate of NEC (0.2%) to early enteral feedings of fresh human milk, both maternal and/or donor milk, at 1, 2, or 3 days postpartum (Springer, 1997). Similar low rates of NEC were reported by the neonatal intensive care unit (NICU) at Ostra Sjukhuset in Göteborg, Sweden. Infants are fed either maternal or banked milk for the first time within the first 6–12 hours of life. They are fed 2–3 ml every 3 hours, increasing the amount slowly until they are on full enteral feedings, usually at 5–6 days of age. This NICU averages 800–900 admissions each year. However, its population of premature infants is somewhat different from that found in a U.S. NICU. In Göteborg, all surgical cases, sick term newborns, and cardiac care patients go to other hospitals. Nevertheless, the Göteborg NICU sees only one or two cases of NEC a year, also a rate of 0.2% (Arnold, 1999), compared to an average U.S. NEC rate of about 10%. While some may view a 10% NEC rate as negligible and too small for concern, any rate of NEC over what would naturally occur in an exclusively human milk-fed population is unacceptable. Physicians constantly work towards reducing rates of NEC in their NICUs because of its added costs and its short- and long-term impact on growth and development in the infant.

Early minimal feedings and a rapid advance to full enteral feedings (FEF) have also been associated with a lower incidence of late-onset sepsis (LOS) in preterm infants. Ronnestad and colleagues (2005) conducted a prospective study of all preterm infants born in Norway in 1999 and 2000. Infants weighing less than 1000 g at birth or who were less than 28 weeks' gestation were enrolled in the study. Sixty percent of infants were started on minimal enteral nutrition within a few hours of life, usually at 1 to 2 cc every 2 to 3 hours. By the third day of life, 95% had begun enteral feeding. This was increased by 0.5 to 1.0 cc every 6 to 8 hours as tolerated until FEF was achieved. Either banked donor milk or the mother's own milk was fed. Within 14 days of delivery, nearly 80% of infants were receiving FEF. The relative risk of LOS increased from day 8 to day 14 if FEF had not been established. Compared to later establishment of FEF, there was approximately a fourfold reduction in LOS if FEF was established within the second week of life. Tyson and Kennedy (2005), in their systematic review, found similar evidence; trophic feedings and larger feedings led to a significantly faster establishment of FEF as well as reduction in hospital stay.

Ronnestad et al. (2005) had a 4% incidence of NEC in their study. In the Sisk, Lovelady, Dillard, Gruber, and O'Shea study (2007), enteral feeding within the first 14 days of life that contained at least 50% human milk was associated with a sixfold decrease in the odds ratio for NEC. Could the Sisk findings have been improved upon if enteral feeding had been started within the first 3 days of life? The delay in beginning enteral feedings with human milk that is still seen in so many NICUs appears to be another case of carryover from the formula feeding model, where delay in beginning enteral feeds with formula was protective (Lucas & Cole, 1990).

Fortification

Low-birth-weight and very-low-birth-weight infants have nutritional requirements that differ from and are in excess of those of full-term infants. This is partly because of nutrient malabsorption secondary to immaturity of their digestive systems. Yet growth is of paramount concern because of the desire to match the intrauterine accretion rates for growth. The composition of milk from preterm mothers differs from that of term mothers for about the first 2 to 4 weeks postpartum (Atkinson, Anderson, & Bryan, 1980) and preterm milk is usually defined as being the milk that is pumped within the first month postpartum by a mother who has delivered at or before 36 weeks' gestation (Luukkainen, Salo, & Nikkari, 1994). Preterm milk is higher in many nutrients than the preterm infant needs, but as the course of lactation proceeds, these nutrients become less concentrated as the milk approaches the composition of term milk, even though the infant still has need for higher amounts. The needs of the infant are better met if human milk is fortified, but fortification has both positive and negative aspects.

There are several mechanisms by which human milk can better meet the nutritional needs of the preterm infant. Current practice in neonatology is that all human milk, including donor milk, is fortified before being fed to low-birth-weight and very premature infants. This provides premature infants with the extra protein, calcium, and phosphorus that they require. Short-term outcomes of infants fed human milk with these additives are faster growth—increase in weight, length, and head circumference—and better bone mineralization (Wight & Morton, 2008). However, no research has been done about either when to initiate fortification or how fast to advance it, according to Wight and Morton (2008; see also for a broad discussion of fortification issues).

Do I Really Want to Feed My Baby That?

The two most commonly used commercial preparations from the formula industry, the so-called human milk fortifiers, are made from cow's milk and are not made out of human milk components as the name might imply. Species specificity of the milk has therefore been altered. These fortifiers are in a powdered or liquid form, depending on the manufacturer. Several cases of infant death from meningitis have been traced to *Enterobacter sakazakii* contamination of powdered formulas, and some NICUs have ceased using the powdered fortifier (powders cannot be made sterile). In the spring of 2008, the Illinois Department of Health issued an alert that a case of preterm death from meningitis had been linked to the use of powdered fortifier. The ready-to-feed variety replaces the volume of human milk fed; therefore, infants fed this product receive smaller doses of human milk and its beneficial properties. Lenati, O'Connor, Hebert, Farber, and Pagotto (2008) found that the intrinsic antibacterial properties of human milk were not adequate to inhibit the growth of *E. sakazakii*, which survived for up to 12 days at 10°C in fortified human milk.

In addition to the risk of enterobacterial infection, the use of commercial bovine preparations to fortify human milk can impair the anti-infective properties of the milk. Quan, Yang, Rubinstein, Lewiston, Stevenson, et al. (1994) found significant decreases in lysozyme content and IgA specific for *Escherichia coli* when fortifiers were added to fresh frozen milk. Jocson, Mason, and Schanler (1997) also noted an increase in bacterial growth during 24 hours of refrigeration when commercial fortifier was added to human milk, although this increase was not large. Differences were statistically significant, however, when fortified milk was refrigerated for 72 hours. More recent studies have shown mixed conclusions about increased bacterial growth in human milk in the presence of fortifiers (Santiago, Codipilly, Potak, & Schanler, 2005, no growth; Askin & Diehl-Jones, 2002, growth), but rates of sepsis and NEC do not appear to increase (Berseth, Van Aerde, Gross, Stolz, Harris, et al., 2004; Schanler, Lau, Hurst, & Smith, 2005). Askin and Diehl-Jones (2002) and Lessaris, Forsythe, and Wagner (2000) found decreases in epidermal growth factor and transforming growth factor-β in fortified human milk, both of which play roles in imunodefense (see **Box 2-3**).

Addition of fortifiers to human milk may increase its osmolality after storage and warming to levels that exceed current recommended limits of osmolality for premature infants (De Curtis, Candusso, Pieltain, & Rigo, 1999; Fenton and Belik, 2002; Srinivasan, Bokiniec, King, Weaver, & Edwards, 2004) and may increase the risk of NEC (Janjindamai & Chotsampancharoen, 2006). When cow's-milk-based fortifiers are used, there is also the added potential for allergic reactions to cow's milk protein. Marinelli (personal communication, 2003) has observed an increased incidence of cow's-milk protein allergy at discharge from the NICU since the use of such fortifiers has become so pervasive.

Box 2-3 A Fortifier Made out of What?

Penny was the mother of preterm twin boys born at 29 weeks' gestation in the autumn of 2002. The boys were in the level 3 NICU of a large New England teaching hospital. The resident neonatologist told Penny that he wanted to add fortifier to her milk so that the boys would gain weight faster. He recommended the powdered human milk fortifier as it would not displace the volume of her milk that each twin would receive. Penny was concerned about this because she and her husband are both allergic to cow's milk protein, and given the vulnerable and permeable state of her infants' gastrointestinal tracts, she did not want to expose them to cow's milk protein for at least the first year of life. She expressed this concern to the neonatologist, who hastened to explain that these fortifiers were not made out of cow's milk but of human milk components.* Penny expressed her skepticism and the neonatologist went off to find the nutritional information about the fortifier to show her, pointing out the presence of lactoferrin and lysozyme in the contents. A closer reading of the nutritional information showed that the listed contents *included* the components of the 25 cc of human milk to which the fortifier is added! The human milk components were listed as if they were in the packet! Marketing spiels for fortifiers made by formula companies need to be met with skepticism by parents and health professionals alike. The boys were fed medium-chain triglycerides, vitamins, and minerals, including calcium and phosphorus.

* Fortifiers made out of human milk were not available commercially in 2002.

Other Methods of Fortification

Some European milk banks have the ability to fractionate and lyophilize (i.e., freeze dry) human milk. Past research has focused on using these fractionated and lyophilized components to fortify either maternal or donor milk on an individualized basis (Hylmo, Polberger, Axelsson, Jakobsson, & Raiha, 1984; Polberger, Raiha, Juvonen, Moro, Minoli, et al., 1999). Polberger et al. (1999) analyzed maternal and donor milk feedings daily for protein content. Then either a bovine whey protein fortifier or a human milk protein fraction was added to bring the total protein content for each infant to 3.5 g/kg. Both groups demonstrated similar biochemical and growth results. This research has now been applied by a commercial company in the United States that is manufacturing a fortifier made exclusively out of human milk protein. Chan, Lee, and Rechtman have found that addition of this human milk-based fortifier does not affect the antibacterial activity of the milk to which it is added (2007). A recent abstract presented at the 2009 Society for Pediatric Research annual meeting also found significant decreases in NEC (p=0.05), surgical NEC (p=0.007), and death or NEC (p=0.04) when comparing the use of the human milk-based fortifier with bovine-based fortifiers. Length of stay, rates of growth, and incidence of sepsis were similar in the two groups (Sullivan, Schanler, Abrams, Ehrenkranz, & HHMF Study Group, 2009).

Other types of fortification can be found in vegetable oils (sources of essential fatty acids), polycose (carbohydrates in liquid form), and simple minerals such as calcium and phosphorus, which are added to improve bone mineralization.

One trend that is being seen more frequently is the analysis of individual feedings of a mother's milk to determine on an individual basis how much fortifier to use. In Scandinavia, full-spectrum infrared analysis of maternal milk (as well as donor milk) determines the protein, fat, and carbohydrate content of donor milk (Michaelsen, Skafte, Badsberg, & Jorgensen, 1990; Arnold, 1999; de Halleux, Close, Stalport, Studzinski, Habibi, et al., 2007). Individual milk feedings can then be analyzed and fortified appropriately to produce milk with the desired levels of protein, fats, and carbohydrates to meet the requirements of a specific preterm infant. A slightly different methodology, near infrared reflectance analysis, was used in another study to monitor nitrogen and fat content of human milk in the NICU so that it could be individually fortified. It was found to be a fast and reliable method (Corvaglia, Battistini, Paoletti, Aceti, Capretti, et al., 2008). Individualized fortification with protein and minerals was also used in a German study that compared a high volume of intake of fortified human milk (200 cc/kg/day) with feeding preterm formula to healthy infants born at less than 28 weeks' gestation. Infants fed the larger amounts of fortified human milk had similar outcomes for growth as the preterm formula-fed group. All fell between the 25th and 50th percentiles of intrauterine growth expectations (Doege & Bauer, 2007).

Several other types of milk manipulation appear in the literature (see **Box 2-4** for one method). Martinez, Desai, Davidson, Nakai, and Radcliffe (1987) used ultrasonic homogenization of expressed milk to prevent fat from

Box 2-4 What About Using the Mother's Hindmilk?

By definition, the foremilk is the milk that comes off at the beginning of the feeding or expression session, and the hindmilk is what comes off at the end. It is a temporal descriptor primarily used in research, so that scientists looking at milk composition know what part of the feeding they are talking about. Researchers have found that when women express their milk using a pump, fat content increases over the course of the expression. If a mother pumps for 15 minutes on a regular schedule, the milk she collects during the last half of the expression will be higher in fat than the first half of the expression. First described by Valentine, Hurst, and Schanler (1994) as a technique to get premature infants to gain weight better on their mothers' own milk, mothers were asked to express for the first 2–3 minutes of a feeding, set that milk aside and then the rest of the milk from that expression, which would be higher in fat content, was fortified with a cow's-milk-based fortifier and fed to the infant. Compared to foremilk, the hindmilk showed a significantly higher energy and fat content, and babies fed a diet of 60% hindmilk feedings had a significant weight increase although head circumference and body length did not increase to the same degree.

This technique was adopted in many U.S. NICUs without further study until recently. In a feasibility study from Nigeria, mean weight gain for 16 preterm infants weighing less than 1800 g at birth exceeded intrauterine standards for growth without the use of additional fortification (Slusher et al., 2003). In another study from Nigeria (Ogechi, William, & Fidelia, 2007), preterm infants who were small for gestational age and were fed unfortified hindmilk gained weight at more than double the rate of infants fed composite expressed milk (milk that had not been separated into foremilk and hindmilk fractions). Those appropriate for gestational age also gained weight more rapidly than composite control subjects, but the differences in rate of weight gain were less dramatic. Similar to Valentine's findings, head circumference and body length were not significantly different from the composite groups. The authors also found that the lipid content was approximately 1.6 times higher in hindmilk than in the composite milk. They recommend this technique of hindmilk feeding to achieve better weight gain and shorten hospital stays for preterm infants.

Box 2-4 What About Using the Mother's Hindmilk? (*continued*)

Another study looking at nutrient composition of hindmilk in mothers of infants born less than 28 weeks' gestation found higher concentrations of retinol (1.6 times), β-tocopherol (1.6 times), γ-tocopherol (1.5 times), fat (1.7 times), energy (1.3 times), and nitrogen (1.05 times) than in foremilk (Bishara, Dunn, Merko, & Darling, 2008). As a result of these higher concentrations, vitamin A and E intakes of infants fed hindmilk fortified with the so-called human milk fortifiers exceeded recommended upper level intakes. Since fat-soluble vitamins are not excreted the way water-soluble vitamins are, they can build to toxic levels if fed at too high concentrations. This may be a cause for concern in the preterm infant. Perhaps using multiple techniques and methods of fortification simultaneously should be reconsidered. If intake volumes of species-specific milk were increased and less fortification used, would there be less risk of obesity and Type I diabetes later in life?

As with other types of fortification, the message such techniques may give to mothers is that their milk is inadequate, deficient, imperfect, and not good enough, and that the mothers are somehow at fault. Steps should be taken to reassure mothers that their milk is exactly what their babies need, and why the babies need more nutrient content. Efforts should also be made to explain to mothers that as their babies grow, the needs for extra nutrients will diminish and their milk really will be perfect for their babies.

adhering to feeding tubes. Premature Brazilian infants with an average birth weight of 1400 g were fed pasteurized ultrasonically homogenized banked donor milk; they gained an average of 5 g/day more than their counterparts receiving milk that had not been homogenized (Martinez, 1989). The group receiving the homogenized donor milk also had significantly greater gains in length, tricipital skinfold, and subscapular skinfold (Martinez & Desai, 1995; Rayol, Martinez, Jorge, Gonçalves, & Desai, 1993). Furthermore, they achieved intrauterine growth rates and hospital stays were shortened (Martinez, 1989). Martinez and Desai (1995) also report the use of a human milk formula, a modification of banked donor milk from term mothers in which excess lactose is precipitated out while leaving other nutrients in concentrated form. These are then diluted, homogenized, and pasteurized for later use.

SUMMARY

The preterm infant, especially when born very early and very small, faces tremendous challenges in trying to gain weight, increase head circumference and brain growth, and develop in a timely fashion. When nutrition is inadequate for the preterm infant, deficits occur in development and the potential for long-term problems increases. Preterm formula appears to give these fragile babies an edge in terms of more rapid growth, but given the hazards of formula feeding, the infant's more permeable and porous gut, and the association of formula feeding with chronic disease later in life, are we doing these vulnerable infants a service by getting them to just grow faster? It appears that there has to be a balance. Human milk is the feeding of choice for not only improving short-term outcomes such as a decrease in NEC and sepsis but also for improving long-term outcomes and decreasing the incidence of chronic disease. Therefore, an adequate supply of human milk needs to be available, and preterm infants need to be fed aggressively to make the biggest impact in immediate growth.

Mothers make the very best milk for their own infants in the majority of cases. In the absence of a mother's own milk, donor milk should be accessed. Maintaining a supply of milk for the mother of a preterm infant is difficult, however, as we have seen in Bonnie's case in Chapter 1. Every effort, therefore, should be made in order to improve the milk supply in a NICU by first supporting individual mothers in their quest to establish and maintain an ample milk supply and then to establish breastfeeding once the infant is able to feed at the breast. How do we do this and make a difference for the Bonnies and their babies in our own communities?

Several models have been implemented in Scandinavia for baby-friendly NICUs. Based on the World Health Organization's Ten Steps to Successful Breastfeeding, these practice sets promote breastfeeding and the use of human milk, protect its use, and support the mother optimally. What follows in Part III of this book is a model developed by the American Breastfeeding Institute (ABI) for the United States to which every hospital with a NICU should subscribe. The ABI Ten Steps are listed in **Table 2-2**. If Bonnie and her newly born infant had had a hospital NICU like the one outlined in the policies and procedures in Table 2-2, she most likely would have been successful in achieving her goals of supplying more milk to her son and transitioning him to the breast.

Table 2-2 The ABI Ten Steps to a Breastfeeding-Friendly NICU

Every neonatal intensive care and special care nursery will complete the following steps.
Step 1: Have a current written evidence-based breastfeeding policy that is routinely communicated to all NICU staff.
Step 2: Educate and train all staff in the specific knowledge and skills necessary to implement this policy.
Step 3: Inform all women and their partners at risk for delivering or who have already delivered a preterm or compromised infant of the benefits of providing human milk.
Step 4: Facilitate bonding and maternal competency from the moment of birth.
Step 5: Enable mothers to begin early milk expression and provide ongoing education and support to promote adequate milk supply.
Step 6: Give preterm and compromised babies only human milk unless *medically* contraindicated.
Step 7: Promote early and continued skin-to-skin contact for mothers and their premature or compromised infants with full mechanical breastmilk expression.
Step 8: Foster early developmentally appropriate initiation and transition to full breastfeeding.
Step 9: Use ethical evidence-based breastfeeding practices free of conflicts of interest.
Step 10: Foster the establishment of NICU/SCN breastfeeding support groups and postdischarge community programs and refer mothers to them.

REFERENCES

Amin, S., Merle, K., Orlando, M., Dalzell, L., & Guillet, R. (2000). Brainstem maturation in premature infants as a function of enteral feeding type. *Pediatrics, 106*(2 Pt. 1), 318–322.

Arnold, L. D. W. (1997). A brief look at drip milk and its relation to donor human milk banking. *Journal of Human Lactation, 13*(4), 323–324.

Arnold, L. D. W. (1999). Donor milk banking in Scandinavia. *Journal of Human Lactation, 15*(1), 55–59.

Arnold, L. D. W. (2002). Human milk for fragile infants. In K. Cadwell (Ed.), *Reclaiming breastfeeding for the United States: Protection, promotion and support* (pp. 137–159). Sudbury, MA: Jones and Bartlett.

Arnold, L. D. W. (2005). Donor human milk banking: Creating public health policy in the 21st century. Doctoral dissertation, Union Institute and University.

Ashraf, R., Jalil, F., Zaman, S., Karlberg, J., Khan, S., Lindblad, B., et al. (1991). Breast feeding and protection against neonatal sepsis in a high risk population. *Archives of Disease in Childhood, 66*(4), 488–490.

Askin, D., & Diehl-Jones, W. (2002). Effects of human milk fortifier on bacterial growth and cytokines in breast milk. *Proceedings of the Annual Meeting, 5*(1), 10–18.

Atkinson, S., Anderson, G., & Bryan, M. (1980). Human milk: Comparison of the nitrogen composition in milk from mothers of premature and full-term infants. *American Journal of Clinical Nutrition, 33*(4), 811–815.

Auricchio, S., Follo, D., deRitis, G., Giunta, A., Marzorati, D., Prampolini, L., et al. (1983). Does breast feeding protect against the development of clinical symptoms of celiac disease in children? *Journal of Pediatric Gastroenterology and Nutrition, 2*(3), 428–433.

Baldwin, E., & Vance, M. (2009). *Summary of breastfeeding legislation in the US*. Retrieved May 29, 2009, from http://www.llli.org/Law/LawBills.html

Benhamou, P.-H., Cheikh, A., Francoual, C., Kalach, N., DeBoisseau, D., & Dupont, C. (1998). Possible protection by breast-feeding against severe esophageal and gastric lesions in the neonate. *Biology of the Neonate, 73*(5), 337–339.

Berseth, C., Van Aerde, J., Gross, S., Stolz, S., Harris, C., & Hansen, J. (2004). Growth, efficacy, and safety of feeding an iron-fortified human milk fortifier. *Pediatrics, 114*(6), e699–e706.

Bishara, R., Dunn, M., Merko, S., & Darling, P. (2008). Nutrient composition of hindmilk produced by mothers of very low birth weight infants born at less than 28 weeks gestation. *Journal of Human Lactation, 24*(2), 159–167.

Bisquera, J., Cooper, T., & Berseth, C. (2000). Impact of necrotizing enterocolitis in very low birthweight infants on morbidity, length of hospitalization, and hospital charges. *Pediatric Research, 47*, 304A.

Bisquera, J., Cooper, T., & Berseth, C. (2002). Impact of necrotizing enterocolitis on length of stay and hospital charges in very low birth weight infants. *Pediatrics, 109*(3), 423–428.

Cadwell, C. (2002). Defining breastfeeding research. In K. Cadwell (Ed.), *Reclaiming breastfeeding for the United States: Protection, promotion, and support* (pp. 81–89). Sudbury, MA: Jones and Bartlett.

Cadwell, K., & Turner-Maffei, C. (2002). *Breastmilk and diabetes: Understanding the connection*. East Sandwich, MA: Health Education Associates.

Cameron, N., Pettifor, J., De Wet, T., & Norris, S. (2003). The relationship of rapid weight gain in infancy to obesity and skeletal maturity in childhood. *Obesity Research, 11*(3), 457–460.

Chan, G., Lee, M., & Rechtman, D. (2007). Effects of a human milk-derived human milk fortifier on the antibacterial actions of human milk. *Breastfeeding Medicine, 2*(4), 205–208.

Chen, Y., Yu, S., & Li, W.-X. (1988). Artificial feeding and hospitalization in the first 18 months of life. *Pediatrics, 81*(1), 58–62.

Corvaglia, L., Battistini, B., Paoletti, V., Aceti, A., Capretti, M., & Faldella, G. (2008). Near infrared reflectance analysis to evaluate human milk's nitrogen and fat content in neonatal intensive care unit. *Archives of Disease in Childhood, Fetal and Neonatal Edition, 93*(5), F372–F375.

Davis, M., Savitz, D., & Graubard, B. (1988, August 13). Infant feeding and childhood cancer. *The Lancet, 2*(8607), 365–368.

De Curtis, M., Candusso, M., Pieltain, C., & Rigo, J. (1999). Effect of fortification on the osmolality of human milk. *Archives of Disease in Childhood, Fetal and Neonatal Edition, 81*(2), F141–F143.

de Halleux, V., Close, A., Stalport, S., Studzinski, F., Habibi, F., & Rigo, J. (2007). Advantages of individualized fortification of human milk for preterm infants. *Archives of Pediatrics, 14*(Suppl. 1), S5–S10.

Dell, S., & To, T. (2001). Breastfeeding and asthma in young children: findings from a population-based study. *Archives of Pediatric and Adolescent Medicine, 155*(11), 1261–1265.

Dewey, K., Heinig, M., & Nommsen-Rivers, L. (1995). Differences in morbidity between breast-fed and formula-fed infants. *Journal of Pediatrics, 126*(5 Pt. 1), 696–702.

Doege, C., & Bauer, J. (2007). Effect of high volume intake of mother's milk with an individualized supplementation of minerals and protein on early growth of preterm infants < 28 weeks of gestation. *Clinics in Nutrition, 26*(5), 581–588.

Duncan, B., Holberg, C., Wright, A., Martinez, F., & Taussig, L. (1993). Exclusive breast-feeding for at least 4 months protects against otitis media. *Pediatrics, 91*(5), 867–872.

Eid, E. (1970). Follow-up study of physical growth of children who had excessive weight gain in first six months of life. *British Medical Journal, 2*(5701), 74–76.

Ellestad-Sayed, J., Coodin, F., Dilling, L., & Haworth, J. (1979). Breast-feeding protects against infection in Indian infants. *Canadian Medical Association Journal, 120*(3), 295–298.

Fenton T., & Belik, J. (2002). Routine handling of milk fed to preterm infants can significantly increase osmolality. *Journal of Pediatric Gastroenterology and Nutrition, 35*(3), 298–302.

Forman, M., Graubard, B. Hoffman, H., Beren, R., Harley, E., & Bennett, P. (1984). The Pima infant feeding study: Breastfeeding and gastroenteritis in the first year of life. *American Journal of Epidemiology, 119*(3), 335–349.

Freudenheim, J., Marshall, J., Graham, S., Laughlin, R., Vena, J., & Bandera, E. (1994). Exposure to breast milk in infancy and the risk of breast cancer. *Epidemiology, 5*(3), 324–331.

Gdalevich, M., Mimouni, D., & Mimouni, M. (2001). Breast-feeding and the risk of bronchial asthma in childhood: A systematic review with meta-analysis of prospective studies. *Journal of Pediatrics, 139*(2), 261–266.

Gerstein, H. (1994). Cow's milk exposure and type I diabetes mellitus. A critical overview of the clinical literature. *Diabetes Care, 17*(1), 13–19.

Hamosh, M. (1994). Digestion in the premature infant: The effects of human milk. *Seminars in Perinatology, 18*(6), 485–494.

Hasselbalch, H., Jeppesen, D., Engelmann, M., Michaelsen, K., & Nielsen, M. (1996). Decreased thymus size in formula-fed infants compared with breastfed infants. *Acta Padeiatrica, 85*(9), 1029–1032.

Hay, W., Lucas, A., Heird, W., Ziegler, E., Levin, E., Grave, G., et al. (1999). Workshop summary: Nutrition of the extremely low birth weight infant. *Pediatrics, 104*(6), 1360–1368.

Haynes, S. (2003, November). *Findings from the national focus groups that will direct the national media campaign.* Paper presented at the "Childbearing and breastfeeding women: Improving outcomes through optimizing practice" conference, Natick, MA.

Horwood, L., & Fergusson, D. (1998). Breastfeeding and later cognitive and academic outcomes. *Pediatrics, 101*(1), E9.

Hylander, M., Strobino, D., Pezzullo, J., & Dhanireddy, R. (2001). Association of human milk feedings with a reduction in retinopathy of prematurity among very low birth weight infants. *Journal of Perinatology, 21*(6), 356–362.

Hylmo, P., Polberger, S., Axelsson, I., Jakobsson, I., & Raiha, N. (1984). Preparation of fat and protein from banked human milk: its use in feeding very-low-birth-weight infants. In A. Williams & J. Baum (Eds.), *Human milk banking: Vol. 5. Nestle Nutrition Workshop Series* (pp. 55–61). New York: Vevey/Raven Press.

Janjindamai, W., & Chotsampancharoen, T. (2006). Effect of fortification on osmolality of human milk. *Journal of the Medical Association of Thailand, 89*(9), 1400–1403.

Jocson, M., Mason, E., & Schanler, R. (1997). The effects of nutrient fortification and varying storage conditions on host defense properties of human milk. *Pediatrics, 100*(2 Pt. 1), 240–243.

Karjalainen, J., Martin, J., Knip, M., Ilonen, J., Robinson, B., Savilahti, E., et al. (1992). A bovine albumin peptide as a possible trigger of insulin dependent diabetes mellitus. *New England Journal of Medicine, 327*(5), 302–307.

Koletzko, B., Dodds, P., Akerblom, H., & Ashwell, M. (Eds.). (2005). *Early nutrition and its later consequences: New opportunities—perinatal programming of adult health.* New York: Springer Dorbrecht.

Koletzko, S., Sherman, S., Corey, M., Griffiths, A., & Smith, C. (1989). Role of infant feeding practices in development of Crohn's disease in childhood. *British Medical Journal, 298*(6688), 1617–1618.

Kosloske, A. (2001). Breast milk decreases the risk of neonatal necrotizing enterocolitis. In B. Woodward & H. Draper (Eds.), *Immunological properties of human milk: Vol. 10. Advances in nutrition research* (pp. 123–137). New York: Kluwer Academic/Plenum Publishers.

Lenati, R., O'Connor, D., Hebert, K., Farber, J., & Pagotto, F. (2008). Growth and survival of Enterobacter sakazakii in human breast milk with and without fortifiers as compared to powdered infant formula. *International Journal of Food Microbiology, 122*(1–2), 171–179.

Lessaris, K., Forsythe, D., & Wagner, C. (2000). Effect of human milk fortifier on the immunodetection and molecular mass profile of transforming growth factor-alpha. *Biology of the Neonate, 77*(3), 156–161.

Lucas, A. (1994). Role of nutritional programming in determining adult morbidity. *Archives of Disease in Childhood, 71*(4), 288–290.

Lucas, A., & Cole T. (1990). Breast milk and neonatal necrotising enterocolitis. *The Lancet, 336*(8730), 1519–1523.

Lucas, A., Morley, R., Cole, T., & Gore, S. (1994). A randomized multicentre study of human milk versus formula and later development in preterm infants. *Archives of Disease in Childhood, 70*(2), F141–F146.

Lucas, A., Morley, R., Cole, T., Lister, G., & Leeson-Payne, C. (1992). Breast milk and subsequent intelligence quotient in children born preterm. *The Lancet, 339*(8788), 261–264.

Lucas, A., Sarson, D., Blackburn, A., Adrian, T., Aynsley-Green, A., & Bloom, S. (1980). Breast vs. bottle: Endocrine responses are different with formula feeding. *The Lancet, 1*(8181), 1267–1269.

Luukkainen, P., Salo, M., & Nikkari, T. (1994). Changes in the fatty acid composition of preterm and term human milk from 1 week to 6 months of lactation. *Journal of Pediatric Gastroenterology and Nutrition, 18*(3), 355–360.

Martin, J., Trink, B., Daneman, D., Dosch, H., & Robinson, B. (1991). Milk proteins in the etiology of insulin-dependent diabetes mellitus (IDDM). *Annals of Medicine, 23*(4), 447–452.

Martinez, F. (1989, October). *Growth of premature neonates fed banked pasteurized human milk homogenized by ultrasonication.* Paper presented at the annual meeting of the Human Milk Banking Association of North America, Vancouver, British Columbia.

Martinez, F., & Desai, I. (1995). Human milk and premature infants. In A. Simopoulos, J. Dutra de Oliveira, & I. Desai (Eds.), *Behavioral and metabolic aspects of breastfeeding: Vol. 78. World review of nutrition and diet* (pp. 55–73). Basel, Switzerland: Karger.

Martinez, F., Desai, I., Davidson, A., Nakai, S., & Radcliffe, A. (1987). Ultrasonic homogenization of expressed human milk to prevent fat loss during tube feeding. *Journal of Pediatric Gastroenterology and Nutrition, 6*(4), 593–597.

Mason, T., Rabinovich, C., Fredrickson, C., Amorosa, K., Reed, A., Stein, L., et al. (1995). Breast feeding and the development of juvenile rheumatoid arthritis. *Journal of Rheumatology, 22*(6), 1166–1170.

McKinney, P., Parslow, R., Gurney, K., Law, G., Bodansky, H., & Williams, R. (1999). Perinatal and neonatal determinants of childhood type 1 diabetes. A case-control study in Yorkshire, U.K. *Diabetes Care, 22*(6), 928–932.

Michaelsen, K., Skafte, L., Badsberg, J., & Jorgensen, M. (1990). Variation in macronutrients in human bank milk: Influencing factors and implications for human milk banking. *Journal of Pediatric Gastroenterology and Nutrition, 11*(2), 229–239.

Mimouni Bloch, A., Mimouni, D., Mimouni, M., & Gdalevich, M. (2002). Does breastfeeding protect against allergic rhinitis during childhood? A meta-analysis of prospective studies. *Acta Paediatrica, 91*(3), 275–279.

Monteiro, P., Victora, C., Barros, F., & Monteiro, L. (2003). Birth size, early childhood growth and adolescent obesity in a Brazilian birth cohort. *International Journal of Obesity, 27*(10), 1274–1282.

Morley, R., & Lucas, A. (1994). Influence of early diet on outcome in preterm infants. *Acta Paediatrica, 405*(Suppl.), 123–126.

Oddy, W. (2000). Breastfeeding and asthma in children: Findings from a West Australia study. *Breastfeeding Reviews, 8*(1), 5–11.

Oddy, W., Peat, J., & de Klerk, N. (2002). Maternal asthma, infant feeding, and the risk of asthma in childhood. *Journal of Allergy and Clinical Immunology, 110*(1), 65–67.

Ogechi, A., William, O., & Fidelia, B. (2007). Hindmilk and weight gain in preterm very low birth-weight infants. *Pediatrics International, 49*(2), 156–160.

Ong, K., Ahmed, M., Emmet, P., Preece, M., & Dunger, D. (2000). Association between postnatal catch-up growth and obesity in childhood: Prospective cohort. *British Medical Journal, 320*(7240), 967–971.

Paradise, J., Elster, B., & Tan, L. (1994). Evidence in infants with cleft palate that breast milk protects against otitis media. *Pediatrics, 94*(6 Pt. 1), 853–860.

Pettitt, D., Forman, M., Hanson, R., Knowler, W., & Bennett, P. (1997). Breastfeeding and incidence of non-insulin-dependent diabetes mellitus in Pima Indians. *The Lancet, 350*(9072), 166–168.

Pettitt, D., & Knowler, W. (1998). Long-term effects of the intrauterine environment, birth weight, and breast-feeding in Pima Indians. *Diabetes Care, 21*(Suppl. 2), B138–B141.

Pikwer, M., Bergstrom, U., Nilsson, J., Jacobsson, L., Berglund, G., & Turesson, C. (2008). Breast-feeding, but not use of oral contraceptives, is associated with a reduced risk of rheumatoid arthritis. *Annals of Rheumatoid Disease, 68*(4), 526–530.

Pisacane, A., de Luca, U., Criscuolo, L., Vaccaro, F., Valiente, A., Inglese, A., et al. (1996). Breast feeding and hypertrophic pyloric stenosis: Population based case-control study. *British Medical Journal, 312*(7033), 745–746.

Pisacane, A., de Luca, U., Vaccaro, F., Valiente, A., Impagliazzo, N., & Caracciola, G. (1995). Breast-feeding and inguinal hernia. *Journal of Pediatrics, 127*(1), 109–111.

Pisacane, A., Graziano, L., Mazzarella, G., Scrapellino, B., & Zona, G. (1992). Breast-feeding and urinary tract infection. *Journal of Pediatrics, 120*(1), 87–89.

Pisacane, A., Graziano, L., Zona, G., Granata, G., Dolezalova, H., Cafiero, M., et al. (1994). Breast feeding and acute lower respiratory infection. *Acta Paediatrica, 83*(7), 714–718.

Polberger, S., Raiha, N., Juvonen, P., Moro, G., Minoli, I., & Warm, A. (1999). Individualized protein fortification of human milk for preterm infants: Comparison of ultrafiltrated human milk protein and a bovine whey fortifier. *Journal of Pediatric Gastroenterology and Nutrition, 29*(3), 332–338.

Quan, R., Yang, C., Rubinstein, S., Lewiston, N., Stevenson, D., & Kerner, J., Jr. (1994). The effect of nutritional additives on anti-infective factors in human milk. *Clinics in Pediatrics, 33*(6), 325–328.

Raisler, J., Alexander, C., & O'Campo, P. (1999). Breast-feeding and infant illness: A dose-response relationship? *American Journal of Public Health, 89*(1), 25–30.

Ravelli, A., van der Meulen, J., Osmond, C., Barker, D., & Bleker, O. (2000). Infant feeding and adult glucose tolerance, lipid profile, blood pressure, and obesity. *Archives of Disease in Childhood, 82*(3), 248–252.

Rayol, M., Martinez, F., Jorge, S., Gonçalves, A., & Desai, I. (1993). Feeding premature infants banked human milk homogenized by ultrasonic treatment. *Journal of Pediatrics, 123*(6), 985–988.

Rees, C., Pierro, A., & Eaton, S. (2007). Neurodevelopmental outcomes of neonates with medically and surgically treated necrotizing enterocolitis. *Archives of Disease in Childhood, Fetal and Neonatal Edition, 92*(3), F193–F198.

Rigas, A., Rigas, B., Glassman, M., Yen, Y-Y., Lan, S. J., Petridou, E., et al. (1993). Breast-feeding and maternal smoking in the etiology of Crohn's disease and ulcerative colitis in childhood. *Annals of Epidemiology, 3*(4), 387–392.

Rogan, W., & Gladen, B. (1993). Breast-feeding and cognitive development. *Early Human Development, 31*(3), 181–193.

Rolland-Cachera, M. (2005). Rate of growth in early life: A predictor of later health? In B. Koletzko, P. Dodds, H. Akerblom, & M. Ashwell (Eds.), *Early nutrition and its later consequences: New opportunities; Vol. 569. Advances in experimental medicine and biology.* (pp. 35–39). New York: Springer Dordrecht.

Ronnestad, A., Abrahamsen, T., Medbo, S., Reigstad, H., Lossius, K., Kaaresen, P., et al. (2005). Late-onset septicemia in a Norwegian national cohort of extremely premature infants receiving very early full human milk feeding. *Pediatrics, 115*(3), e269–e276.

Russell, R., Green, N., Steiner, C., Meikle, S., Howse, J., Poschman, K., et al. (2007). Cost of hospitalization for preterm and low birth weight infants in the United States. *Pediatrics, 120*(1), e1–e9.

Ruuska, T. (1992). Occurrence of acute diarrhea in atopic and nonatopic infants: The role of prolonged breastfeeding. *Journal of Pediatric Gastroenterology and Nutrition, 14*(1), 27–33.

Sadauskaite-Kuehne, V., Ludvigsson, J., Padaiga, Z., Jasinskiene, E., Samuelsson, U. (2004). Longer breastfeeding is an independent protective factor against development of type I diabetes mellitus in childhood. *Diabetes and Metabolic Research Review, 20*(2), 150–157.

Santiago, M., Codipilly, C., Potak, D., & Schanler, R. (2005). Effect of human milk fortifiers on bacterial growth in human milk. *Journal of Perinatology, 25*(10), 647–649.

Schanler, R., Lau, C., Hurst, N., & Smith, E. (2005). Randomized trial of donor human milk versus preterm formula as substitutes for mothers' own milk in the feeding of extremely premature infants. *Pediatrics, 116*(2), 400–406.

Sharpe, G. (2002, May 31). Donor milk in the NICU. Presentation at "Breastfeeding premature infants: A blueprint for success" conference, Natick, MA.

Shu, X-O., Clemens, J., Zheng, W., Ying, D. M., Ji, B. T., & Jin, F. (1995). Infant breastfeeding and the risk of childhood lymphoma and leukemia. *International Journal of Epidemiology, 24*(1), 27–32.

Singhal, A., Cole, T., Fewtrell, M., Deanfield, J., & Lucas, A. (2004). Is slower early growth beneficial for long-term cardiovascular health? *Circulation, 109*(9), 1108–1113.

Singhal, A., Cole, T., Fewtrell, M., & Lucas, A. (2004). Breastmilk feeding and lipoprotein profile in adolescents born preterm: Follow-up of a prospective randomized study. *The Lancet, 363*(9421), 1571–1578.

Singhal, A., Cole, T., & Lucas, A. (2001). Early nutrition in preterm infants and later blood pressure: Two cohorts after randomised trials. *The Lancet, 357*(254), 413–419.

Singhal, A., Farooqi, I., O'Rahilly, S., Cole, T., Fewtrell, M., & Lucas, A. (2002). Early nutrition and leptin concentrations in later life. *American Journal of Clinical Nutrition, 75*(6), 993–999.

Singhal, A., Fewtrell, M., Cole, T., & Lucas, A. (2003). Low nutrient intake and early growth for later insulin resistance in adolescents born preterm. *The Lancet, 361*(9363), 1089–1097.

Singhal, A., Morley, R., Cole, T., Kennedy, K., Sonksen, P., Isaacs, E., et al. (2007). Infant nutrition and stereoacuity at age 4–6 y. *American Journal of Clinical Nutrition, 85*(1), 152–159.

Sisk, P., Lovelady, C., Dillard, R., Gruber, K., & O'Shea, T. (2007). Early human milk feeding is associated with a lower risk of necrotizing enterocolitis in very low birth weight infants. *Journal of Perinatology, 27*, 428–433.

Slusher, T., Hampton, R., Bode-Thomas, F., Pam, S., Akor, F., & Meier, P. (2003). Promoting exclusive feeding of own mother's milk through the use of hindmilk and increased maternal milk volume for hospitalized low birth weight infants (< 1800 grams) in Nigeria: A feasibility study. *Journal of Human Lactation, 19*(2), 191–198.

Springer, S. (1997). Human milk banking in Germany. *Journal of Human Lactation, 13*(1), 65–68.

Srinivasan, L., Bokiniec, R., King, C., Weaver, G., & Edwards, A. (2004). Increased osmolality of breast milk with therapeutic additives. *Archives Disease in Childhood, Fetal and Neonatal Edition, 89*(6), F514–F517.

Sullivan, S., Schanler, R., Abrams, S., Ehrenkranz, R., & HHMF Study Group. (2009). *A randomized controlled trial of human vs. bovine-based human milk fortifiers in extremely preterm infants.* Retrieved May 29, 2009, from http://www.prolacta.com/docs/pas_abstract_2009.pdf

Thorsdottir, I., Birgisdottir, B., Johannsdottir, I., Harris, D., Hill, J., Steingrimsdottir, L., et al. (2000). Different beta-casein fractions in Icelandic versus Scandinavian cow's milk may influence diabetogenicity of cow's milk in infancy and explain low incidence of insulin-dependent diabetes mellitus in Iceland. *Pediatrics, 106*(4), 719–724.

Thureen, P., & Hay, W. (2001). Early aggressive nutrition in preterm infants. *Seminars in Neonatology, 6*(5), 403–415.

Toschke, A., Grote, V., Koletzko, B., & von Kries, R. (2004). Identifying children at high risk for overweight at school entry by weight gain during the first 2 years. *Archives of Pediatric and Adolescent Medicine, 158*(5), 449–452.

Tyson, J., & Kennedy, K. (2005). Trophic feedings for parenterally fed infants. *Cochrane Database Systematic Reviews, 20*, CD000504.

United States Breastfeeding Committee. (2002). *Economic benefits of breastfeeding* [Issue paper]. Raleigh, NC: Author.

United States Breastfeeding Committee. (2005). State legislation that protects, promotes, and supports breastfeeding. Retrieved May 29, 2009, from http://www.usbreastfeeding.org/LinkClick.aspx?link=Publications%2fState-Legislation-Inventory-Analysis-2005-USBC.pdf&tabid=70&mid=388

Valentine, C., Hurst, N., & Schanler, R. (1994). Hindmilk improves weight gain in low-birth-weight infants fed human milk. *Journal of Pediatric Gastroenterology and Nutrition, 18*(4), 474–477.

Victora, C., Smith, P. Vaughan, J., Nobre, L., Lombardi, C., Teixeira, A., et al. (1989). Infant feeding and deaths due to diarrhea: A case-control study. *American Journal of Epidemiology, 129*(5), 1032–1041.

Virtanen, S., Rasanen, L., Ylonen, K., Aro, A., Clayton, D., Langholz, B., et al. (1993). Early introduction of dairy products associated with increased risk of IDDM in Finnish children. The Diabetes in Childhood in Finland Study Group. *Diabetes, 42*(12), 1786–1790.

Vohr, B., Poindexter, B., Dusick, A., McKinley, L., Wright, L., Langer, J., et al., for the NICHD Neonatal Research Network. (2006). Beneficial effects of breast milk in the neonatal intensive care unit on the developmental outcome of extremely low birth weight infants at 18 months of age. *Pediatrics, 118*(1), 115–123.

von Kries, R., Koletzko, B., Sauerwald, T., von Mutius, E., Barnert, D., Grunert, V., et al. (1999). Breast feeding and obesity: Cross sectional study. *British Medical Journal, 319*(7203), 147–150.

Wallensteen, M., Lindblad, B., Zetterstrom, R., & Persson, B. (1991). Acute C-peptide, insulin and branched chain amino acid response to feeding in formula and breast fed infants. *Acta Paediatrica Scandinavia, 80*(2), 143–148.

Wight, N., & Morton, J. (2008). Human milk, breastfeeding, and the preterm infant. In T. Hale & P. Hartmann (Eds.), *Textbook of human lactation* (pp. 215–253). Amarillo, TX: Hale Publishing, L.P.

Young, T., Martens, P., Taback, S., Sellers, E., Dean, H., Cheang, M., et al. (2002). Type 2 diabetes mellitus in children: Prenatal and early infancy risk factors among native Canadians. *Archives of Pediatric and Adolescent Medicine, 156*(7), 651–656.

Yu, V. (2005). Extrauterine growth restriction in preterm infants: Importance of optimizing nutrition in neonatal intensive care units. *Croatian Medical Journal, 46*(5), 737–743.

Ziegler, E., Thureen, P., & Carlson, S. (2002). Aggressive nutrition of the very low birth weight infant. *Clinics in Perinatology, 29*(2), 225–244.

Part III

Policies to Improve Human Milk Use in the NICU: A Ten-Step Framework

chapter three

Implementing NICU Breastfeeding Support: Policies and Procedures: Step 1

CAN THERE BE BABY-FRIENDLY NICUS?

The Ten Steps to Successful Breastfeeding, upon which the Baby-Friendly Hospital Initiative (BFHI) is based, are a method of improving maternity care practices in hospitals and providing continuity of care so that breastfeeding gets off to a good start and the mother and baby's right to breastfeed is not denied. While the BFHI is intended primarily for those practices that impact healthy, term newborns, there are aspects of the Ten Steps that cover what to do if the baby and mother are separated during the maternity stay for legitimate medical reasons of illness, prematurity, and/or low birth weight. Step 1, the establishment of an evidence-based breastfeeding policy, and Step 2, education of the staff on implementing the policy, should be standard in any pediatric or neonatal unit. Step 3, educating mothers prenatally about the benefits of breastfeeding, is also important when working with any mother, but with mothers who deliver preterm, there is less time to provide the basic knowledge with which a mother can exercise an informed choice about infant feeding, and the importance of human milk for her particular baby's circumstances must be underlined. Step 5 maintains that mothers should know how to establish and maintain a milk supply, even when separated from their infants—perhaps the step most pertinent to the NICU mother and the reality of a milk supply for her infant. Step 10 also has applications for the NICU and pediatric unit in the establishment of support systems for mothers who have hospitalized infants.

Merewood, Philipp, Chawla, and Cimo (2003) found that implementing the Baby-Friendly Hospital Initiative had a spillover effect in the NICU. Boston Medical Center, a tertiary care inner city hospital serving a multiracial and largely impoverished minority population, was awarded the Baby-Friendly™ designation in 1999. According to Merewood and colleagues (2003), during the site visit in which Baby-Friendly status was evaluated, the NICU was also inspected to determine if it met the same standards as other units for those steps that were applicable, including whether it was purchasing specialty formulas at fair market value (Step 6). Breastfeeding rates (i.e., mothers supplying their own milk) for all NICU babies during the first week of feeding increased substantially in the 4-year period of comparison from before implementation of the BFHI to after implementation (34.6% [1995] to 74.4% [1999]). Additionally, among U.S.-born Blacks, the racial minority with the lowest breastfeeding rates in the United States, breastfeeding in the NICU increased from 34.5% (1995) to 64% (1999) and for Blacks born outside the United States from 27% (1995) to 81% (1999). During the second week of feeding, those receiving any of their mother's milk rose from 27.9% (1995) to 65.9% (1999) and those receiving *only* their mother's milk rose from 9.3% to 39% in 1999. It is clear that implementing the Ten Steps in the maternity setting had a positive impact on breastfeeding rates in the NICU.

> Thus, the importance of a hospital system that is designed (by following the Ten Steps) to support breastfeeding and ease the complicated NICU situation is critical in vulnerable, low income women who may lack the resources and the ability to advocate for themselves and for their infants. (Merewood et al., 2003, p. 170)

APPLICATION OF BFHI MODELS TO NICUS IN OTHER SETTINGS

It is obvious from Bonnie's story in Chapter 1 of this book, as well as other women's stories, that there is a need for initiatives similar to the Ten Steps for the NICU geared specifically to the mother and baby who are potentially physically separated from each other for long periods of time. In Scandinavia, hospitals have become interested in developing and implementing steps for NICU settings that promote, protect, and support breastfeeding just as the BFHI does in maternity settings. In Denmark, the National Breastfeeding Centre developed a series of Ten Steps to Successful Breastfeeding of

Preterm Infants, which was adopted by the National Board of Health in 2006. In Sweden, Nyqvist and Kylberg (2008) have suggested 13 Steps for NICU practice based on interviews with mothers who had previously had infants in the NICU. **Table 3-1** shows a side-by-side comparison of the BFHI Ten Steps for term newborns; these two Scandinavian proposals for the NICU, and the American Breastfeeding Institute (ABI)'s Ten Steps delineated at the end of Chapter 2.

In the United States, Spatz (2004) has also suggested Ten Steps for promoting and protecting breastfeeding in NICU populations. These Ten Steps (see **Box 3-1**) are similar to the steps presented in Table 3-1. However, they highlight important practice elements of breastfeeding management and support rather than the broader principles espoused by others (see Table 3-1).

RESPECT: THE UNDERPINNING OF HUMANE PERINATAL CARE

A reexamination of Bonnie's story in Chapter 1 demonstrates how poor continuity of care can be in NICU settings. Bonnie's story is not unique. I have been told of similar experiences in very different parts of the United States. Nurses and doctors disagree; what is done on one shift is undone on the next; different nurses have different non–evidence-based explanations for the same situation; there are no evidence-based policies in place that dictate how and when to do something. When continuity of care is lacking, the outcome is that mothers of preterm infants are ignored and disrespected. Their requests for assistance are disregarded, their informed choices are thwarted, and obstacles that prevent them from learning how to be a mother are placed in their way every day. Mothers live under the threat that at any time they could request something that would make the NICU staff think that they are bad mothers and suggest that social services be called, perhaps for foster care placement of the baby. These elements of care show a lack of respect for the mother (and family) and often a violation of ethical principles (see Chapter 17). Lack of respect from hospital staff can mean that mothers are unnecessarily separated from their babies not just physically, but emotionally as well.

From the results of Nyqvist and Kylberg's 2008 survey of former special care nursery (SCN) mothers, it would appear that lack of respect and empathy for the mother is not just a U.S. phenomenon. I believe that sensitivity, empathy, and respect for the mother and her important nurturing role should underpin *every* action taken in the NICU. Everyone wants what is best for the baby—most of all, the mother. She needs to be respected as an individual who has her baby's best interests at heart. She should be the ultimate decision

Table 3-1 Side-by-Side Comparison of Three Models Based on the WHO/UNICEF Model

Principle	*WHO/UNICEF Ten Steps to Successful Breastfeeding for the Healthy Term Newborn*	*ABI's Ten Steps for the NICU/SCN*	*Nyqvist and Kylberg (2008) Swedish Mothers' 13 Steps*	*Danish Ten Steps to Successful Breastfeeding of Preterm Infants*
Development of a breastfeeding policy	Step 1. Have a written breastfeeding policy that is routinely communicated to all healthcare staff.	Step 1. Have a current written evidence-based breastfeeding policy that is routinely communicated to NICU staff.	Step 1. Have a written breastfeeding policy, adapted to infants who require neonatal care, that is routinely communicated to all concerned staff and to parents.	Step 1. The hospital has a strategy on breastfeeding preterm infants based on updated knowledge.
Staff training	Step 2. Train all healthcare staff in skills necessary to implement this policy.	Step 2. Educate and train all staff in the specific knowledge and skills necessary to implement this policy.	Step 3. Educate and train all staff in the specific knowledge and skills necessary to implement this policy.	Step 2. The healthcare staff is able to translate the strategy into good clinical practices.
Prenatal breastfeeding education	Step 3. Inform all pregnant women about the benefits and management of breastfeeding.	Step 3. Inform all women and their partners at risk for delivering or who have already delivered a preterm or compromised infant of the benefits of providing human milk.	Step 4. Inform all pregnant women about initiation of lactation and breastfeeding in the event that the infant is born preterm or ill.	
The immediate postpartum period: bonding and breastfeeding	Step 4. Help mothers to initiate breastfeeding within 30 minutes after birth.[a]	Step 4. Facilitate bonding and maternal competency from the moment of birth.		
Establishing and maintaining milk supply	Step 5. Show mothers how to breastfeed and maintain lactation even if they should be separated from their infants.	Step 5. Enable mothers to begin early milk expression and provide ongoing education and support to promote adequate milk supply.	Step 6. Inform, encourage, and support mothers in early initiation and establishment of breast milk expression and maintenance of milk production.	Step 6. The mother is encouraged to establish and maintain milk production by expression.

Table 3-1 (*Continued*)

Principle	*WHO/UNICEF Ten Steps to Successful Breastfeeding for the Healthy Term Newborn*	*ABI's Ten Steps for the NICU/SCN*	*Nyqvist and Kylberg (2008) Swedish Mothers' 13 Steps*	*Danish Ten Steps to Successful Breastfeeding of Preterm Infants*
Exclusive use of human milk	Step 6. Give [breastfed] newborn infants no food or drink other than breast milk, unless medically indicated.	Step 6. Give preterm and compromised babies only human milk unless *medically* contraindicated.	Step 8. Give the infant the mother's own milk as first choice, and pasteurized donor milk as second choice, fortified when indicated.	
Mother–infant contact	Step 7. Practice rooming in—allow mothers and infants to remain together 24 hours a day.	Step 7. Promote early and continued skin-to-skin contact for mothers and their premature or compromised infants with full mechanical breastmilk expression.	Step 5. Encourage early, continuous, and prolonged skin-to-skin care (kangaroo mother care) without unwarranted restrictions, and offer opportunities for mothers to remain together with their infants 24 hours a day.	Step 4. Parents are encouraged to have skin-to-skin contact with their infant.
Baby-led feeding	Step 8. Encourage breastfeeding on demand.[b]	Step 8. Foster early developmentally appropriate initiation and transition to full breastfeeding.	Step 7. Encourage and support mothers in early initiation of breastfeeding, with infant stability as the only criterion. Give mothers individual support. Step 9. Encourage breastfeeding on demand as early as possible, with semidemand breastfeeding as a transitional strategy for preterm infants (the mother nurses when an infant shows	Step 3. Parents are prepared to breastfeed a preterm infant. Step 5. The mother gets the support and information she needs to facilitate breastfeeding. Step 7. The mother is guided in positioning and attachment of the infant at the breast.

(*continues*)

Table 3-1 *(Continued)*

Principle	*WHO/UNICEF Ten Steps to Successful Breastfeeding for the Healthy Term Newborn*	*ABI's Ten Steps for the NICU/SCN*	*Nyqvist and Kylberg (2008) Swedish Mothers' 13 Steps*	*Danish Ten Steps to Successful Breastfeeding of Preterm Infants*
			signs of interest, and in addition offers her infant the breast in order to reach a breastfeeding frequency per 24 hours that is sufficient for adequate infant milk intake.	
Pacifier use	Step 9. Give no artificial teats or pacifiers (also called dummies or soothers) to breastfeeding infants.		Step 10. Offer the infant a pacifier for relief of pain, stress, and anxiety, and for stimulating the uptake of nutrients during tube feeding. Introduce bottle-feeding when there is a reason.	Step 9. Parents are prepared to continue breastfeeding/milk expression after discharge.
Ethical practice		Step 9. Use ethical evidence-based breastfeeding practices free of conflicts of interest.	Step 2. Treat every mother with sensitivity, empathy, and respect for her maternal role. Support her in taking informed decisions about milk production and breastfeeding according to her own wishes.	
Breastfeeding protection and support	Step 10. Foster the establishment of breastfeeding support groups and refer mothers to them on discharge from the hospital or clinic.	Step 10. Foster the establishment of NICU/SCN breastfeeding support groups and postdischarge community programs, and refer mothers to them.	Step 11. Provide a family-centered and supportive physical environment. Step 12. Support the father's presence without	Step 8. Parents are encouraged to use their social network. Step 10. Parents are supported if they choose not

Table 3-1 (*Continued*)

Principle	*WHO/UNICEF Ten Steps to Successful Breastfeeding for the Healthy Term Newborn*	*ABI's Ten Steps for the NICU/SCN*	*Nyqvist and Kylberg (2008) Swedish Mothers' 13 Steps*	*Danish Ten Steps to Successful Breastfeeding of Preterm Infants*
Breastfeeding protection and support (cont.)			restrictions, as the mother's main supporter and the infant's caregiver. Step 13. Plan the infant's discharge by early transfer of the infant's care in the neonatal unit to the parents. Inform the mother about where she can obtain breastfeeding support after discharge by staff or members of breastfeeding support groups with adequate knowledge.	to breastfeed or if they are unable to make breastfeeding work.

[a] The U.S. BFHI has an evidence-based exemption from the 30-minute time limit. Based on research, the time frame has been extended to 1 hour.

[b] Should be read as "on cue."

Box 3-1 Ten Steps to Promote and Protect Breastfeeding in the NICU

1. Informed decision making on the part of the mother
2. Establishment and maintenance of milk supply through frequent milk expression
3. Management of breastmilk supplies: storage, handling, labeling, etc.
4. Methods of feeding of human milk and transitioning from one method to another
5. Frequent skin-to-skin care opportunities
6. Use of nonnutritive sucking at the breast for familiarization and facilitation of learning
7. Transition to breast with early and frequent opportunities
8. Measuring milk transfer using test weighing procedures
9. Planning and preparation for discharge
10. Appropriate follow-up post-discharge

Source: Adapted from Spatz, 2004.

maker about the baby's care, and she should be respected and the recipient of appropriate information with which to make decisions.

But rather than be included as one of a series of steps, this respectful behavior on the part of staff should be developed into a mission statement of the special care unit and prominently posted throughout the NICU so that staff and parents can see it easily and often (see **Box 3-2**). Belittling the mother and her milk supply, denying her skin-to-skin contact with her baby, threatening her because of disagreement with a staff member who dislikes the mother's insistence on certain practices and describes the mother as a troublemaker is the antithesis of Step 2 in Nyqvist and Kylberg's steps (2008).

It is important, however, to acknowledge that nurses, physicians, and other NICU staff are busy and stressed themselves, particularly in situations of short staffing. Emergencies arise consistently in the NICU setting and babies' needs are immediate and may be life threatening. Staff must respond to these emergencies. Nerves become frayed, people get overtired, and staff may be short tempered. We are all human, and sometimes say things we shouldn't say or wish we hadn't said. However, if the mother was given more responsibility for the care of her infant, staff would be less harried and pressured and would begin to respect the mother as an integral part of the care team, as found by Levin's experience in Estonia (Chalmers & Levin, 2001). A better balance ensures that the mother is included in the

Box 3-2 Sample Mission Statement

It is the mission of this special care unit to:

- Provide sensitive, empathetic, and respectful care of babies and their mothers in our unit.
- Deliver evidence-based quality care to ensure the healthiest outcomes of our patients.
- Include parents in the care and nurturing of their baby.
- Speak softly and kindly and provide appropriate information, encouragement, and support to parents of babies in our care.

care of the infant simultaneously with completing all necessary procedures. The mother is not just the anonymous producer of milk; she is the baby's nurturer and caregiver.

STEP 1: CREATING A BREASTFEEDING POLICY SPECIFIC FOR THE NICU

According to Cadwell and Turner-Maffei (2009), the cornerstone of continuity of care is evidence-based policies that are routinely practiced uniformly so that mothers get consistent information across the multidisciplinary continuum of healthcare providers that the mother and her baby may encounter. For example, the effects of absent policy or lack of policy enforcement are seen in Bonnie's case, especially the inconsistent information given to her about skin-to-skin care and why she could/could not hold her baby skin to skin. Bonnie reports that one of the reasons for the inconsistencies was that the doctors and nurses could not agree on skin-to-skin contact—when to have it, for how long, how frequently to have it, who should have it, what criteria for readiness should be used, etc. An evidence-based policy was needed to address these practices.

Hospitals have policies about everything including purchasing sterile gauze pads, counting instruments after a surgical procedure, how often to weigh babies, and when to give the vitamin K or eye ointment after birth. Why should breastfeeding be any different? Detailed policies, protocols, and procedures should be easily available to staff and to mothers. Written policies and procedures guide an organization and enable consistent, evidence-based practice. Updating policies with new evidence-based information as it becomes available is vital to protecting, promoting, and supporting breastfeeding. Following established and agreed-upon policies protects employees against liability as well. Finally, when there are established policies and procedures in place, an individual must have a very good reason for not following them, otherwise disciplinary action can be taken against the employee. Without the policy, disciplinary action is not possible. The World Health Organization documents the need for written policies to effect change and sustain it. Written policies and the accompanying protocols and procedures act as a road map for the activities of an organization (WHO, 1998).

To create policies, a multidisciplinary task force must be created. This task force should include members of the staff who are negative about breastfeeding. In doing the research to find articles that will help with the creation of a new policy, a staff member with doubts or who is negative may learn something and become more positive about the policy. This also gives the team that develops the policy ownership of the policy and means that it is more likely to be followed. If the policy is something that many people have worked on together and created out of consensus, it is also much more apt to be implemented.

As the team engages in the process of examining articles for the development of a new breastfeeding policy, it also reexamines current policies for conflicts. For example, in a newborn nursery for term infants, the staff is working on a new policy on supplementation of breastfed infants with only medically acceptable reasons for doing so. However, there may be a longstanding policy that states that all infants must be fed a bottle of sugar water at 2 hours of age in an effort to prevent hypoglycemia. If continued, this practice could be counterproductive to achieving the goal of early and frequent breastfeeding without unnecessary supplementation. If the existing policy is not revised or deleted entirely, then each staff member could choose which practice to follow and lack of consistent information and continuity of care would continue. A model policy covering this step is given in **Appendix 3-1**.

SUMMARY

Consistent information and communication with mothers and families is the key to providing continuity and quality of care. This can only be accomplished through evidence-based practice that is implemented uniformly and respected across every department that mothers interact with in the daily care of their hospitalized baby. Underlying this policy should be respect for the family unit, in particular the mother and her baby, so a mission statement that reflects respect should be developed. All of these components need to be clearly communicated to mothers at all times, and the mission statement and breastfeeding policy should be posted for easy access for both parents and staff.

REFERENCES

Cadwell, K., & Turner-Maffei, C. (2009). *Continuity of care in breastfeeding: Best practices in the maternity setting*. Sudbury, MA: Jones and Bartlett.

Chalmers, B., & Levin, A. (2001). *Humane perinatal care*. Tallinn, Estonia: TEA Publishers.

Merewood, A., Philipp, B., Chawla, N., & Cimo, S. (2003). The Baby-Friendly Hospital Initiative increases breastfeeding rates in a U.S. neonatal intensive care unit. *Journal of Human Lactation, 19*(2), 166–171.

Nyqvist, K., & Kylberg, E. (2008). Application of the Baby-Friendly Hospital Initiative to neonatal care: Suggestions by Swedish mothers of very preterm infants. *Journal of Human Lactation, 24*(3), 252–262.

Spatz, D. (2004). Ten steps for promoting and protecting breastfeeding for vulnerable infants. *Journal of Perinatal and Neonatal Nursing, 18*(4), 385–396.

World Health Organization (WHO). (1998). *Evidence for the ten steps to successful breastfeeding*. Geneva, Switzerland: Author.

Appendix 3-1

STEP 1

Have a current written evidence-based breastfeeding policy that is routinely communicated to all NICU staff.

Policies 1.1–1.3

Title

Development of a breastfeeding policy for the NICU/SCN.

Purpose

Evidence-based policies and procedures on the use of human milk and breastfeeding that are separate from other NICU policies should be developed. These policies need to be readily accessible and routinely communicated to all healthcare staff to ensure continuity of care and consistency of information given to mothers. Policies should be reviewed in an ongoing manner and revised when appropriate to ensure that procedures and protocols are evidence-based and current.

Supportive Data

The World Health Organization (1998) documents the need for written policies to effect change and sustain it. Lack of policy leads to inconsistency in staff practices. This leads to lack of continuity of care and gives mothers conflicting and confusing messages. Periodic review of policies highlights where they are no longer evidence-based and where conflicts with other, older existing policies may occur. Non–evidence-based policies need to change to benefit breastfeeding mothers and their premature and/or compromised NICU/SCN babies.

Rationale

Written policies and procedures give direction to an organization and ensure consistent, evidence-based practice. Updating policies with new evidence-based information as it becomes available is vital to protecting, promoting, and supporting breastfeeding and/or the provision of human milk to premature and/or compromised infants in the NICU/SCN. Following established and agreed-upon policies and procedures decreases institution and employee liability because mothers and families have been given information that is not conflicting. Frequent access to policies by staff is important to an understanding of and consistency in compliance with policies. Responsibility for policies should be shared and interdisciplinary so that parties affected by the policies have ownership of them and are more likely to comply with them.

Scope

The policies cover NICU/SCN personnel including medical director, nursing director, nursing supervisors, licensed staff, ancillary staff, and volunteers.

Policy 1.1

The unit should maintain current, written, evidence-based policies and procedures to address the implementation of the Ten Steps that facilitate breastfeeding and the provision of human milk when a mother makes an informed decision to do so for her hospitalized baby.

Elements of the NICU Policy Manual

NICU/SCN breastfeeding policies should include (but not be limited to) the following:

- Education and training of all NICU/SCN employees
- Education of pregnant and postpartum women
- Distribution of educational materials
- Support to mothers in early and ongoing milk expression/breastfeeding
- Assistance for parents with the establishment of early skin-to-skin contact
- Assistance for mothers with developmental progression from skin-to-skin contact to exclusive breastfeeding
- Assistance for mothers with lactation problems
- Education of mothers in the use of electric breast pumps
- Education of mothers on proper collection and storage of human milk
- Labeling procedures for expressed/pumped milk
- Procedures for transporting human milk to the NICU/SCN
- Use of donor milk if mother's own milk is unavailable or a supplement is needed
- Transitioning the baby to the breast
- Procedures for the use of alternate feeding methods, gadgets, and devices
- Development of unit-based breastfeeding support groups

- Establishment of working relationships with community organizations that offer support for breastfeeding/pumping mothers
- Use of proprietary materials that are not evidence-based, e.g., pump company collection/storage information

Procedure 1.1.1
Form a multidisciplinary committee to develop policies and procedures. The lactation committee should include, but not be limited to, personnel from neonatology, NICU/SCN nursing, pharmacy, infection control, respiratory therapy, social work, dietitics/nutrition, as well as one or more lactation consultants.

Procedure 1.1.2
Review the research literature on topics to be included and write policies that address each of the Ten Steps, including the aforementioned issues, incorporating evidence-based research into the policy.

Procedure 1.1.3
Examine existing policies for information and practices that conflict with successful implementation of the breastfeeding policy being developed.

Policy 1.2

A designated healthcare provider should be responsible for providing easy access to the policy as a reference to all staff who care for mothers and their premature and/or compromised infants in the NICU/SCN. The policy is communicated to prospective new employees, newly hired employees in their orientation, and at other times to all staff as determined by the healthcare facility.

Procedure 1.2.1
The policy manual should be visible and accessible in the NICU/SCN at all times.

Procedure 1.2.2
Staff should demonstrate knowledge of the location of the policy manual, and which sections are pertinent to their particular job descriptions.

Policy 1.3

Policies should be reviewed on a regular basis for accuracy and currency.

Procedure 1.3.1
Group process that is interdisciplinary should be used to routinely review and revise current policies and to create new policies when additional evidence-based information becomes available.

REFERENCES

World Health Organization (WHO). (1998). *Evidence for the ten steps to successful breastfeeding*. Geneva, Switzerland: Author.

chapter four

Step 2: Staff Training for Improved Skills and Competency in Assisting Breastfeeding Mothers

If we return to Bonnie's story from Chapter 1 and examine it for staff competency, we find multiple instances in both hospitals where demonstration of knowledge and skills by staff would have supported Bonnie in the establishment and maintenance of her milk supply.

In the first hospital, where Bonnie gave birth, the nurses did not demonstrate knowledge about the use of the pump or where to obtain one in the community. Instructions were not given on how to use the pump. Collection of milk in case of mother–baby separation is a basic competency for all community hospital staff, according to WHO and UNICEF, because they do and will care for mothers who have given birth to babies who are too small, fragile, or sick to nurse or who are separated from their mothers because they are transported to tertiary facilities, sometimes at great distances away. It is incumbent on nurses and other staff who help mothers through this initial separation to have the skills and resources in order to assist the mother in the initiation of an abundant supply of milk or to collect and store her milk.

Hand expression is an excellent way to initiate and maintain lactation in case of separation and every nurse who works with mothers and babies should be able to teach mothers this technique according to WHO and UNICEF. In resource adequate settings such as the United States, nurses who work with mothers and babies should be able to assist the mother in locating breast pumps—even on holidays. Nurses should also be competent in the use of commonly available pumps and be able to instruct mothers in the proper use of the pump and how to establish a routine of pumping or milk expression (how soon after the birth to begin, whether or not milk should be collected during the night, how many times a day, how to store the milk properly, etc.).

In the first hospital, a nurse told Bonnie to wear a supportive bra 24 hours a day to prevent engorgement—the sole piece of (mis)information given. Perhaps this is something that was done in that hospital in the past; however, information about prevention of engorgement has changed dramatically in the ensuing years, yet in Bonnie's case, which began in late 2007, this particular nurse was still practicing a skill set from the 1950s!

In the second hospital, NICU nurses appeared to believe that it was someone else's role to help the mother. They made no effort to give Bonnie information, waiting for the postpartum lactation specialist to pay Bonnie a visit. There was no designated lactation specialist whose competencies included the specialized skills required to support NICU mothers; instead the hospital lactation specialist responsible for helping mothers of healthy term babies was enlisted. This lactation specialist lacked current general lactation knowledge as well, dismissing Bonnie's complaint about the size of the pump flange being too tight and thereby causing pain and compromising the amount of milk collected and future milk supply.

In addition, the knowledge base of the NICU nurses was inadequate, as they misinformed Bonnie that her baby could become lactose intolerant if Bonnie drank too much cow's milk; that fortification of human milk could only be done with a bovine milk-based fortifier; and that bottle-feeding was less stressful physiologically than breastfeeding when the opposite has been described in well-done research. The staff appeared to lack competency in the process of transitioning the baby from gavage (tube) feedings to the breast; the lactation specialist who delivered the nursing pillow failed to help with positioning or any real assistance of a practical nature. Another lactation specialist was not competent in the standard of use of a nipple shield for premature infants.

NICU staff had deficiencies in the knowledge and skills required to assist the mother in the practice of skin-to-skin (STS) contact, a standard of care for premature infants. Current and historical research demonstrates the benefits of STS care—increasing milk supply, increasing the duration of breastfeeding, and achieving better physiological stabilization for the infant. They appeared to lack the necessary competencies for transporting the baby to the mother's chest. The neonatologists also were unaware of the myriad benefits of STS contact. The unit had no policies or procedures describing or encouraging the practice.

When hospital personnel are competent with adequate knowledge, training, and skills, staff skills would better support the mother in her goals. Education is only as effective as the policy that backs up the practice of the skill set, as seen in Chapter 3.

> ...*policy and practice changes should be implemented in tandem with training*. Winikoff and Baer [1980] examined research studies in an early systematic review of the literature in order to understand which medical practices promoted optimal breastfeeding outcomes. They reported that education without policy and practice change did not significantly change breastfeeding outcome. One of the least influential practices was education of healthcare providers alone, without policy change, hence the recommendation that education should include clinical skills and the construction of policy that supports best practice. (Cadwell & Turner-Maffei, 2009, p. 230)

Both of the hospitals that were described in Bonnie's case demonstrated deficiencies in policy, knowledge, and skills necessary to translate knowledge into practice. Even in the case of the lactation specialists, whose knowledge should have been more current and evidence-based in the field of lactation compared to the NICU nurses, it appears that the competency skills required to implement the knowledge were missing, such as proper use of the nipple shield, how to transition the baby to the breast, etc. This is a poignant reminder that staff training should consist of both elements—learning from the literature and demonstrating this learning by doing—and that policy should be current and evidence-based.

Table 4-1 describes the four different versions of Step 2—dealing with staff training and education. It is notable that all clearly include the statement that skills must be present as part of the education, not just knowledge. Translation of knowledge into being able to actually counsel and help mothers overcome problems is paramount.

This is also everyone's job. As Cadwell and Turner-Maffei (2009) point out, to achieve continuity of care it is vital that everyone have the same skill set rather than concentrating knowledge and skills in the hands of a few.

> Spreading the responsibility for breastfeeding care throughout the facility's staff assures that needed service will be available vertically

Table 4-1 Side-by-Side Comparison of Three Models

Principle	*WHO/UNICEF Ten Steps to Successful Breastfeeding for the Healthy Term Newborn*	*ABI's Ten Steps for the NICU/SCN*	*Nyqvist and Kylberg (2008) Swedish Mothers' 13 Steps*	*Danish Ten Steps to Successful Breastfeeding of Preterm Infants*
Staff training	Step 2. Train all healthcare staff in skills necessary to implement this policy.	Step 2. Educate and train all staff in the specific knowledge and skills necessary to implement this policy.	Step 3. Educate and train all staff in the specific knowledge and skills necessary to implement this policy.	Step 2: The healthcare staff is able to translate the strategy into good clinical practices.

> and horizontally. ... [F]acilities that concentrate competence, knowledge and skill meet overwhelming obstacles in providing continuity of breastfeeding care. In this model, the breastfeeding caregiver spends the majority of their work time helping mothers and babies to overcome obstacles to breastfeeding created by care practices that do not favor optimal breastfeeding. (p. 20)

STAFF TRAINING IN LACTATION MANAGEMENT: FROM SCHOOL TO WORKPLACE

Academic Training

Cadwell and Turner-Maffei (2009) have recently reviewed the literature on the effectiveness of breastfeeding and lactation management training, beginning with professional education in medical schools, nursing schools, and dietetics training programs. By their own report, physicians in the fields of obstetrics, pediatrics, and family medicine find that training is inadequate, both in medical school and in residency programs (Freed, Clark, Sorenson, Lohr, Cefalo, & Curtis, 1995; Goldstein & Freed, 1993; Howard, Shaffer, & Lawrence, 1997; Schwartz, 1995; Williams & Hammer, 1995). This lack of training and knowledge means that some physicians, despite having positive beliefs about breastfeeding, rely on personal breastfeeding experience. There is lack of consistent information from one discipline to another (Barnett, Sienkiewicz, & Roholt, 1995) and these inconsistencies translate into lack of counseling skills and clinical skills to resolve breastfeeding problems (Freed, Clark, Lohr, & Sorenson, 1995).

In several studies of dietitians, dietitians were found to have a keener interest in breastfeeding than nurses, as well as a greater knowledge base (Bagwell, Kendrick, Stitt, & Leeper, 1993), but were the least likely to provide assistance and information to mothers (Helm, Windham, & Wyse, 1997). Breastfeeding information given to mothers by nurses on obstetric units was consistently outdated (Lewinski, 1992), reflecting lack of proper training in academic programs. Philipp and Merewood (2004) examined a number of pediatric textbooks for accuracy and consistency of breastfeeding information and found that when information on the topic was present, it frequently was inaccurate, inconsistent, and highly variable from one textbook to another.

Postgraduate Training: Continuing Education and Skills Training in Maternity Settings

An Irish study that examined breastfeeding rates in several rural maternity units found that breastfeeding rates were lowest in the units where staff thought they had sufficient knowledge because they had frequent in-service meetings and printed information on infant feeding from formula company representatives. The unit with the best breastfeeding rates had a staff member with postgraduate training in breastfeeding skills and management (Becker, 1992). Many U.S. hospitals still receive much of their information and training about breastfeeding from formula company representatives who pay for special educational offerings as well as lavish food.

When specific breastfeeding training is conducted in hospitals and community settings around the world, we see that training sessions that incorporate didactic material with practical problem solving and clinical experience are the most successful. They not only improve the knowledge base of the participants, but also the practice and the provision of appropriate assistance to mothers (Davies-Adetugbo & Adebawa, 1997; Hillenbrand & Larsen, 2002; Valdes et al. 1995; see also Cadwell & Turner-Maffei, 2009). The success of these training programs is reflected in increased breastfeeding duration rates and rates of exclusivity of breastfeeding (Cattaneo & Buzzetti, 2001; Taddei, Westphal, Venancio, Bogus, & Souza, 2000; Vittoz, Labarere, Castell, Duran, & Pons, 2004).

Training Specific to Breastfeeding in the NICU

In response to mothers expressing their dissatisfaction with the inconsistent advice and negative attitudes about breastfeeding that undermined their efforts to breastfeed and supply their milk, Siddell, Marinelli, and Froman (2003) examined the relationship between nurses' demographic variables and their preintervention knowledge and attitudes towards breastfeeding in the NICU setting. A second research question examined whether attending an education session on infant feeding theory and techniques made a difference in NICU nurses' knowledge and attitudes about breastfeeding.

Topics in the 8-hour curriculum included, but were not limited to, a discussion of the benefits of breastfeeding/human milk for the preterm infant, milk composition, physiology and anatomy of lactation, as well as NICU-specific topics including the mechanics of establishing a milk supply using a breast pump, fortification of human milk, the development of feeding behaviors in the preterm infant, the role of kangaroo care (skin-to-skin contact), and the use of different devices and gadgets intended to help transition the infant to the breast from tube feeding. Participants had opportunities to practice positioning techniques and determine solutions to latch-on difficulties. A panel of former NICU mothers gave the nurses feedback on what attitudes and practices helped them to succeed and which were barriers to success.

The results demonstrated that specific breastfeeding education can change knowledge and attitudes about breastfeeding in NICU nurses. However, other results were more puzzling. Nurses with the most life experience and longest tenure in the NICU were the least likely to have attitudes that were pro-breastfeeding and pro–baby-focused care, suggesting that those nurses who could benefit most from additional breastfeeding specific training are those that have been on the job the longest. Sidell and colleagues (2003) also reported that it cannot be assumed that NICU nurses have had adequate breastfeeding training, as most appear to rely on skills acquired on the job for helping mother–infant dyads. They suggest that training needs to be offered "on a recurrent basis to enhance and maintain positive attitudes about breastfeeding" (p. 299) and that querying a prospective employee about his or her attitudes and knowledge about breastfeeding should be part of a job interview to ensure that the new employee will be a good fit in a breastfeeding environment.

Spatz (2005) developed a multifaceted approach to improve knowledge and practice in a children's hospital in order to promote and support breastfeeding for all vulnerable and ill infants in the hospital. The comprehensive hospital-wide system included the following elements:

- The development of a continuous quality-improvement team to monitor and address problems with human milk storage and handling
- A hospital-wide survey of nurses' knowledge about management of human milk and the development of a Web-based competency test
- The establishment of a hospital-wide breastfeeding committee
- The development of breastfeeding resource binders for each unit
- Educational programs for nurses and residents (for nurses: 2 days, 16 hours, offered four times a year during both day and night shifts)
- An interdisciplinary clinical consensus program on the feeding of human milk to the high-risk infant

This program is seen as an integral part of providing family-centered care.

Bernaix, Schmidt, Arrizola, Iovinelli, and Medina-Poelinez (2008) found that intermittent, short educational programs that included practical how-tos and motivational encouragement for nursing staff were effective in improving NICU nurses' lactation knowledge and attitudes about breastfeeding. Furthermore, improvement was maintained over time, and the atmosphere in the NICU improved significantly following implementation of the educational intervention. A 4-hour educational intervention was designed with a lecture and discussion format that included practical strategies for discussing the provision of milk with mothers in the NICU and skin-to-skin care. Nurses' intentions, attitudes, and beliefs about supporting the mothers' attempts to provide milk were surveyed both before the intervention and 3 months later. Lactation knowledge, beliefs, and attitudes of nurses improved from moderately positive to very positive. Two groups of mothers were also surveyed—one group before and one group after the educational intervention to determine their perceptions of breastfeeding support. There was statistically significant improvement in the mothers' perceptions of lactation support in the postintervention group. The authors conclude:

> Studies have indicated that a change in attitude and an improved knowledge base regarding lactation by NICU nurses can positively influence the supportive atmosphere and culture of a unit ... Such positive changes in culture were mirrored in this study even though there was only 50% nurse involvement. Periodic attendance to educational programs like the one tested in this study, therefore, should be *mandated* [italics added] for all NICU nurses. (Bernaix et al., 2008, p. 444)

ELEMENTS OF SUCCESSFUL TRAINING

As seen in Bonnie's case, many of the individuals involved in her care and that of her baby not only seemed to lack information but also lacked skills. One of the elements of successful training is the inclusion of practical clinical experience, either through role playing or through direct patient contact with a preceptor. In 2006, WHO and UNICEF revised their criteria for hospital staff in Baby-Friendly hospitals. Any staff person whose primary responsibility is the care of breastfeeding mothers and infants, whether in the NICU or not, should have a minimum of 20 hours of training that includes didactic, practical, and counseling strategies for assisting mothers with breastfeeding (UNICEF/WHO, 2006). While competencies in the NICU for assisting mothers may be somewhat different from those to assist mothers with healthy term infants, they are no less important, and may be more challenging for both mother and healthcare provider in the NICU. Lack of competency frequently results in the sometimes inappropriate substitution of a gadget or device, as in the case of the nursing pillow when Bonnie wanted help with transitioning her baby to the breast.

In their review of the literature, Cadwell and Turner-Maffei (2009) found that the most effective training programs included the following points:

- Didactic material by itself was insufficient.
- Practical on-the-job experience was the most valuable learning activity (Cantrill, Creedy, & Cooke, 2003).
- Training should provide competency verification in the practice setting (Sloper, McKean, & Baum, 1975).
- Training should be directed at changing attitudes as well, mitigating the effects of negative personal experiences of the staff.
- Staff training should be mandatory.
- Refresher training may be needed if improvements are to be maintained.

SUMMARY

Appendix 4-1 provides ABI's model policy for lactation training in the NICU based on the specific skill sets which physicians, nurses, dietitians, etc. need to assist mothers who wish to provide their own milk and then breastfeed their hospitalized babies. The model policy addresses each one of the major points in this chapter:

- Continuity of care is best addressed by having all staff trained in the evidence-based basics of lactation support. This leaves specialist staff the time to focus energies on the more problematic cases requiring lactation support.
- Training is most successful in changing staff attitudes and beliefs as well as practices when it includes didactic material, practical skills, and counseling techniques.
- Demonstration and verification of skills need to be part of the culture of education.
- Training needs to be ongoing. Staff need refresher courses and new hires need training during orientation to maintain continuity of care.
- Training needs to be mandatory.

Had all of these things been in place for Bonnie and her baby, the messages Bonnie would have received and her experience with her fragile, premature, hospitalized infant would have been very different. Optimally, Bonnie would have understood herself to be a valued member of the team caring for her son, and staff would have viewed Bonnie as an asset rather than a threat to either their knowledge or to her infant. The situation would not have devolved into an adversarial one fueled by lack of evidence-based policy and staff training.

REFERENCES

Bagwell, J., Kendrick, O., Stitt, K., & Leeper, J. (1993). Knowledge and attitudes toward breastfeeding: Differences among dietitians, nurses, and physicians working with WIC clients. *Journal of the American Dietetic Association, 93*(7), 801–804.

Barnett, E., Sienkiewicz, M., & Roholt, S. (1995). Beliefs about breastfeeding: A statewide survey of health professionals. *Birth, 22*(1), 15–20.

Becker, G. (1992). Breastfeeding knowledge of hospital staff in rural maternity units in Ireland. *Journal of Human Lactation, 8*(3), 137–142.

Bernaix, L., Schmidt, C., Arrizola, M., Iovinelli, D., & Medina-Poelinez, C. (2008). Success of a lactation education program on NICU nurses' knowledge and attitudes. *Journal of Obstetric, Gynecologic, and Neonatal Nursing, 37*(4), 436–445.

Cadwell, K., & Turner-Maffei, C. (2009). *Continuity of care in breastfeeding: Best practices in the maternity setting.* Sudbury, MA: Jones and Bartlett.

Cantrill, R., Creedy, D., & Cooke, M. (2003). How midwives learn about breastfeeding. *Australian Journal of Midwifery, 16*(2), 11–16.

Cattaneo, A., & Buzzetti, R. (2001). Effects on rates of breast feeding of training for the Baby Friendly Hospital Initiative. *British Medical Journal, 323*(7325), 1358–1362.

Davies-Adetugbo, A., & Adebawa, H. (1997). The Ife South Breastfeeding Project: Training community health extension workers to promote and manage breastfeeding in rural communities. *Bulletin of the World Health Organization, 75*(4), 323–332.

Freed, G., Clark, S, Lohr, J., & Sorenson, J. (1995). Pediatrician involvement in breastfeeding promotion: A national study of residents and practitioners. *Pediatrics, 96*(3 Pt. 1), 490–494.

Freed, G., Clark, S., Sorenson, J., Lohr, J., Cefalo, R., & Curtis, P. (1995). National assessment of physicians' breast-feeding knowledge, attitudes, training and experience. *Journal of the American Medical Association, 273*(6), 472–476.

Goldstein, A., & Freed, G. (1993). Breastfeeding counseling practices of family practice residents. *Family Medicine, 25*(8), 524–529.

Helm, A., Windham, C., & Wyse, B. (1997). Dietitians in breastfeeding management: An untapped resource in the hospital. *Journal of Human Lactation, 13*(3), 221–225.

Hillenbrand, K., & Larsen, P. (2002). Effect of an educational intervention about breastfeeding on the knowledge, confidence, and behaviors of pediatric resident physicians. *Pediatrics, 110*(5), e59.

Howard, C., Shaffer, S., & Lawrence, R. (1997). Attitudes, practices, and recommendations by obstetricians about infant feeding. *Birth, 24*(4), 240–246.

Lewinski, C. (1992). Nurses' knowledge of breastfeeding in a clinical setting. *Journal of Human Lactation, 8*(3), 143–148.

Philipp, B., & Merewood, A. (2004). The baby-friendly way: The best breastfeeding start. *Pediatric Clinics of North America, 51*(3), 761–783.

Schwartz, K. (1995). Breastfeeding education among family physicians. *Journal of Family Practice, 40*(3), 297–298.

Siddell, E., Marinelli, K., Froman, R., & Burke, G. (2003). Evaluation of an educational intervention on breastfeeding for NICU nurses. *Journal of Human Lactation, 19*(3), 293–302.

Sloper, K., McKean, L., & Baum, J. (1975). Factors influencing breastfeeding. *Archives of Disease in Childhood, 50*(3), 165–170.

Spatz, D. (2005). Report of a staff program to promote and support breastfeeding in the care of vulnerable infants at a children's hospital. *Journal of Perinatal Education, 14*(1), 30–38.

Taddei, J., Westphal, M., Venancio, S., Bogus, C., & Souza, S. (2000). Breastfeeding training for health professionals and resultant changes in breastfeeding duration. *Sao Paulo Medical Journal, 118*(6), 185–191.

UNICEF & World Health Organization (UNICEF/WHO). (2006). *Baby-Friendly Hospital Initiative: Revised, updated, and expanded for integrated care. Section 4: Hospital self-appraisal and monitoring*. Retrieved May 29, 2009, from http://www.who.int/nutrition/publications/infantfeeding/9789241595018_s4.pdf

Valdes, V., Pugin, E., Labbok, M., Perez, A., Catalan, S., Aravena, R., et al. (1995). The effects on professional practices of a three-day course on breastfeeding. *Journal of Human Lactation, 11*(3), 185–190.

Vittoz, J., Labarere, J. Castell, M., Duran, M., & Pons, J. (2004). Effect of a training program for maternity ward professionals on duration of breastfeeding. *Birth, 31*(4), 302–307.

Williams, E., & Hammer, L. (1995). Breastfeeding attitudes and knowledge of pediatricians-in-training. *American Journal of Preventive Medicine, 11*(1), 26–33.

Winikoff, B., & Baer, E. (1980). The obstetrician's opportunity: Translating "breast is best" from theory to practice. *American Journal of Obstetrics and Gynecology, 138*(1), 105–117.

Appendix 4-1

STEP 2

Train all staff in the necessary skills to implement the policy.

Policies 2.1–2.5

Title

Staff training

Purpose

To ensure that all NICU/SCN healthcare staff receives training in the evidence-based skills necessary for practice.

Supportive Data

Implementation of evidence-based policies can occur only through adequate training of staff.

Rationale

Adequate training of staff will promote consistency of information given to mothers and continuity of care within the NICU/SCN. It is everyone's obligation to be informed and trained in the policies so that relevant basic support may be given to mothers even though the setting may have an individual whose sole job is lactation support. This frees the specialist to concentrate on problems and concerns that are out of the ordinary. However, having a lactation specialist whose sole job description is to help breastfeeding/expressing mothers protects that individual from having her focus drawn away by other duties, services, or responsibilities (e.g., the staff nurse who is also the lactation specialist being pulled from lactation duties to fill staff nurse duties).

Scope

The policies cover all NICU/SCN personnel including the medical director, nursing director, nursing supervisors, licensed staff, ancillary staff, and volunteers.

Policy 2.1

A designated healthcare professional (or team/committee) should be responsible for assessing needs, planning, implementing, evaluating, and updating competency-based training for all NICU/SCN healthcare staff.

Procedure 2.1.1
Training should differentiate the level of competency required and/or needed based on the staff function and responsibility.

Procedure 2.1.2
All training should be documented by the designated trainer for each individual on the staff.

Procedure 2.1.3
All new staff should be initially trained during orientation.

Procedure 2.1.4
Once all staff are initially trained, assessment of skills and competencies should occur on an ongoing basis (e.g., during yearly evaluations).

Procedure 2.1.5
Staff should be required to demonstrate competency by a combination of written tests and return demonstrations.

Procedure 2.1.6
A copy of the curricula or course outlines for competency-based training of NICU staff should be available for review.

Policy 2.2

All postpartum and NICU/SCN staff should have a basic level of knowledge regarding lactation physiology and breastfeeding support, as evidenced by competencies, including, but not limited to, classroom instruction of mothers, bedside observation and assessment of mother–baby dyads during breastfeeding sessions, and counseling techniques.

Policy 2.3

Whenever possible, NICU/SCN staff position(s) with sole responsibility for lactation should be developed (e.g., lactation specialists). Besides supporting and assisting breastfeeding NICU mothers and babies, duties may include chairing committees/task forces that develop breastfeeding policies in the NICU.

Policy 2.4

Training should include, but not be limited to:

- The benefits of human milk for premature and/or vulnerable infants and their mothers
- The establishment and maintenance of a milk supply during mother-infant separation
- The use and care of breast pumps
- Milk collection and storage techniques
- Skin-to-skin contact
- Developmental breastfeeding skills
- Alternative feeding methods
- Troubleshooting
- Procuring and handling banked donor milk
- Appropriate discharge follow-up and lactation support

Policy 2.5

Skills necessary for assisting mothers in using and maintaining breast pumps, placing special needs babies at the breast, use of alternative feeding methods, and transitioning to full breastfeeding should be required and competencies assessed on an annual basis.

chapter five

Step 3: Informing Mothers of Preterm Infants About the Need for Their Milk

PRENATAL EDUCATION OF MOTHERS

Step 3 of the Ten Steps to Successful Breastfeeding for term infants (**Table 5-1**) states that in order for breastfeeding to succeed, mothers should be educated about the benefits of breastfeeding during the prenatal period. Usually this responsibility falls to the childbirth educator who may or may not incorporate breastfeeding education into her childbirth class series. However, Cadwell & Turner-Maffei (2009) cite poor attendance at childbirth and prenatal classes as a barrier, with fewer than 20 percent of delivering families attending educational offerings in many facilities. Obstetrical care providers also bear responsibility for including discussions of breastfeeding in their interactions with pregnant women, although Taveras et al. (2004) report that frequently, because of the manner in which the information is presented, many women do not hear this information when it is given by their obstetrical care providers—it is not client centered and specific to the individual mother's concerns. Prenatal care providers may also have a lack of comfort discussing the topic prenatally because of insecurity in their own knowledge base (Cadwell & Turner-Maffei, 2009).

A study by the CDC of mothers of term infants concluded that the mother's perception of her prenatal physician's and hospital staff's attitudes related to infant feeding choices was a strong predictor of later breastfeeding. After controlling for mother's prenatal breastfeeding intentions, father's feeding preference, and demographic and psychosocial variables, adjusted

Table 5-1 Side-by-Side Comparison of Three Models

Principle	*WHO/UNICEF Ten Steps to Successful Breastfeeding for the Healthy Term Newborn*	*ABI's Ten Steps for the NICU/SCN*	*Nyqvist and Kylberg (2008) Swedish Mothers' 13 Steps*	*Danish Ten Steps to Successful Breastfeeding of Preterm Infants*
Prenatal breast-feeding education	Step 3. Inform all pregnant women about the benefits and management of breastfeeding.	Step 3. Inform all women and their partners at risk for delivering or who have already delivered a preterm or compromised infant of the benefits of providing human milk.	Step 4. Inform all pregnant women about initiation of lactation and breastfeeding in the event that the infant is born preterm or ill.	Step 2: The healthcare staff is able to translate the strategy into good clinical practices.

analyses indicated that no preference regarding infant feeding by hospital staff was a significant risk factor for failure to breastfeed after 6 weeks (DiGirolamo, Grummer-Strawn, & Fein, 2003). Every effort must therefore be made by prenatal care providers to ensure that all pregnant women are aware of the benefits of breastfeeding and/or providing human milk and of the potential health risks of formula. Breastfeeding is the method of feeding that is preferred by the healthcare provider. Not only should the message be presented in a manner that is conducive to the mother remembering it, but also it must be given at every interaction of prenatal care providers and expectant mothers. There should be no misunderstanding on the part of the mother about the breastfeeding messages that she has heard during pregnancy, and if the same message is repeated numerous times, the potential for remembering is greater.

This is also true for the population of preterm and/or compromised babies. Messages about the importance of human milk and breastfeeding should be incorporated early in prenatal care so that the mother who delivers early will receive some of the information. Antepartum hospital stays are opportunities for dispelling myths (e.g., "I can't breastfeed because I have a premature infant"), for stressing the importance of the mother's own milk for her infant, and for providing anticipatory guidance regarding procedures to ensure a full milk supply and safe storage and use of pumped and/or donor milk. The unique benefits of human milk for the preterm infant *must* be stressed to the mother who is threatening to deliver early.

For women identified as being at risk for preterm birth, a prenatal consultation with a neonatologist has been shown to be effective. Halamek (2001) found that women and their partners appreciated information that would help them make difficult decisions, and that a focused and thorough consultation with the neonatologist helped to ease the transition from obstetrical to neonatal team care. Another study by Paul, Epps, Leef, & Stefano (2001) evaluated whether mothers found the prenatal consult to be useful and comforting. Mothers less than 30 weeks gestation were less likely to feel comforted by the consultation than mothers who were further along than 30 weeks gestation. However, 84% indicated the consult was useful, and 71% were comforted by the consultation. Yee & Sauve (2007) evaluated the antenatal consultation for women already hospitalized pending a preterm delivery in a tertiary center. Ninety-two percent of the women answering a questionnaire about what they remembered from the consultation thought that the consultation was helpful in increasing their knowledge about what might happen if their baby were born prematurely. The most important topics for which information was requested were information about their infants' chances of survival; what possible medical problems the infant might experience, including a risk of disability; types of medical treatments that might be used; and breastfeeding. In general, respondents to the survey were satisfied with the information they received but remained anxious and wanted more opportunities to share their feelings and talk about the baby and their interactions with him when he arrived.

Currently, depending on how early the mother of a preterm infant delivers, she may or may not have heard much of this information. If the obstetrical care provider plans to include this material late in the last trimester of prenatal care, it may be too late and the mother may have already delivered. If this is the case, then it is up to the neonatologist and lactation care providers in the NICU to ensure that mothers who give birth early know the importance of providing their own milk and that having human milk available is imperative to the optimal physical health and development of the preterm infant. Even if the mother finds the idea of putting the infant to the breast abhorrent, making expressed milk available should be encouraged, at least during the infant's hospital stay.

Better outcomes are achieved, both short term and long term, when a mother establishes her milk supply early and provides her milk long term. For example, preterm infants who are fed human milk demonstrate higher scores on the Bayley Mental Development Index, Psychomotor Development Index, and the Behavior Rating Scale at 18 months of age (Vohr et al., 2006). The likelihood of rehospitalization is also decreased in a dose-dependent way. The authors calculated the mean volume of human milk per kilogram per day ingested during hospitalization and divided the infants into quintiles of human milk ingestion. After adjusting for confounders in each group, analysis demonstrated a 14% difference in Behavior Rating Scale between the groups with the highest and lowest volume of milk ingestion. Significant differences in scores on the Mental Development Index, Psychomotor Development Index, Behavior Rating Scale, and in rehospitalization rates during the first year of life were found only for the highest human milk consumption quintile (> 80th percentile) compared to no breastmilk. For every 10 cc/kg/day increase in human milk ingestion, scores increased. Vohr et al. (2006) suggest that significant savings in special educational needs could be realized if human milk consumption was increased in the NICU. These differences persisted at 30 months corrected age (Vohr et al., 2007). (See **Table 5-2**.) The authors conclude:

Table 5-2 Comparison of Bayley Scores in Breastmilk-Fed (BM) Infants at 18 and 30 Months of Age vs. No Breastmilk (No BM)

	No BM—18 months	*BM > 80th quintile—18 months*	*No BM—30 months*	*BM > 80th quintile—30 months*
Bayley MDI (mean)	75.8	87.3; p < 0.0044*	76.5	89.7; p = 0.0326
Bayley PDI (mean)	81.3	89.4; p = 0.0027*	78.4	90.2; p = 0.0639
Behavior scale—total percentage	45.6	58.8; p = 0.0281*	52.6	66.1; p = 0.2129
Rehospitalization (any reason)	30.2% (< 1 yr)	12.7% (< 1 year); p = 0.0460*	60.0% (to 30 months)	53.3% (to 30 months) p = 0.0238

* Value significantly different from no breastmilk value at p < 0.01.

Source: Data extracted from Vohr et al., 2006, and Vohr et al., 2007.

> On the basis of findings of persistent effects of BM [breastmilk] on cognition at 30 months CA [corrected age], we reiterate our recommendation that efforts must be made to introduce all of the mothers to the benefits of BM. Efforts should be initiated not only by the obstetrician, neonatologist, lactation consultant, and primary care provider but should begin before pregnancy with supports after discharge from the birthing hospital. To optimize efforts, the introduction of the concept of breastfeeding can be considered in elementary school as part of healthy living education. (Vohr et al., 2007, p. e958)

Introduction of breastfeeding education in elementary school is beyond the scope of this book, but the quotation above highlights the importance of having a variety of hospital staff participate in educating the mother about the benefits of breastfeeding, both before and after the birth of her premature infant. Responsibility for education should not fall only to the lactation specialist. In this regard, a retrospective case-control study examined the duration of human milk/breastfeeding in mothers who received a prenatal consultation within 2 weeks prior to the preterm delivery from a neonatologist compared with a group that did not receive a prenatal consultation. Mothers received a mean of 2.5 visits, each lasting 10–20 minutes, in which the benefits and importance of human milk were discussed, along with practical information about milk expression and support. Mothers in both groups received the same type of lactation support in the NICU after birth from the on-service staff. The only difference was the prenatal neonatologist's consultation. In the group that had the prenatal consultation, the rates of human milk feeding in the NICU and at discharge were significantly higher in the intervention group. Full breastfeeding postdischarge was also significantly higher in the group that received the consultation. (See **Table 5-3**.) The authors conclude that the "... surprisingly large effect of prenatal consultation suggests that the hours and days immediately before preterm delivery may be of critical importance in influencing maternal planning regarding the feeding ..." of her preterm infant (Friedman, Flidel-Ramon, Lavie, & Shinwell, 2004, p. 777).

Elements of effective prenatal education programs usually contain several approaches and do not rely on just printed materials. For the mother of a preterm infant, these elements are no less important: at least 1 one-on-one visit from the neonatologist, which may be followed up with other staff reinforcing the initial teaching in either individual or group sessions; following

Table 5-3 Effects of Prenatal Consultation on Human Milk Feeding and Breastfeeding

	PC	*Control*	*p value*
HMF—in hospital (d, mean)	37 ± 34	15 ± 19	0.001
Formula only—in hospital (d, mean)	6 ± 11	26 ± 32	0.0001
HMF—% feeding at discharge	65%	24%	0.0001
Formula only—% feeding at discharge	24%	52%	0.001
BF after discharge (d, mean)	60 ± 57	21 ± 32	0.0001
Partial BF after discharge (d, mean)	2 ± 5	5 ± 16	0.008

PC = prenatal consult; HMF = human milk feeding; BF = breastfeeding; d = duration, in days.

Source: Data extracted from Friedman et al., 2004.

structured protocols so that the same information is given by all who have contact with the mother; and "practical, behavioral skills training and problem solving in addition to didactic instruction" (Cadwell & Turner-Maffei, 2009, p. 42). A model policy for achieving this step in the Ten Steps for the NICU/SCN appears in **Appendix 5-1**.

The Preterm Mother: More Than a Milk Dispenser

As a mother moves through gestation she has changing mental images of what her baby is going to be like. At around 4 months of gestation the fetus becomes more real to the mother, especially with the use of ultrasound technology. Fingers and toes and body parts can be easily identified, heartbeats and motion can be seen on ultrasound, and the mother begins to feel the first flutterings of fetal movement. Suddenly the baby seems real and begins to take on a personality of its own. Between the 4th and the 7th months of gestation, the images that the mother has of her infant-to-be grow in "richness, quantity, and specificity" (Stern, 1995, pp. 22–23). The mother may choose to learn the sex of the baby. She may notice that she is getting kicked in the ribs often, she can see the motion of the baby in her abdomen, and perhaps she imagines that this baby will be a soccer player. The size of the fetus's feet on ultrasound contribute to this image. Between the 7th and 9th months of gestation, these mental images become less clear and specific. Stern states that the most plausible reason is so that mothers protect the baby-to-be and themselves from a discordance between reality and a specific mental image, thus preventing disappointment from being too acute when reality is different (Stern, 1995, p. 23). A mother who gives birth prematurely, however, may still be in the phase of clear and specific mental images of her baby. When her baby arrives early she must reconcile the reality of her baby's condition and immaturity with her mental representation of the fetus—a very discordant and jarring experience.

Mothers (and fathers) experience shock, panic, denial, anger, and sadness, which affect the way they interact with the baby, hospital staff, other family members and friends (Manginello & DiGeronimo, 1991). In a review of postpartum mood disorders (Driscoll, 2008, p. 9), women with histories of infertility or pregnancy loss have higher rates of postpartum depression. Experiencing multiple births and very preterm deliveries also contribute to significant depressive symptoms and higher maternal depression scores on the Edinburgh Postnatal Depression Scale. It would seem that the population of mothers with infants in the NICU would qualify for having multiple risk factors, especially if assisted reproductive technologies have resulted in higher order multiples that are born very prematurely. Women with depression, shock, panic, denial, and anger cannot react in the same way to information from external sources, as all their energies are focused inward on their own emotions. In order to become effective members of the care team, women's mental and physical health needs must also be met, and the NICU must focus on not just the baby but also the mother. Frequently the mother is discharged from the hospital several days after the birth and then viewed by the nursery staff as a milk dispenser. NICUs cannot assume that the mother is good to go days after the birth even though she has been discharged. Effective and comprehensive care requires that NICUs cannot behave as if the baby is the only concern. For example, the mother may be physically weak if she has been on bed rest while trying to prevent the preterm birth. One mother had to call for a wheelchair to pick her up in the parking lot when she found she did not have the energy to walk to the NICU. A mother also may be emotionally labile and vulnerable and still require care, albeit of a different sort from prenatally. What mothers need to be effective members of the care team for their babies is mental health support, physical therapy, and social work support services in a continuous fashion. Only in this way will we have competent, bonded mothers who can hear, understand, and assimilate information provided to them.

THE BENEFITS OF HUMAN MILK FOR THE PRETERM INFANT

The benefits of human milk as delineated in this section are based in evidence completed with breastfed infants as the subjects. They may not automatically be true for the infant who is fed expressed milk from his own mother without ever being put to the breast[1] or for the infant who receives a steady diet of banked donor human milk (see Chapter 13 for a discussion of use of banked donor milk in premature infants). Storage and handling of milk, including freezing, exposure to light and air, and pasteurization in the case of banked donor milk, all impact milk composition. Studies proving that benefits are the same have not been published. For purposes of the discussion in this book, and since we have no compelling research indicating the converse, the assumption will be made that outcomes are comparable and that the losses due to storage and handling are balanced by the acute need of the fragile infant and therefore have a minimal impact on the benefits of human milk feeding for infants.

By definition, preterm infants have not undergone the full 40 weeks of gestation and are therefore immature in every organ and system. Iron stores, normally laid down in the third trimester of gestation, are shortchanged. The preterm infant therefore has critical needs that the term infant does not have. Furthermore, the preterm infant must mature his organs and systems while he is learning how to suck, swallow, and breathe, often with technological assistance. He is also expected to grow as if he were still in utero, a challenge given that the mother is no longer nourishing him, keeping him oxygenated, and keeping him warm. The characteristics of human milk that help the infant achieve maturation are species specificity, disease protection, digestibility, bioavailability, and bioactivity. A review of the specific components and biochemistry of human milk and their benefits can be found in Lawrence and Lawrence (2005, pp. 105–170).

Species Specificity

From animal studies we know that *species specificity* of the milk is very important. Zoos know that it is important to try to get the colostrum (first

[1] The act of breastfeeding itself has benefits for the infant that are primarily social and psychological as well as developmental. Researchers looking at specific diseases and conditions tend to separate the act from the product delivered, but in the long run, it is the whole package that is important to the full development of the infant. It is therefore important to transition the preterm infant to the breast as soon as possible so that the benefits of the breastfeeding process may be experienced and losses in milk quality due to expression, storage, and handling may be minimized.

milk) from the mother to feed her offspring, otherwise the offspring is at high risk of dying. Horse breeders bank horse colostrum so that if a mare dies during the birth the foal can be saved and the breeding investment can also be saved (Sullivan, 1997).[2] Historically, calves died of scours if they did not get bovine colostrum, but scours can now be treated with antibiotics. The veterinarians at Sea World in Orlando, Florida, freeze dolphin colostrum and milk to have on hand in case a dolphin is rejected at birth or is orphaned. No two animal species have the same milk composition. Each is individually tailored to provide optimal growth and development of that species' infants. Therefore the milk that is best suited to the offspring's needs is its own species' milk.

As newborns and infants, humans do not do well on the milks of other animals or substitutes made from plants. Goat's milk has a very high solute load that can lead to kidney damage. Cow's milk is much more difficult to digest, even when its proteins have been modified, as is the case with formula. Individuals may mount superimmune responses that take the form of allergies in response to the modified cow's milk proteins as well as the proteins found in soy formulas. When we receive our own species' milk, however, we are programmed appropriately.

At birth, we must rapidly adapt physiologically to extrauterine life. Human colostrum plays an important role in this transition by providing a thick, sticky fluid that coats the lining of the gut, protecting it from early exposure to pathogens and antigens. Colostrum contains extremely high levels of immune proteins that are specific to the baby's environment. The mother has made antibodies to germs that are found in her home and environment and these antibodies are transmitted to the baby through the colostrum and milk. An infant's first feeding of colostrum becomes its first vaccination, and it is immunized against the organisms that it will come in contact with at home. This immunological protection continues for the duration of breastfeeding, even as the composition of the milk changes somewhat. As the baby weans, is started on solids, or begins a child care experience, periods where there are increased exposures to potential pathogens, this immunological protection becomes even more essential. For the preterm infant who

[2] From the April 1997 issue of *Horse America*, an equine news magazine, comes the following: "Bill Richey is a Santa Ana area horseman in California who is reacting to personal loss in an innovative way. After losing a 1996 Quarter Horse foal due to complications from using a manufactured colostrum product, Richey has begun a colostrum bank for use in emergencies.... Nancy King successfully began another colostrum bank in Northern California." (p. 7)

may experience a lengthy stay in the hospital with its own peculiar array of pathogens, mothers make antibodies specific to the organisms found in the hospital environment,[3] and therefore the use of a mother's own expressed milk in the hospital setting is preferred. Using colostrum as oral care for the premature infant who is not feeding by mouth is also an effective method of protecting the infant's oral mucosa from infection (Marinelli & Hamelin, 2005; Narayanan, Prakash, Verma, & Gurjal, 1983).

Colostrum also contains growth factors and hormones that foster proliferation of the absorptive cells lining the gut. Thickening of the gut wall also occurs, and tight junctions between the absorptive cells are created, making it difficult for any pathogens or antigens to which the infant is exposed to penetrate the gut wall. With proliferation of cells there is a corresponding increase in the surface area available for absorption, so utilization of digested nutrients and growth become more effective. Interruption of human milk feeding during this critical period may have lifelong consequences in terms of greater susceptibility to gastrointestinal tract illness and nutrient absorption. Because their gastrointestinal systems are even more immature than their term counterparts, premature infants benefit even more from the ability to absorb more nutrients and grow more rapidly.

Closure of the gut is an extremely important development that occurs in the first few weeks of infancy with species-specific feeding, and it is important because it helps prevent pathogens and harmful molecules from crossing the mucosal intestinal barrier. An increase in closure (decrease in permeability) is an indication that the gut is maturing. According to Taylor, Basile, Ebeling, and Wagner (2009), infants who received >75% of their feedings as human milk had significantly lower intestinal permeability on days 7, 14, and 30 of life when compared to infants whose feedings contained minimal or no human milk. Receiving any milk compared to only infant formula, a significant difference in permeability existed on days 7 and 14 but not day

---

[3] Frequent contact through touching, kissing, nuzzling, and skin-to-skin holding of the baby allows the mother to ingest or inhale germs in the baby's environment. In the mother's body, lymphoid cells found in the lining of the gut or respiratory system have the ability to migrate to the breast. These cells then initiate production of antibodies specific to the antigen in the mother's gastrointestinal tract or lungs. The specific antibody is then secreted in the milk and the baby is protected in this fashion (Lawrence & Lawrence, 2005, pp. 173–174; Newman, 1995). This is referred to in the literature as either the gut-associated immunocompetent lymphoid tissue (GALT), bronchial-associated lymphoid tissue (BALT), or mucosal associated lymphoid tissue (MALT). Many other immune components of milk complement this production of specific immunoglobulins in a much less focused and broad-spectrum manner.

30. This study once again demonstrates the importance of species specificity in feeding.

Colostrum also facilitates the establishment of a beneficial bacterium in the gut, *Lactobacillus bifidus*. Bifidobacteria help the gut to maintain an acid pH by excreting an acetic acid buffer (Bullen, 1981). These beneficial bacteria also become part of the immunoprotection system since by maintaining an acid gut pH, they are making it impossible for pathogenic bacteria (which require a more basic environment for survival) to colonize the gut. Once established in the gut, these bifidobacteria offer protection for the lifetime of the individual. What an individual's gut is colonized with shortly after birth will remain the major bacterial flora. The early introduction of formula can interfere at a critical period and negatively impact the establishment of these bacteria and the proper pH (Bullen, Tearle, & Stewart, 1977). Developmentally, it is appropriate for the preterm infant to receive colostrum from its mother when it first starts receiving oral feedings, even if these feedings are only minimal. This primes the gut properly and establishes the correct pH and bacterial colonization.

Colostrum is also a potent laxative and helps stimulate gut motility in the term baby. Physiologically, the laxative effect stimulates the movement of meconium (fetal fecal material that is not excreted in utero unless the baby is in distress during birth) and helps to reduce the risk of neonatal jaundice. Preterm infants have a much higher risk of becoming jaundiced because of the extreme immaturity of the liver. Early enteral[4] feeding of colostrum is therefore an important part of caring for these infants and may help to reduce the degree of jaundice they experience.

Disease Protection

Immune factors such as the immunoglobulins, lactoferrin, and lysozyme are important to infants and children whose immune systems are either too

[4] Parenteral feeding is the intravenous administration of amino acids, fats, carbohydrates, vitamins, trace minerals, electrolytes, and fluids. Babies fed in this manner for long periods of time can suffer liver problems and have a high mortality rate. Enteral feeding is accomplished whenever the baby absorbs nutrients through the gastrointestinal tract. In preterm infants who cannot suck, enteral feeding is accomplished via a tube that goes through the nose or mouth directly into the stomach or jejunum. Many neonatologists now accept that it is physiologically unnatural for preterm babies not to be fed something enterally within hours of birth. In utero, these babies have been swallowing amniotic fluid. Minimal enteral (trophic) feeds are encouraged in many NICUs (in conjunction with parenteral feeding) so that the gut remains primed and does not atrophy. As enteral feedings are advanced in volume and frequency, parenteral feedings are withdrawn.

immature to function or have been compromised in some way by disease or genetics. For example, human milk is the optimal source of immunoglobulin A (IgA) for patients with IgA deficiency. The immunoglobulins protect the baby from disease. Some of these immunoglobulins, such as secretory immunoglobulin A (sIgA), prevent adhesion of pathogens to the gut wall by forming a protective coating. In one study, Eibl, Wolf, Furnkranz, and Rosenkranz (1988) used human IgA-IgG extracted from serum as a therapy to try to prevent NEC in a small population of nonbreastfed, premature infants. In the group that received the oral preparation, there were no cases of NEC as opposed to nine cases in the control group not receiving the therapy.

Equally important are the anti-infective nutrients in human milk. Nutrients found in human milk frequently have roles other than nutrition. These other anti-infective factors include complex carbohydrates such as mucins, oligosaccharides, and glycans with antibacterial and antiviral properties (Habte et al., 2007; Newburg, 2008; Newburg, Ruiz-Palacios, & Morrow, 2005; Yolken et al., 1992), lipids with antiviral properties (Isaacs & Thormar, 1990), and carbohydrates that prevent bacterial and parasitic adhesion.

Digestibility

Over the course of lactation, the composition of human milk changes to meet the changing needs of a growing infant. Early in life, the infant needs to have an easily digestible source of nutrition because the gastrointestinal (GI) tract must learn how to function in an extrauterine environment. As the GI tract matures, it can handle nutrients that are more difficult to digest. Milk proteins are divided into whey and casein fractions. The whey proteins are found in the liquid portion of the milk and are much more easily digested than the solid casein fraction. In human milk, the immune proteins constitute most of the whey portion of the milk. In early lactation (colostrum), the whey:casein ratio is 90:10 (Kunz & Lonnerdal, 1992) but gradually shifts over the course of lactation to 50:50. This gradual shift is ideal for the maturational curve that the GI tract must undergo in an extrauterine environment. Formulas for term infants, however, usually have a whey:casein ratio of 60:40, exactly the reverse of what would be most beneficial to the infant. Preterm formulas have cow's milk whey as a source of protein; however, digestibility may be reduced because of lack of species specificity (Jensen et al., 1995, p. 854).

This adaptive whey:casein ratio causes less metabolic stress in infants. For an infant who must spend a great deal of energy trying to grow and mature in an extrauterine environment when it should have still been in utero, extra metabolic stress detracts from growth. Energy that could be spent on growth is now being utilized for thermoregulation, breathing, digesting, etc. If less metabolic stress is placed on the infant by providing easily digestible and utilizable nutrients, then the extra energy can be utilized to achieve more growth.

Besides the species specificity of the nutrients themselves, increased digestibility of human milk comes in part from the enzymes that are important components in human milk that complement the baby's own digestive enzymes. According to Hamosh (1994), the newborn infant, especially the preterm infant, is deficient in pancreatic lipase and bile salts needed for proper digestion of fats. However, even very premature babies can absorb about 95% of human milk fat, compared with only 83–85% absorption of fats in special preterm formulas whose fats have been modified and blended to improve absorption. This is because human milk contains important enzymes that digest fat—milk digestive lipase (previously referred to as bile salt stimulated lipase, bile salt dependent lipase, or bile salt stimulated esterase) and lipoprotein lipase. These enzymes complement the baby's own gastric lipase and make fat digestion and absorption extremely efficient in the absence of pancreatic enzymes (Hamosh, 1994). Other enzymes in human milk, such as milk amylase (involved in breakdown of carbohydrates) and proteases (which break down proteins) also facilitate absorption and complement the infant's own digestive enzymes or lack thereof (Hamosh, 1994).

Bioavailability

While it may appear that human milk is low in some components when compared to formulas, this may be because the component in formula is not species specific and is in a form that is not bioavailable to the baby. For example, iron appears in human milk in relatively low concentrations, but nearly all of the iron can be utilized by the baby. Milk from the mothers of preterm infants appears to be higher in iron than the milk from mothers of term infants, a distinct advantage to the preterm infant because he has not been able to lay down optimal iron stores in the shortened third trimester of gestation. The form of iron in infant formulas is not as bioavailable or as easily metabolized, and formula companies must add many times more iron to the formula in order to get the same amount of absorption as in a human milk-fed infant.

Excess iron may have harmful consequences in infants. In a study of healthy Chilean children that spanned 10 years, the children fed the high-iron formulas had IQ scores that were 11 points lower than the scores of the children fed low-iron, regular formulas. The children fed the high-iron formulas also scored lower on tests for spatial memory, visual motor integration, visual perception, and motor coordination. While there were some benefits of the high-iron formulas seen in children who were iron deficient at birth, this was not the case for babies who were iron replete. According to a review by Griffin and Abrams (2008), negative consequences of too much iron in infancy (through the first year) include: an increase in infections; gastrointestinal intolerance; adverse effects on absorption of other essential minerals (zinc and copper) due to imbalances of ratios of one to another; and possibly an increase in SIDS, although the evidence for this is weak. Extra iron may serve as a nutritional substrate for pathogens that require iron in their life cycle, thus setting infants up for more infections. Other components in formula may actually interfere with absorption of certain nutrients. For example, plant compounds called phytates naturally occur in soy formula and prevent the absorption of zinc and selenium, minerals essential to the functioning of the infant's immune system (Lonnerdal, Bell, Hendrickx, Burns, & Keen, 1988). The American Academy of Pediatrics Committee on Nutrition does not recommend the use of soy formula for use in either the term or preterm population (Bhatia, Greer, & the Committee on Nutrition, 2008).

Bioactivity

The final advantage to human milk is that all of its components work together in a synergistic fashion to provide the baby with optimal nutrition and optimal disease protection when immune systems are immature, no matter what the baby's age. Many of the component systems within human milk are complementary to one another, producing a redundancy for optimal health. There are numerous ways to protect the infant and provide optimal nutrition. Taking similar chemical reagents off the shelf and mixing them together does not provide this bioavailability and bioactivity, as we see when formula companies try to put additives into formula. A good example of this is the latest addition of the long-chain polyunsaturated fatty acids (LC-PUFAs), arachidonic acid (ARA), and docosahexaenoic acid (DHA). Both of these LC-PUFAs occur naturally in human milk and are involved in the development of visual acuity and blood platelet membrane formation. But research looking at formula where these two LC-PUFAs have been added shows no additional benefit to infants in improved visual acuity or developmental scores—the human-milk-fed infants have a distinct advantage in nearly every study (Simmer, 2004; Simmer & Patole, 2004). Clearly, the bioactivity of the DHA and ARA depends on it occurring naturally and not being extracted from genetically engineered algae and soil fungi and then added to a milieu that is different. Despite the research evidence to the contrary, formula manufacturers are adding ARA and DHA (both of which have a relatively short shelf life and become rapidly inactive) to formula and phasing out formulas that do not contain these fatty acids. This means that consumers will be forced to pay higher prices for a formula that works no better than the older versions.

TRANSLATING THE BENEFITS FOR MOTHERS

In combination with the studies cited in Table 2-1, the aforementioned benefits of human milk for the preterm infant can be used in discussions with mothers prenatally and postpartum. They can be recombined and simplified so that mothers under a great deal of stress from the birth of a preterm infant can understand them. They may need to be said in various ways several times before the mother comprehends them and remembers them if she is postpartum, which is why it is imperative for prenatal healthcare providers to begin to incorporate this type of information into their earliest prenatal contacts with mothers-to-be. Increasing knowledge among pregnant women about the importance of breastfeeding and/or providing human milk provides the basis for informed consent and achieves an ethical goal of autonomy. Women are able to make informed decisions when presented with evidence-based information before a crisis occurs and can therefore improve the health outcomes of their infants, whether they are born healthy or sick and preterm.

The importance of providing human milk to their specific infant should be routinely communicated to women identified as being at risk for delivering prematurely or who have already delivered a premature and/or compromised infant. The consequences of not providing their milk should also be provided. As more women are presented with the importance of breastfeeding/providing their own milk for their premature or ill infants, they will also contribute to an increase in the incidence of breastfeeding and help achieve the nation's goals for breastfeeding initiation and duration. Infants will also achieve better health outcomes.

With over 530,000 preterm infants born in the United States each year (national preterm birth rate of 12.7%), an increase of about 20% since 1990, the costs of prematurity are estimated at more than $26 billion per year, according to the March of Dimes (2008). While breastmilk cannot prevent preterm birth, it can mitigate many of the effects of preterm birth and provide vulnerable infants with a better start in life than if they were fed formula. Hospital stays are shorter when preterm infants are fed human milk and morbidity with long-term costs attached is reduced. Therefore, every effort must be made to ensure that every pregnant woman is made aware of the benefits of breastfeeding and/or providing human milk and of the potential health risks of formula to preterm and/or compromised babies.

REFERENCES

Bhatia, J., Greer, F., & the Committee on Nutrition, American Academy of Pediatrics. (2008). Use of soy protein-based formulas in infant feeding. *Pediatrics, 121*(5), 1062–1068.

Bullen, C. (1981). Infant feeding and faecal flora. In A. Wilkinson (Ed.), *Immunology of infant feeding* (pp. 41–53). New York: Plenum Press.

Bullen, C., Tearle, P., & Stewart, M. (1977). The effect of "humanized" milks and supplemented breast feeding on the faecal flora of infants. *Journal of Medical Microbiology, 10*(4), 403–413.

Cadwell, K., & Turner-Maffei, C. (2009). Prenatal and perinatal education regarding infant feeding. In *Continuity of care in breastfeeding: Best practices in the maternity setting* (pp. 37–47). Sudbury, MA: Jones and Bartlett.

DiGirolamo, A., Grummer-Strawn, L., & Fein, S. (2003). Do perceived attitudes of physicians and hospital staff affect breastfeeding decisions? *Birth, 30*(2), 94–100.

Driscoll, J. (2008). *Women's moods: Psychiatric disorders during the postpartum period.* Unit No. 16: Lactation consultant series two. Schaumburg, IL: La Leche League International.

Eibl, M., Wolf, H., Furnkranz, H., & Rosenkranz, A. (1988). Prevention of necrotizing enterocolitis in low-birth-weight infants by IgA-IgG feeding. *New England Journal of Medicine, 319*(1), 1–7.

Friedman, S., Flidel-Ramon, O., Lavie, E., & Shinwell, E. (2004). The effect of prenatal consultation with a neonatologist on human milk feeding in preterm infants. *Acta Paediatrica, 93*(6), 775–778.

Griffin, I., & Abrams, S. (2008). *Iron metabolism in human milk-fed infants.* Lactation Consultant Series Two, Unit 11. Schaumburg, IL: La Leche League International.

Habte, H., Kotwal, G., Lotz, Z., Tyler, M., Abrahams, M., Rodriques, J., et al. (2007). Antiviral activity of purified human breast milk mucin. *Neonatology, 92*(2), 96–104.

Halamek, L. (2001). The advantages of prenatal consultation with a neonatologist. *Journal of Perinatology, 21*(2), 116-120.

Hamosh, M. (1994). Digestion in the premature infant: the effects of human milk. *Seminars in Perinatology, 18*(6), 485–494.

Isaacs, C., & Thormar, H. (1990). Human milk lipids inactivate enveloped viruses. In S. Atkinson, L. Hanson, & R. Chandra (Eds.), *Human lactation 4: Breastfeeding, nutrition, infection and infant growth in developed and emerging countries* (pp. 161–174). St. John's, Newfoundland, Canada: ARTS Biomedical Publisher.

Jensen, R., Couch, S., Hansen, J., Lien, E., Ostrom, K., Bracco, U., et al. (1995). Infant formulas. In R. Jensen (Ed.), *Handbook of milk composition* (pp. 835–855). New York: Academic Press, Inc.

Kunz, C., & Lonnerdal, B. (1992). Re-evaluation of the whey protein/casein ration of human milk. *Acta Paediatrica, 81*(2), 107–112.

Lawrence, R., & Lawrence, R. (2005). *Breastfeeding: A guide for the medical profession.* Philadelphia: Elsevier Mosby.

Lonnerdal, B., Bell, J., Hendrickx, A., Burns, R., & Keen, C. (1988). Effect of phytate removal on zinc absorption from soy formula. *American Journal of Clinical Nutrition, 48*(5), 1301–1306.

Manginello, F., & DiGeronimo, T. (1991). *Your premature baby: Everything you need to know about the childbirth, treatment, and parenting of premature infants.* New York: John Wiley & Sons, Inc.

March of Dimes. (2008). *Nation gets a "D" as March of Dimes releases premature birth report card.* Retrieved December 1, 2008, from http://www.marchofdimes.com/printableArticles/22684_42538.asp

Marinelli, K., & Hamelin, K. (2005). Breastfeeding and the use of human milk in the neonatal intensive care unit. In M. MacDonald, M. Mullet, & M. Seshia (Eds.), *Avery's neonatology: Pathophysiology and management of the newborn* (6th ed., pp. 413–444). Philadelphia: Lippincott Williams & Wilkins.

Narayanan, I., Prakash, K., Verma, R., & Gujral, V. (1983). Administration of colostrum for the prevention of infection in the low birth weight infant in a developing country. *Journal of Tropical Pediatrics, 29*(4), 197–200.

Newburg, D. (2009). Neonatal protection by an innate immune system of human milk consisting of oligosaccharides and glycans. *Journal of Animal Science, 87*(Suppl. 13), 26–34.

Newburg, D., Ruiz-Palacios, G., & Morrow, A. (2005). Human milk glycans protect infants against enteric pathogens. *Annual Review of Nutrition, 25*, 37–58.

Newman, J. (1995). How breast milk protects newborns. *Scientific American Magazine, 273*(6), 76–79.

Paul, D., Epps, S., Leef, K., & Stefano, J. (2001). Prenatal consultation with a neonatologist prior to preterm delivery. *Journal of Perinatology, 21*(7), 431-437.

Simmer, K. (2004). Longchain polyunsaturated fatty acid supplementation in infants born at term (Cochrane Review). In *The Cochrane Library* (Issue 4). Chichester, UK: John Wiley & Sons, Ltd.

Simmer, K., & Patole, S. (2004). Longchain polyunsaturated fatty acid supplementation in preterm infants (Cochrane Review). In *The Cochrane Library*, Issue 4. Chichester, UK: John Wiley & Sons, Ltd.

Stern, D. (1995). *The motherhood constellation.* New York: Basic Books.

Sullivan, J. (1997, April). Milk train. *Horse America*, p. 7.

Taveras, E, Li, R., Grummer-Strawn, L., Richardson, M., Marshall, R., Rego, V., et al. (2004). Mothers' and clinicians' perspectives on breastfeeding counseling during routine preventive visits. *Pediatrics, 113*(5), e405–e411.

Taylor, S., Basile, L., Ebeling, M., & Wagner, C. (2009). Intestinal permeability in preterm infants by feeding type: Mother's milk versus formula. *Breastfeeding Medicine, 4*(1), 11–15.

Vohr, B., Poindexter, B., Dusick, A., McKinley, L., Higgins, R., Langer, J., et al. (2007). Persistent beneficial effects of breast milk ingested in the neonatal intensive care unit on outcomes of extremely low birth weight infants at 30 months of age. *Pediatrics, 120*(4), e953–e959.

Vohr, B., Poindexter, B., Dusick, A., McKinley, L., Wright, L., Langer, J., et al. (2006). Beneficial effects of breast milk in the neonatal intensive care unit on the developmental outcome of extremely low birth weight infants at 18 months of age. *Pediatrics, 118*(1), e115–e123.

Yee, W., & Sauve, R. (2007). What information do parents want from the antenatal consultation? *Paediatrics and Child Health, 12*(3), 191–196.

Yolken, R., Peterson, J. Vonderfecht, S., Fouts, E., Midthun, K., & Newburg, D. (1992). Human milk mucin inhibits rotavirus replication and prevents experimental gastroenteritis. *Journal of Clinical Investigation, 90*(5), 1984–1991.

Appendix 5-1

STEP 3

Inform all women at risk for delivering or who have already delivered a preterm and/or compromised infant and their partners of the benefits of providing human milk.

Policies 3.1–3.5

Title

Prenatal and postpartum education for parents of NICU babies.

Purpose

Mothers at risk for delivering or who have already delivered premature and/or compromised infants should be encouraged to learn about the benefits and importance of providing human milk to their infants. Consequences of not providing their milk should also be explained.

Supportive Data

Increasing knowledge among pregnant women about the importance of breastfeeding and/or providing human milk provides the basis for informed consent and achieves an ethical goal of autonomy. Women are able to make informed decisions when presented with evidence-based information and can therefore improve the health outcomes of their infants. As more women are presented with the importance of breastfeeding/providing their own milk for their premature or ill infants they will also contribute to an increase in the incidence of breastfeeding and help achieve the nation's goals for breastfeeding initiation and duration. Infants will also achieve better health outcomes.

Rationale

Every effort must be made to ensure that all pregnant women are aware of the benefits of breastfeeding and/or providing human milk and of the potential health risks of formula to preterm and/or compromised babies. Antepartum hospital stays are opportunities for dispelling myths (e.g., "I can't breastfeed because I have a premature infant") and for providing anticipatory guidance regarding procedures to ensure a full milk supply and safe storage and use of pumped and/or donor milk. After controlling for a mother's prenatal breastfeeding intentions, father's feeding preference, and demographic and psychosocial variables, a study by the CDC concluded that the mother's perceptions of her prenatal physician's and hospital staff's attitudes on infant feeding was a strong predictor of later breastfeeding. In high-risk settings such as NICUs, neonatologists also have a strong influence on mothers and their choice to and success at providing milk for their preterm infants.

Scope

The policies apply to all NICU/SCN personnel including the medical director, neonatologists, nursing director, nursing supervisors, licensed staff, ancillary staff, and volunteers.

Policy 3.1

Expectant mothers identified as at risk for delivering a premature and/or compromised infant requiring special care (e.g., those mothers in an antepartum monitoring unit or whose babies have prenatally identified birth anomalies on ultrasound) should receive oral, written, and audiovisual education about the benefits and importance of breastfeeding and/or providing human milk to their special-needs infants.

Procedure 3.1.1
Prior to the birth of the infant, the neonatologist should visit personally with each high-risk mother and introduce the importance of the provision of human milk and breastfeeding. Physicians and other hospital staff should periodically reinforce the benefits of human milk to expectant at-risk mothers in short messages designed for memory retention.

Procedure 3.1.2
Individualized culturally sensitive education on the documented barriers and/or contraindications to breastfeeding or providing human milk and other special medical conditions should be given to pregnant women at risk for preterm delivery when indicated.

Policy 3.2

Expectant mothers and fathers identified as at risk for a preterm or complicated delivery, either outpatient or in antepartum units should be visited by a

NICU/SCN lactation specialist and oriented to breastfeeding, collection/storage policies and procedures, and about what to expect while the baby is hospitalized.

Policy 3.3

Mothers who have unexpectedly delivered a preterm or sick infant should be given information about the importance and benefits of providing their own milk as soon as possible after the birth of the baby.

Procedure 3.3.1
The neonatologist should visit personally with each new mother of an infant in the NICU and introduce the importance of the provision of human milk and breastfeeding. Physicians and other hospital staff should periodically reinforce the benefits of human milk to expectant at-risk mothers.

Policy 3.4

Antepartum, NICU/SCN, and postpartum units should have culturally appropriate videotapes, DVDs, or closed-circuit television programs delineating the benefits of human milk for their infants. These media presentations should be unbiased by commercial interests.

Policy 3.5

The NICU/SCN should provide appropriate written materials for the extended family of a NICU baby on the benefits of human milk for their premature or sick infant. These materials should emphasize the feasibility of both providing human milk and breastfeeding. Materials should not be biased by commercial interests.

Procedure 3.5.1
Educational materials should be written at a seventh-grade reading level or lower as per individual hospital policy.

Procedure 3.5.2
Educational materials should be accurately translated and available in the languages of the hospital's population.

Procedure 3.5.3
Education should include but not be limited to:

- Benefits of breastfeeding the premature and/or compromised infant
- Risks of not breastfeeding or providing human milk
- Basic lactation management for establishing and maintaining a full milk supply
- Skin-to-skin/kangaroo care
- Potential for full breastfeeding or just short-term milk provision
- Dietary concerns
- Medical concerns
- Psychosocial and sociocultural barriers
- Family support
- Mothers' return to work

chapter six

Step 4: Helping Preterm Mothers Mother Through Increased Mother–Infant Contact

"Birth is more than just the physical beginning of a new life—it is also the start of the psychosocial development of the newborn infant together with its family." (De Chateau, 1988, p. 21)

In Step 4 of the Ten Steps to Successful Breastfeeding for the healthy, term infant, the requirement is to assist mothers and babies to breastfeed within the first 30 minutes of life (see **Table 6-1**). This step was based on the research of Widstrom and others (1990), which demonstrated that healthy, term babies have a predictable pattern of self-attachment to the breast and that, if left unseparated from the mother and skin to skin with her, they will crawl to the breast and self-attach in the first minutes of life. The expectation for this step was clarified by WHO and UNICEF in 2006 in a revision of the Baby-Friendly Hospital Initiative. The original wording of the step remains the same, but the following explanation has been added to standards and criteria for the Baby-Friendly Hospital designation:

> This Step is now interpreted as: Place babies in [skin-to-skin] contact with their mothers immediately following birth for at least an hour and encourage mothers to recognize when their babies are ready to breastfeed, offering help if needed. (Cadwell & Turner-Maffei, 2009, p. 52)

Healthy, term infants are very competent little people who can elicit mothering behaviors from the mother by the simple act of nuzzling the breast or licking it. Babies who had the opportunity to touch or lick the areola or the nipple in the first half hour of life elicited different behaviors from their mothers than babies who did not have this opportunity. In the first 4 days postpartum, more mothers talked to their babies and left them in the nursery for only short periods of time when the infants had the nipple/areolar contact (Widstrom et al., 1990). Extra contact in the first hour after delivery compared to routine separation elicited different maternal behaviors in the mother, and babies cried less at 36 hours postpartum (de Chateau & Wiberg, 1977a). The same mother/infant couplets were followed at 3 months of age, and those with the extra hour of contact spent more time kissing and talking to their infants. The infants smiled more and cried less often than the control subjects with routine separation (de Chateau & Wiberg, 1977b) Mother–baby interaction in the first hours postpartum that comes with skin-to-skin contact has positive effects on both the mother's and infant's physiology as well as psychology, providing improved temperature regulation for the baby, increased homeostasis in the infant, decreased stress in both mother and baby, increased maternal attachment behaviors, and improved breastfeeding outcomes (see Cadwell & Turner-Maffei, 2009; Moore, Anderson, & Berman, 2007).

For the preterm infant, the frequent need for lifesaving interventions and stabilization at birth complicate the process, and mothers and babies are separated out of medical necessity in many cases, losing that initial contact period. Assisting the mothers of preterm infants to achieve a closer relationship with their infants and become a better parent is the goal of ABI's Step 4 of the Ten Steps for the Baby-Friendly NICU (Table 6-1). The goal is to facilitate bonding and begin the acquisition of parenting skills from as close to the moment of birth as possible.

PSYCHOLOGICAL STATUS OF MOTHERS OF PRETERM INFANTS

Risk Factors, Demographics, and Prevalence of Depressive Symptoms

Mothers of preterm infants are at greater risk for psychological distress than mothers of term infants. New mothers' emotional involvement with the newborn was less when the mother had one or more of the following risk factors: was unemployed, unmarried, had less than a high school education, had previous psychological or obstetrical problems, was depressed, or had an infant

Table 6-1 Side-by-Side Comparison of Three Models

Principle	*WHO/UNICEF Ten Steps to Successful Breastfeeding for the Healthy Term Newborn*	*ABI's Ten Steps for the NICU/SCN*	*Nyqvist and Kylberg (2008) Swedish Mothers' 13 Steps*	*Danish Ten Steps to Successful Breastfeeding of Preterm Infants*
The immediate postpartum period: bonding and breast-feeding	Step 4. Help mothers to initiate breastfeeding within 30 minutes* after birth.	Step 4. Facilitate bonding and maternal competency from the moment of birth.		

* The U.S. BFHI has an evidence-based exemption from the 30-minute time limit. Based on research, the time frame has been extended to 1 hour.

who was premature/sick and was admitted to the NICU. When the mother was depressed *and* had a lower educational level, significantly lower levels of bonding were observed. Being depressed, unemployed, and single were also predictive of negative emotions towards the infant (Figueiredo, Costa, Pacheco, & Pais, 2009).

In the United States, demographic confluence of the population characteristics of poverty, lack of insurance, and low levels of maternal education are reported factors contributing to the high levels of preterm birth observed in states such as Alabama, Louisiana, and Mississippi, the three states in which prematurity rates reached greater than 16.5% of births (Alabama = 16.7%; Louisiana = 16.5%; Mississippi = 18.8%; U.S. average in 2005 = 12.7% of births) (March of Dimes, 2008). In other words, the population most at risk demographically for preterm birth is also the population with the most challenges to becoming a parent and often the fewest support systems.

In a British study, having a preterm multiple birth also resulted in more stress and higher rates of maternal depression. Bryan (2003) reports a higher incidence of maternal depression and child abuse in families with multiple births, and that parents of preterm twins are less responsive to their infants than parents of singleton births. Given that multiple births (especially higher-order multiples) are more common related to an increased access to infertility treatments, this is a risk factor that is relatively recent and is perhaps limited to certain countries.

In a study by Davis, Edwards, Mohay, and Wollin (2003), factors that were associated with postpartum depressive symptoms included the stressful life event of coping with a preterm infant and lack of social support in the NICU as primary contributors. In the unfamiliar, unexpected, and scary environment of high technology and monitors with alarms, parents are stressed beyond their wildest imaginations, and many are beyond their ability to cope. Davis and colleagues (2003) report that some of the greatest sources of distress are the physical appearance of the preterm and very sick infant, fears for the survival of their infant, and separation from the infant. Not being able to touch or hold the baby and being separated from the infant, especially going home and leaving the baby behind in the hospital each day, was reported by mothers to be "the worst," "pretty horrible," and "the toughest" (Bernaix, Schmidt, Jamerson, Seiter, & Smith, 2006, pp. 95–100).

The association of preterm delivery with increased emotional (di)stress and depressive symptoms and inability to respond appropriately to the preterm infant is cross-cultural, and studies from different countries demonstrate similar findings. In a cross-sectional study from Nigeria that employed the Beck Depression Inventory as one measure of depressive symptoms, scores for preterm mothers were higher for levels of emotional stress and depression than those of mothers of term infants (Ukpong, Fatoy, Oseni, & Adewuya, 2003). In Brazil, a higher number of mothers of preterm infants expressed more negative or conflicted feelings about their preterm infants when compared to mothers of term infants. The negative and conflicting emotions were more severe if the infant was smaller at birth, sicker, and in need of more intensive care, and when the hospital stay was longer. These negative and conflicting emotions also correlated with higher levels of anxiety and depression (Padovani, Linhares, Pinto, Duarte, & Martinez, 2008). The levels of state anxiety also decreased after discharge of the infants (Carvalho, Martinez, & Linhares, 2008). Using the Edinburgh Postpartum Depression Scale, a Finnish study found that the prevalence of depression in mothers of infants born at < 32 weeks' gestation or ≤ 1500 g was 12.6%. An inverse relationship was noted between the number of signs of depression and the maternal interactions with preterm infants, suggesting that depression may be a risk factor in the development of maternal–infant interaction (Korja et al., 2008).

Davis et al. (2003) estimate that between 28% and 70% of mothers of preterm infants have significant levels of psychological stress. In their findings, a one-point increase on a stress score increased the risk of depression by 14%. This was the most significant variable associated with symptoms of depression. The mother's perception of support from NICU nurses and depression also reached statistical significance; as perceived nursing support decreased by a point, the risk of depression increased by 6%. Miles, Holditch-Davis, Burchinal, and Nelson (1999) report that at hospital discharge, 45% of mothers studied had scores indicating depression risk. In a more recent study that used an adaptation of the Preterm Parental Distress Model, mean depressive symptom scores during the infant's hospitalization were also high with 63% of mothers having scores of ≥ 16, indicating risk of depression. These depressive scores declined over time after discharge (Miles, Holditch-Davis, Schwartz, & Scher, 2007).

Effects of Depression and Maternal Emotions on Preterm Infants

Mothers' depressive symptoms are a concern because these symptoms have been associated with poorer emotional, cognitive, and developmental outcomes in their infants, irrespective of gestation age. The effects may also last for some time. As reported in Kendall-Tackett (2008), abnormalities in electroencephalograms can be seen in 3- to 6-month-old term children raised by depressed mothers (Field, Diego, Hernandez-Reif, Schanberg, & Kuhn, 2002) and also scored lower on measures of overall intelligence at age 4 (Hay & Kumar, 1995). Low birth weight enhanced the negative effect of maternal depression. Kendall-Tackett (2008) also reports that the negative impact of maternal depression can last into elementary school and manifest itself in more behavioral problems and lower vocabulary scores at age 5 (Brennan et al., 2000). Social competence (e.g., functioning in social relationships, school achievements, chores, hobbies, and other children's activities) was also impaired in children of mothers with depressive symptoms at 8 to 9 years of age in a Finnish study (Luoma et al., 2001).

Mothers who are not securely emotionally attached to their infants also might abandon their newborn babies and simply walk out of the hospital without them after the birth. This was observed firsthand by the author in Romania in 1997, where mothers and their term infants in one hospital were separated and cared for on separate floors. During the routine hospital stay of 7 days, the mothers were sequestered in their dormitory rooms not interacting with or holding their babies in any way, and certainly not breastfeeding! In the 2 weeks prior to our visit, the mothers of 18 babies (half of the delivering population) had simply walked out of the hospital without their infants. In another hospital, we were told by the nurses that a young girl who had a cardiac defect did not like to be picked up. She was lying in an extremely contorted posture, probably from lack of contact. We guessed her age to be about 15–18 months based on her size. She was actually 3 years old, but lack of affection, bonding, and human contact had stunted her growth and created abnormal social and behavioral responses similar to those observed by Harlow in the baby rhesus monkeys who had contact only with unresponsive wire or cloth surrogates.

The premature or sick infant is at greater risk for developmental delays and poorer outcomes because he is less responsive to his environment and has an increased need for appropriate stimulation that the depressed mother may not be able to provide simply because she is depressed (Davis et al., 2003). The mother may not be able to initiate appropriate physical contact with the infant. Physical separation may be lengthy while the infant stabilizes and becomes less fragile. According to Poehlmann and Fiese (2001), the more symptomatic the mothers of preterm infants were, the less securely emotionally attached the infants were to their mothers.

The NICU Environment and Its Contribution: Coping Strategies

Mothers of preterm infants, particularly those who are very preterm, very sick, and extremely low birth weight, are separated from their infants, unable to participate in or feel a part of their care and worried about the infant's survival. Other barriers contribute to separation. The mother may be isolated in her hospital room, unable to get to her baby in the NICU. Inadequate staff may make wheelchair transport of the mother inconvenient, and she may not be able to visit her infant as soon or as often as she would like. She is dependent on others to get her to the NICU, especially if prolonged bed rest has led to muscle atrophy. Once the mother is discharged, she may have other restrictions on her time. She may have other children to care for. She may have to travel a long way between her home and the NICU. She may not have transportation or the funds to get from her home to the NICU for the frequent visits she desires. She may be physically exhausted and not feeling well herself. She may have returned to work in order to save her maternity leave until the baby's discharge. Once in the NICU, she may find herself being told that parents are not welcome at specific times, and access to her infant is restricted. A final barrier may be hospital staff attitudes and behaviors that make mothers feel unwelcome in the NICU environment.

Table 6-2 Mothers' Needs in the NICU

Emotional support
Information
Establishment of a meaningful relationship with their infant (interactional needs)
Learning caregiving
Getting adequate rest
Developing confidence in their ability to parent successfully after discharge

In a qualitative study, Hurst (2001) observed and interviewed in depth 12 mothers of preterm infants, spending a total of 448 hours in observing/interviewing mothers about their own needs in the NICU setting, the actions they took to meet their own needs, and the conditions within the NICU that affected the mothers' actions. Maternal priorities for their own needs are listed in **Table 6-2**. Among the most important was emotional support, from NICU staff as well as family. Hurst points out that many mothers perceive a somewhat adversarial relationship with nurses, believing that nurses do not understand, appreciate, or acknowledge the difficulty and emotional stress of the situation the mothers are in. Mothers also perceive many actions of nurses and other healthcare providers in a negative manner, "ranging from conflicting instructions to intimidation" (p. 66) that prevent mothers from addressing their own needs for information, learning caregiving, and establishing a relationship with the infant. On the other hand, a study by Martinez, Monti Fonseca, and Silna Scochi (2007), where professional staff in the NICU of a public hospital in Mexico were interviewed at length, found that staff felt that presence of the parents interfered with nursing routines, created insecurity among staff who felt supervised by the parents, and elevated concerns about hospital infection. Ambivalence was evident in that staff also acknowledged the need for mother–child interactions to achieve improved clinical stability and recognized that mothers assisted nursing staff in giving routine care to the preterm infant.

Hurst (2001) also found that mothers perceived that their own needs competed with those of their infants, and since the care providers were shared by mother and baby, the mothers did not want to jeopardize their infants' care by being difficult or demanding. The primary needs for the mother were informational in nature and interactional. To fulfill these needs mothers became adept at:

1. Negotiating with healthcare providers to reach an agreement about the care of their babies and themselves.
2. Challenging institutional authority judiciously, deciding when and how to voice concerns and wishes.
3. Using institutional knowledge to challenge institutional authority, such as using knowledge of a hospital policy on human milk storage to challenge conflicting information from a staff member.
4. Using peer experience gleaned from observations and direct conversation with other parents to advocate for themselves and their babies.
5. Seeking a higher authority than the immediate care provider to raise concerns and get questions answered.
6. Creating support systems with other mothers in the NICU.
7. Garnering the support of family and friends.

Hurst's reports of mothers' stories mirror many of Bonnie's experiences. Mothers in the NICU described the nursing staff as being inconsistent in their approaches to caregiving. They described the understanding they got from some nurses about the need to touch their babies, while others felt that touching the baby was at the infant's expense. Hurst terms this *securing meaningful moments*. Securing meaningful moments was extremely difficult and could be impeded by numerous events in the NICU. Mothers described the lack of continuity of care created by large numbers of different care providers. In one mother's case, 65 nurses cared for her infant over a 5-month period (p. 73). Nurse:patient ratios could also impede the ability of mothers to have these meaningful moments because staff were too busy with other babies to provide individual information or support.

Hurst also reports that some mothers experienced conflicting messages between nurses and other healthcare providers and disrespect for the mothers' expert knowledge of their infants. They told the researcher about seeing their babies punished through rough handling after the mother had dared to assert her knowledge, as Bonnie did in the issue of skin-to-skin care. Mothers were made to feel as though they were an inconvenience in the nursery, that phone calls to inquire about the infant's status were treated by nurses as enormous inconveniences and interruptions. They experienced breaches in confidentiality, overhearing nurses talk about themselves or other mothers in derogatory terms in front of others. All of these things threatened the emotional security of the mother. Advocating for herself and her infant can put a mother in a situation such as Bonnie's—threatened with having the baby taken away from her because staff believe she is an unfit mother. Hurst concludes by saying:

> The mothers' evaluations and actions point to the clear need to implement and further develop models of care that explicitly recognize mothers as an important ally and to incorporate a partnership that addresses the needs of the mothers as an essential feature of nursing practice. The mothers' actions in this study conveyed the importance they attributed to promoting and preserving a positive, collaborative partnership with health care providers, particularly nurses. In order to achieve these goals nurses must work in partnership with mothers and families to forge models of care that mutually empower mothers and families and nurses. (Hurst, 2001, p. 80)

METHODS FOR FACILITATING BONDING

Touch

Infants born at very early gestational ages such as 23 or 24 weeks have skin that is very undeveloped and is more like cellophane. It is extremely fragile and extra handling of the infant is avoided whenever possible. However, the mother of an extremely preterm infant is the mother who most needs to bond with her baby. The best way to do this is through touch, even if it is impossible for the baby to be picked up and held. In one Connecticut NICU, nurses and neonatologists encourage mothers of even the smallest, sickest babies to put their hands through the portholes of the isolette and to touch their infants gently without rubbing the skin. Gentle pressure is applied to the top of the head and the soles of the feet simultaneously to make the baby feel more secure. Gentle pressure is applied to the belly. Babies are allowed to hold onto mothers' fingers. This starts immediately after the birth and makes the mother feel that she has something to contribute to the baby's care (K. Marinelli, personal communication, December 7, 2008). As the baby gets older and matures, parents in this NICU are taught ways to massage their infants. Feary (2002) has found that touching premature infants in this way promotes bonding and well-being and provides benefits for parents, babies, and healthcare providers, stating that touch is an essential therapy. Increased cholecystokinin levels from the peripheral nerve stimulation of touch provides feelings of wellness and well-being in both mother and infant as well as growth and maturation in the infant (Furman & Kennell 2000; Uvnas-Moberg, Widstrom, Marchini, & Winberg, 1987). Providing their preterm infants with infant massage also lowered depressed mood scores and anxiety scores in mothers (Feijo et al., 2006).

Kangaroo Mother Care or Skin-to-Skin Care

Kangaroo mother care (KMC) is a specific type of holding that the mother does with the preterm infant. The mother removes clothing barriers from her chest and snuggles the infant between her breasts. The infant is clothed only in a diaper and hat. She then covers both herself and her infant and keeps the baby warm and secure. (A description of the infant benefits of KMC/skin-to-skin (STS) care will be discussed in Chapter 9.) Similar to the little joey in the kangaroo mother's pouch, the baby is kept upright and close to the mother, smelling the breast and hearing the mother's heartbeat. The upright position that is characteristic of the KMC method prevents the weight of the infant's internal organs from pressing on his or her diaphragm and lungs and helps keep the baby's respiratory functions optimal.

In terms of initial bonding of mothers and preterm infants, KMC provides a feeling of closeness that helps mothers' mood states. According to Furman and Kennell (2000), the strong feelings of "guilt about the loss of normal pregnancy, labor and delivery, and feelings of responsibility for their infants' stressful and painful course, and lack of mothering experiences with their baby were ameliorated by the one to one intimate contact" (p. 1282) provided by KMC. Reconciliation and healing occurred when mothers implemented KMC over the course of several weeks (Affonso, Bosque, Wahlbert, & Brady, 1993). Mothers and babies got to know each other. They reported having increased self-esteem and confidence in their ability to care for their babies and more joyous feelings related to the babies. Being able to hold their infants in KMC calmed mothers as well (Roller, 2005), and mothers reported feeling "calmer, stronger, well-coordinated, energetic, contented, tranquil, quick-witted, relaxed, proficient, happy, friendly and clear-headed" in a study by de Macedo, Cruvinel, Lukasova, and D'Antino (2007, p. 344). KMC thus has a positive effect on maternal mood in the NICU. A more positive attitude/mood on the part of the mother may translate into a different dynamic vis-à-vis depressive symptoms in the mother, a hypothesis that needs to be tested.

Tessier et al. (1998) observed a change in the mother's perception of her child when KMC occurred. Mothers who practiced KMC felt better bonded to their infants and more competent as mothers. Mothers were also more responsive to their at-risk infants and changed their behavior towards their infants. At 37 weeks' gestation age, mothers who had experienced KMC touched their babies more, had a more positive affect and read the infants' cues better. Mothers also reported less depression and perceived their infants as being less abnormal. The effects were lasting, and at 3-month and 6-month follow-up, mothers showed increased sensitivity to their infants and provided a better home environment than mothers who had not practiced KMC (Feldman, Eidelman, Sirota, & Weller, 2002).

Even when infants were really sick KMC was useful in establishing a special quality of mother–infant interaction. Neu (1999) conducted a qualitative study on mothers who did KMC when their babies were on ventilators. While the mothers were apprehensive about doing KMC with their infants for fear of harming them or dislodging the ventilator tube, they also yearned to hold the infants. Mothers who continued KMC after the study was completed talked about the supportive environment in the NICU for KMC (i.e., nurses who thought the mothers were doing something wonderful for the baby and who were encouraging) as being a factor in continuing. Mothers who discontinued KMC commented on the lack of nursing support among other barriers such as a crowded environment, lack of privacy, and loss of control (Neu, 1999). Anderson et al. (2003) also found that more support is needed in the NICU for families in order to initiate STS contact early, to prolong the periods of contact, and to reduce maternal stress (Anderson et al., 2003). Neu states:

> Some parents may wish to do skin-to-skin care but feel powerless to make the request. Nursing actions such as providing privacy, expressing a positive attitude toward skin-to-skin care, and offering to assist may alleviate anxiety and provide encouragement for a parent who values the skin-to-skin experience. (1999, p. 163)

Other special circumstances in which KMC has been of benefit to parents have been in the resolution of grief and anxiety from a previous stillbirth (Burkhammer, Anderson, & Chiu, 2004) and in the case of adoptive parents of a critically ill infant born at 27 weeks (Parker & Anderson, 2002). In another case, KMC was used 2 hours postbirth to help a mother overcome postpartum depression. Self-reported depression scores decreased rapidly and had disappeared by 32 hours postbirth (Dombrowski, Anderson, Santori, & Burkhammer, 2001).

WHEN AND HOW TO DO KANGAROO CARE

Depending on the condition of the infant, mothers may be able to begin KMC immediately after the birth. In Colombia, where KMC originated, KMC begins in the delivery room for babies of more mature gestational ages (Ludington-Hoe et al., 1993). In a case report, KMC was begun at 4 hours postbirth in a 32-week, 1953-gram infant (Moran et al., 1999). Many infants born in the United States are much younger gestationally and much more critical than those in other parts of the world. Mothers may not be able to do KMC until the baby's skin develops further, but once exposed to an extrauterine environment, this maturational process appears to speed up and happen on a more rapid time frame than if the baby were still in utero, perhaps within a week (K. Marinelli, personal communication, December 7, 2008). Careful, appropriate touch, as described earlier, can be initiated in these cases. Another means of providing tactile stimulation for the infant is to have the mother learn to do colostrum oral care. This may be an integral part of the bonding process.

There are very few babies for whom KMC is not appropriate. These restrictions are listed in **Table 6-3**. There should be no eminent risk to life for KMC to occur, and the infant should be cardiovascularly stable and not on pressor therapy (K. Marinelli, personal communication, December 7, 2008). This does not mean that babies who have bradycardia and apnea should be excluded from receiving KMC. On the contrary, KMC helps to stabilize these babies further, and they have fewer spells when they are being held in STS contact with the mother.

In order for a baby to be held STS with the mother, the infant must transfer from the incubator to the mother's chest. This transfer can be problematic, causing stress for some infants. Commonly, the mother sits in a chair near the incubator and the nurse transfers the infant to the mother's chest. However, mothers report that they prefer transferring the baby themselves because the infant is handled less and they believe they are actively helping the infant (Neu, 1999). When the mother transfers the baby, the nurse changes the leads and then opens the incubator. The mother leans into

Table 6-3 Criteria for Delaying KMC

Cellophane skin in extremely premature infants
KMC may begin as soon as skin matures and firms up.
Cardiovascular instability (Pressor therapy)

the incubator and transfers the infant to her chest and then sits down. This method features less manipulation of the infant and the infant feels more secure as well (K. Marinelli, personal communication, December 7, 2008). The duration of KMC should be long enough so that the baby experiences infrequent disruptions. The infant can be tube fed while in KMC, and some authors point out an advantage to this because the infant has elevated levels of cholecystokinin and gastrin during KMC that promote better digestion and absorption of nutrients, promoting better growth. A model policy is presented in **Appendix 6-1**.

Rooming in with a Baby in the NICU

Some NICUs have limited rooming-in arrangements, reserved for several days before the baby is discharged. The mother takes care of the baby as she would at home, but she has backup and help if she feels uncertain or has questions. Usually this type of rooming in is of very short duration, perhaps only one or two nights. It is becoming somewhat more common in the United States to see premature infants and their mothers in rooms that are clustered in a pod around a central nursing area. In Uppsala, Sweden, NICU mothers and fathers are allowed to stay with their infants 24 hours a day in the critical care area, moving to a cocare room as soon as the baby is out of immediate danger (Nyqvist, 2009). According to Nyqvist, the presence and support of fathers alleviated the added stress of being alone and having to cope alone. Parents begin to assume more of their infant's routine care together, similar to the model proposed by Levin (Chalmers & Levin, 2001) and cited in Chapter 1. Do these opportunities make a difference in a mother's mental health and her ability to parent?

Erdeve, Arsan, Yigit, et al. (2008) and Erdeve, Arsan, Canpolat, et al. (2009) conducted a study to investigate the effect of rooming in during babies' hospital stay for babies born prior to 34 weeks' gestation compared with not rooming in with liberal visitation policies. At the 3rd month post-discharge, mothers were assessed for postpartum depression, parental stress, and perception of vulnerability. Although not statistically significant, mothers in the rooming-in group demonstrated less postpartum depression (half the rate of the non–rooming-in mothers), less stress, and less vulnerability. The lack of statistical significance led the authors to state that the rooming-in experience did not prevent any of these negative effects on mood because they derived from the fact of having the preterm infant (Erdeve, Arsan, Canpolat, et al., 2009). Mothers who did not have the experience of rooming in, however, had higher utilization of the healthcare system than those mothers who roomed in with their infants (Erdeve, Arsan, Yigit, et al., 2008). The mean number of acute care visits, mean number of phone consultations, and the rehospitalization rate were statistically significantly higher in the group that did not room in. The reasons for seeking additional medical help also differed, with problems primarily related to prematurity, such as feeding difficulties, predominating in the no–rooming-in group. Care by parents "gives the mother an opportunity to assume full responsibility for her preterm infant's care, tests the reality of caregiving, helps her learn about caregiving activities and her infant's patterns of behavior, and confirms her readiness for independent parenting and the infant's readiness for discharge home" (Costello & Chapman, 1998, p. 37).

SUMMARY

Mothers are vulnerable after giving birth prematurely and may experience very strong feelings of disenfranchisement. Their babies cannot be held and cuddled, and experts are responsible for the care of the newly born infant. The mother's feelings of separation are exacerbated by fears and anxiety related to the health of her baby, the severity of his condition, the duration of time her baby will be in the NICU, and the number and severity of setbacks that occur. Mothers understandably may become depressed and angry over their situation. If not allowed opportunities to bond with their babies, we know that their parenting skills and their infants' development may be negatively impacted.

NICU barriers serve to obstruct mothers from assuming their rightful role as mother and caregiver. Examination of these barriers by staff can enable mothers to appropriately participate in infant care and be respected for their desire to learn and feel competent as a parent. To accomplish this, NICU teams must assure that they are providing evidence-based care, removing physical barriers and constraints such as lack of privacy, praising the mother for her efforts so that she will become more confident, and including her in the process as appropriate. Because the mother's mental and emotional health will have a direct impact on the health, development, and well-being of the baby in their care, the healthcare team's perception of the mother as an adjunct to the continued welfare of their patient mandates her inclusion in the plan of care.

REFERENCES

Affonso, D. Bosque, E., Wahlberg, V., & Brady, J. (1993). Reconciliation and healing for mothers through skin-to-skin contact provided in an American tertiary level intensive care nursery. *Neonatal Network, 12*(3), 25–32.

Anderson, G. C. (1991). Current knowledge about skin-to-skin (kangaroo) care for preterm infants. *Journal of Perinatology, 11*(3), 216–226.

Anderson, G., Chiu, S., Dombowski, M., Swinth, J., Albert J., & Wada, N. (2003). Mother-newborn contact in a randomized trial of kangaroo (skin-to-skin) care. *Journal of Obstetric, Gynecologic, and Neonatal Nursing, 32*(5), 604–911.

Bernaix, L., Schmidt, C., Jamerson, P., Seiter, L., & Smith, J. (2006). The NICU experience of lactation and its relationship to family management style. *American Journal of Maternal Child Nursing, 31*(2), 95–100.

Bier, J., Ferguson, A., Morales, Y., Liebling, J., Archer, D., Oh, W., et al. (1996). Comparison of skin-to-skin contact with standard contact in low-birth-weight infants who are breast-fed. *Archives of Pediatric and Adolescent Medicine, 150*(12), 1265–1269.

Brennan, P., Hammen, C., Anderson, M., Bor, W., Najman, J., & Williams, G. (2000). Chronicity, severity, and timing of maternal depressive symptoms: Relationships with child outcomes at age 5. *Developmental Psychology, 36*(6), 759–766.

Bryan, E. (2003). The impact of multiple preterm births on the family. *British Journal of Obstetrics and Gynecology, 110*(Suppl. 20), 24–38.

Burkhammer, M., Anderson, G., & Chiu, S. (2004). Grief, anxiety, stillbirth, and perinatal problems: Healing with kangaroo care. *Journal of Obstetric, Gynecologic, and Neonatal Nursing, 33*(6), 774–782.

Cadwell, K., & Turner-Maffei, C. (2009). *Continuity of care in breastfeeding: Best practices in the maternity setting.* Sudbury, MA: Jones and Bartlett.

Carvalho, A., Martinez, F., & Linhares, M. (2008). Maternal anxiety and depression and development of prematurely born infants in the first year of life. *Spanish Journal of Psychology, 11*(2), 600–608.

Chalmers, B., & Levin, A. (2001). *Humane perinatal care.* Tallinn, Estonia: TEA Publishers.

Costello, A., & Chapman, J. (1998). Mothers' perceptions of the care-by-parent program prior to hospital discharge of their preterm infants. *Neonatal Network, 17*(7), 37–42.

Davis, L., Edwards, H., Mohay, H., & Wollin, J. (2003). The impact of very premature birth on the psychological health of mothers. *Early Human Development, 73*(1–2), 61–70.

de Chateau, P. (1988). The interaction between the infant and the environment: The importance of mother–child contact after delivery. *Acta Paediatrica Scandinavica, 344*(Suppl.), 21–30.

de Chateau, P., Holmberg, H., Jakobsson, K., & Winberg, J. (1977). A study of factors promoting and inhibiting lactation. *Developmental Medicine and Child Neurology, 19*(5), 575–584.

de Chateau, P., & Wiberg, B. (1977a). Long-term effect on mother-infant behaviour of extra contact during the first hour postpartum. I. First observations at 36 hours. *Acta Paediatrica Scandinavica, 66*(2), 137–143.

de Chateau, P. & Wiberg, B. (1977b). Long-term effect on mother–infant behaviour of extra contact during the first hour postpartum. II. A follow-up at three months. *Acta Paediatrica Scandinavica, 66*(2), 145–151.

de Macedo, E., Cruvinel, F., Lukasova, K., & D'Antino, M. (2007). The mood variation in mothers of preterm infants in kangaroo mother care and conventional incubator care. *Journal of Tropical Pediatrics, 53*(5), 344–346.

Dombrowski, M., Anderson, G., Santori, C., & Burkhammer, M. (2001). Kangaroo (skin-to-skin) care with a postpartum woman who felt depressed. *American Journal of Maternal Child Nursing, 26*(4), 214–216.

Erdeve, O., Arsan, S., Canpolat, F., Ertem, I., Karagol, B., Atasay, B., et al. (2009). Does individual room implemented family-centered care contribute to mother–infant interaction in preterm deliveries necessitating neonatal intensive care unit hospitalization? *American Journal of Perinatology, 26*(2), 159–164.

Erdeve, O., Arsan, S., Yigit, S., Armangil, D., Atasay, B., & Korkmaz, A. (2008). The impact of individual room on rehospitalization and health service utilization in preterm infants after discharge. *Acta Paediatrica, 97*(10), 1351–1357.

Feary, A. (2002). Touching the fragile baby: Looking at touch in the special care nursery (SCN). *Australian Journal of Holistic Nursing, 9*(1), 44–48.

Feijo, L., Hernandez-Reif, M., Field, T., Burns, W., Valley-Gray, S., & Simco, E. (2006). Mothers' depressed mood and anxiety levels are reduced after massaging their preterm infants. *Infant Behavior and Development, 29*(3), 476–480.

Feldman, R., Eidelman, A., Sirota, L., & Weller, A. (2002). Comparison of skin-to-skin (kangaroo) and traditional care: Parenting outcomes and preterm infant development. *Pediatrics, 110*(1 Pt. 1), 16–26.

Field, T., Diego, M., Hernandez-Reif, M., Schanberg, S., & Kuhn, C. (2002). Relative right versus left frontal EEG in neonates. *Developmental Psychobiology, 41*(2), 147–155.

Figueiredo, B., Costa, R., Pacheco, A. & Pais, A. (2009). Mother-to-infant emotional involvement at birth. *Maternal Child Health Journal, 13*(4), 539–549.

Furman, L., & Kennell, J. (2000). Breastmilk and skin-to-skin kangaroo care for premature infants: Avoiding bonding failure. *Acta Paediatrica, 89*(11), 1280–1283.

Furman, L., Minich, N., & Hack, M. (2002). Correlates of lactation in mothers of very low birth weight infants. *Pediatrics, 109*(4), e57.

Hay, D., & Kumar, R. (1995). Interpreting the effects of mothers' postnatal depression on children's intelligence: a critique and re-analysis. *Child Psychiatry and Human Development, 25*(3), 165–181.

Hurst, I. (2001). Mothers' strategies to meet their needs in the newborn intensive care nursery. *Journal of Perinatal and Neonatal Nursing, 15*(2), 65–82.

Hurst, N., Valentine, C., Renfro, L., Burns, P., & Ferlic, L. (1997). Skin-to-skin holding in the neonatal intensive care unit influences maternal milk volume. *Journal of Perinatology, 17*(3), 213–217.

Kendall-Tackett, K. (2008). *Postpartum depression and the breastfeeding mother. Part I: Causes and consequences.* Unit 5, Lactation Consultant Series Two. Schaumburg, IL: La Leche League International.

Kirsten, G., Gergman, N., & Hann, F. (2001). Kangaroo mother care in the nursery. *Pediatric Clinics of North America, 48*(2), 443–452.

Korja, R., Savonlahti, E., Ahlqvist-Bjorkroth, S., Stolt, S., Haataja, L., Lapinleimu, H., et al., (2008). Maternal depression is associated with mother-infant interaction in preterm infants. *Acta Paediatrica, 97*(6), 724–730.

Ludington-Hoe, S., Anderson, G., Simpson, S., Hillingsead, A., Argote, L., Medellin, G., et al. (1993). Skin-to-skin contact beginning in the recovery room for Colombian mothers and their preterm infants. *Journal of Human Lactation, 9*(4), 241–242.

Luoma, I., Tamminen, T., Kaukonen, P., Laippala, P., Puura, K., Salmelin, R., et al. (2001). Longitudinal study of maternal depressive symptoms and child well-being. *Journal of the American Academy of Child and Adolescent Psychiatry, 40*(12), 1367–1374.

March of Dimes. (2008). *Nation gets a "D" as March of Dimes releases premature birth report card.* Retrieved December 1, 2008, from http://www.marchofdimes.com/printableArticles/22684_42538.asp

Martinez, J., Monti Fonseca, L., & Silna Scochi, C. (2007). The participation of parents in the care of premature children in a neonatal unit: Meanings attributed by the health team. *Revista Latino-Americana de Enfermagem, 15*(2), 239–246.

Miles, M., Holditch-Davis, D., Burchinal, P., & Nelson, D. (1999). Distress and growth outcomes in mothers of medically fragile infants. *Nursing Research, 48*(3), 129–140.

Miles, M., Holditch-Davis, D., Schwartz, T., & Scher, M. (2007). Depressive symptoms in mothers of prematurely born infants. *Journal of Developmental and Behavioral Pediatrics, 28*(1), 36–44.

Moore, E., Anderson, G., & Berman, N. (2007). Early skin-to-skin contact for mothers and their healthy newborn infants. *Cochrane Database Systematic Reviews, 3*, CD003519.

Moran, M., Radzyminski, S., Higgins, K., Dowling, D., Miller, M., & Anderson, G. (1999). Maternal kangaroo (skin-to-skin) care in the NICU beginning 4 hours postbirth. *American Journal of Maternal Child Nursing, 24*(2), 74–79.

Neu, M. (1999). Parents' perception of skin-to-skin care with their preterm infants requiring assisted ventilation. *Journal of Obstetric, Gynecologic, and Neonatal Nursing, 28*(2), 157–164.

Nyqvist, K. (2009, January). *Baby-friendly neonatal care*. Paper presented at the 2009 International Conference on the Theory and Practice of Human Lactation Research and Breastfeeding Management, Orlando, FL.

Padovani, F., Linhares, M., Pinto, I., Duarte, G., & Martinez, F. (2008). Maternal concepts and expectations regarding a preterm infant. *Spanish Journal of Psychology, 11*(2), 581–592.

Parker L., & Anderson, G. (2002). Kangaroo care for adoptive parents and their critically ill preterm infant. *American Journal of Maternal Child Nursing, 27*(4), 230–232.

Poehlmann, J., & Fiese, B. (2001). The interaction of maternal and infant vulnerabilities on developing attachment relationships. *Developmental Psychopathology, 13*(1), 1–11.

Righard, L., & Alade, M. (1990). Effect of delivery room routines on success of first breast-feed. *The Lancet, 336*(8723), 1105–1107.

Roller, C. (2005). Getting to know you: Mothers' experiences of kangaroo care. *Journal of Obstetric, Gynecologic, and Neonatal Nursing, 34*(2), 210–217.

Salariya, E., Easton, P., & Cater, J. (1978). Duration of breast-feeding after early initiation and frequent feeding. *The Lancet, 2*(8100), 1141–1143.

Tessier, R., Cristo, M., Velez, S., Giron, M., de Calume, Z., Ruiz-Palaez, J., et al. (1998). Kangaroo mother care and the bonding hypothesis. *Pediatrics, 102*(2), e17.

Ukpong, D., Fatoye, F., Oseni, S., & Adewuya, A. (2003). Postpartum emotional distress in mothers of preterm infant: A controlled study. *East African Medical Journal, 80*(6), 289–292.

Uvnas-Moberg, K., Widstrom, A-M., Marchini, G., & Winberg, J. (1987). Release of GI hormones in mother and infant by sensory stimulation. *Acta Paediatrica Scandinavica, 76*(6), 851–860.

Widstrom, A-M., Wahlberg, V., Matthiesen, A-S., Eneroth, P., Uvnas-Moberg, K., Werner, S., et al. (1990). Short-term effects of early suckling and touch of the nipple on maternal behaviour. *Early Human Development, 21*(3), 153–163.

Appendix 6-1

STEP 4

Facilitate bonding and maternal competency from the moment of birth.

Policies 4.1–4.3

Title

Maternal bonding and competency.

Purpose

To provide parents with unlimited access to their hospitalized infants from the moment of birth to facilitate bonding and acquisition of parenting skills, including education and support to initiate skin-to-skin contact with their infants as soon as medically possible.

Supportive Data

Providing parents with opportunities to visit their infants frequently and for unrestricted durations establishes feelings of attachment. Providing opportunities to touch and hold her infant increases a mother's sense of competency in her ability to parent and provide comfort. Being allowed to touch and hold their babies also ameliorates depressive symptoms in mothers of preterm babies and provides a foundation of better mental health. Ideally, the mother should be allowed to room in with her NICU baby and assume elements of routine care as soon as she is physically able. In this model, Levin reports better weight gain as well as immunological benefits of fewer infections, shorter durations of infections, and reduced need for antibiotic therapy (Chalmers & Levin, 2001). This results in the potential for shorter hospital stays and reduced costs. Increased contact, particularly skin-to-skin contact, also increases milk expression and breastfeeding success as well as increased durations of breastfeeding. Infants held skin to skin experience more physiologic stability and faster brainstem maturation.

Rationale

Parents have reported increased closeness to their infants and improved feelings of competence in handling their infants when they are allowed to visit, touch, and hold their babies skin to skin. Visual and tactile contact with her infant allows the mother to recognize the reality of the birth and the need for provision of breastmilk. Early maternal–infant contact (< 1 hour) is associated with increased initiation and duration of breastfeeding in term infants (de Chateau, Holmberg, Jakobsson, & Winberg, 1977; de Chateau & Winberg, 1977a and b; Righard & Alade 1990; Salariya, Easton, & Cater, 1978). Admission to the NICU negatively affects chances of successful breastfeeding because of initial and continuing separation and immaturity of the baby. Being close to one's baby and early and frequent skin-to-skin care are associated with increased amounts of milk, longer duration of breastfeeding, and breastfeeding success (Anderson, 1991; Bier et al., 1996; Furman, Minich, & Hack, 2002; Hurst, Valentine, Renfro, Burns, & Ferlic, 1997; Kirsten, Gergman, & Hann, 2001), and it is an easy, economical, safe, and necessary practice.

Scope

The policies apply to all NICU/SCN personnel including medical director, nursing director, nursing supervisors, licensed staff, ancillary staff, and volunteers.

Policy 4.1

Mothers delivering at less than 37 weeks' gestation should have the opportunity to see, touch, and/or hold their infants in the delivery room as both the infant's and mother's conditions warrant.

Procedure 4.1.1
Appropriately trained staff should attend deliveries of infants less than 37 weeks' gestation and promote early maternal bonding as the infant's and/or mother's medical condition allows.

Procedure 4.1.2
All awake mothers should be given the opportunity to see, if possible touch, and at best to hold their premature and/or compromised infants skin to skin prior to transfer to the NICU/SCN.

Policy 4.2

All babies not requiring immediate life-saving intervention (e.g., intubation, CPR, vascular access, cardiopulmonary stabilization, immediate surgery, etc.) should be allowed skin-to-skin contact before being transferred to the NICU/SCN.

Procedure 4.2.1

The infant is brought to the mother's chest in labor and delivery or recovery as soon as the baby's condition allows and the mother is prepared. Privacy should be provided. If mother is too ill to hold her baby, or unconscious, offer the opportunity for skin-to-skin contact to the father.

- Document vital signs before initiating skin-to-skin contact (axillary temperature, respirations, heart rate, and O_2 saturation).
- NICU/SCN staff lifts baby and places the infant gently against the mother's unclothed chest.
- Position the infant so the mother supports the baby's buttocks and back with her hands, tucking lower extremities into flexion. The infant is covered with the mother's shirt/gown or warmed blanket to prevent chilling. The head and neck are positioned to protect the airway.
- Document vital signs 15 minutes after initiating skin-to-skin contact and per routine care thereafter.
- NICU/SCN staff will remain available to family for support and assistance.
- Document vital signs upon return to infant's bed.
- Document description of baby's and mother's tolerance of skin-to-skin contact.
- Terminate skin-to-skin contact immediately at parent's request or if infant exhibits sustained desaturations, color changes, respiratory distress, heart rate instability, unrelenting irritability, or other signs of intolerance noted by parents or staff.

Procedure 4.2.2

If the baby is stable during maternal skin-to-skin contact and has no contraindications to immediate breastfeeding (extreme prematurity, possible GI anomalies) the baby should be offered an attempt at nuzzling/feeding at the breast prior to transfer to the NICU/SCN.

Policy 4.3

For infants requiring lifesaving measures at birth, the mother should be allowed to be at the baby's bedside whenever she is able/wants to, without restriction. Unnecessary barriers should not be placed between the mother and her infant.

Procedure 4.3.1

The mother should be encouraged to touch and hold her baby skin to skin in a continuous manner as soon as medically possible to facilitate physiological stability, improve body temperature, establish bonding, and improve maternal mental health.

REFERENCES

Anderson, G. C. (1991). Current knowledge about skin-to-skin (kangaroo) care for preterm infants. *Journal of Perinatology, 11*(3), 216–226.

Bier, J., Ferguson, A., Morales, Y., Liebling, J., Archer, D., Oh, W., et al. (1996). Comparison of skin-to-skin contact with standard contact in low-birth-weight infants who are breast-fed. *Archives of Pediatric and Adolescent Medicine, 150*(12), 1265–1269.

Chalmers, B., & Levin, A. (2001). *Humane perinatal care.* Tallinn, Estonia: TEA Publishers.

de Chateau, P., Holmberg, H., Jakobsson, K., & Winberg, J. (1977). A study of factors promoting and inhibiting lactation. *Developmental Medicine and Child Neurology, 19*(5), 575–584.

de Chateau, P., & Wiberg, B. (1977a). Long-term effect on mother-infant behaviour of extra contact during the first hour postpartum. I. First observations at 36 hours. *Acta Paediatrica Scandinavica, 66*(2), 137–143.

de Chateau, P. & Wiberg, B. (1977b). Long-term effect on mother–infant behaviour of extra contact during the first hour postpartum. II. A follow-up at three months. *Acta Paediatrica Scandinavica, 66*(2), 145–151.

Furman, L., Minich, N., & Hack, M. (2002). Correlates of lactation in mothers of very low birth weight infants. *Pediatrics, 109*(4), e57.

Hurst, N., Valentine, C., Renfro, L., Burns, P., & Ferlic, L. (1997). Skin-to-skin holding in the neonatal intensive care unit influences maternal milk volume. *Journal of Perinatology, 17*(3), 213–217.

Kirsten, G., Gergman, N., & Hann, F. (2001). Kangaroo mother care in the nursery. *Pediatric Clinics of North America, 48*(2), 443–452.

Righard, L., & Alade, M. (1990). Effect of delivery room routines on success of first breast-feed. *The Lancet, 336*(8723), 1105–1107.

Salariya, E., Easton, P., & Cater, J. (1978). Duration of breast-feeding after early initiation and frequent feeding. *The Lancet, 2*(8100), 1141–1143.

chapter seven

Step 5: Establishing and Maintaining a Milk Supply for the NICU Infant

THE DECISION TO PROVIDE MILK: "IS IT TOO LATE TO CHANGE MY MIND?"

The effects of healthcare provider (HCP) encouragement on breastfeeding initiation were investigated in one retrospective U.S. survey representative of a cross-section of the population (Lu, Lange, Slusser, Hamilton, & Halfon, 2001). Women who were encouraged by their HCP to breastfeed were more than 4 times as likely to initiate breastfeeding than the group that received no encouragement. In populations of women who are traditionally less likely to breastfeed, encouragement by the HCP was even more significant. Breastfeeding initiation increased by greater than threefold in low-income, young, less-educated women, by nearly fivefold in Black women, and by nearly elevenfold in single women.

Traditionally, women who deliver preterm, very-low-birth-weight infants also initiate breastfeeding at much lower rates than women who have delivered healthy term infants (Miracle, Meier, & Bennett, 2004a, 2004b; Ryan, Wenjun, & Acosta, 2002; Sisk, Lovelady, & Dillard, 2004). The same demographic factors for choosing bottle-feeding, e.g., low income, less education, and belonging to a racial or ethnic minority (primarily women of African descent born in the United States), are also risk factors for premature delivery. States with large African American populations and large low-income populations are states with the highest rates of prematurity and the lowest breastfeeding initiation rates (See CDC, 2008a, 2008b; March of Dimes, 2008). In the United Kingdom, Lucas et al. (1988)

found similar factors at play in the decision to provide maternal milk for low-birth-weight infants. Less maternal education, lower social class (indicative of income level), single marital status, age less than 20 years, higher parity, and smoking during the first and especially the second trimester of pregnancy were predictive of choosing to formula feed.

Ideally, the decision to breastfeed or express milk for a hospitalized infant is made prior to the delivery of the infant. As discussed in Chapter 5, Step 3, a prenatal visit from the neonatologist makes a difference in the mother's choice whether or not to provide her own milk. But if a mother delivers unexpectedly and has already made the decision to feed formula, is there a possibility of changing her mind? In the study conducted by Miracle et al. (2004b), women who chose initially to formula feed gave the following reasons for their decisions:

- Lack of role models—no one in their families had ever breastfed so they assumed that they would formula-feed also.
- A belief that breastfeeding would be painful—they had heard horror stories from relatives and friends who attempted breastfeeding and had difficulties.
- Lack of knowledge about breastfeeding and a belief that formula and human milk were equivalent.

When they were told about the special characteristics of their milk and the difference between human milk and formula for their babies, the 21 mothers in the study changed their minds about expressing for their infants, with most starting expression within 48 hours after delivery. One mother who was not told about the differences until she went to see her baby for the first time asked, "Is it too late to change my mind?"

Of note in this study is the sample population—women who according to their demographics were unlikely to choose breastfeeding—71% were African American and 62% were low income. According to Miracle, Meier, and Bennett (2004b), in the United States, African American women are three times more likely than White women to deliver a premature low-birth-weight infant, and low-income women of all ethnicities are twice as likely to do so as women of higher socioeconomic status. Yet a simple intervention of talking to the mother about *her* importance in helping to feed her baby convinced a group that would be most unlikely to initiate breastfeeding to change their minds and begin to supply their milk to their NICU babies. The personal connection made by the HCP with the individual mother in this discussion is very powerful. Women remember the name of the person and what he/she looked like when the discussion is personalized (Miracle et al., 2004b). The results of this study indicate several things:

- Even women who have chosen to formula feed their babies if born full term want HCPs to discuss the benefits of human milk with them and give them enough information with which to make an informed choice.
- Mothers receiving personalized information from an HCP are more likely to initiate lactation—even those least likely to do so because of their demographic features.
- Professional encouragement for initiating lactation did not make mothers feel coerced or guilty because the information given was factual and concentrated on the short term and getting the baby off to a good start (as opposed to discussing long-range goals such as breastfeeding for a year).

Mothers' decisions *can* be changed, to the benefit of both infants and mothers.

In a follow-up paper, suggestions were made that are intended to help nurses and other HCPs feel more comfortable in having these types of discussions with mothers (Rodriguez, Miracle, & Meier, 2005). These suggestions are highlighted in **Table 7-1** and answer the following questions:

- How should I introduce the topic when it's not what the mother really wanted?
- Will I make the mother feel guilty or pressured with this discussion?
- What kinds of questions should I expect from mothers? How do I answer them? I am *not* an expert on breastfeeding.
- How do I help the mother get started with pumping when she doesn't plan on breastfeeding?
- What do I say when asked about alternatives to long-term pumping?

PRINCIPLES OF ESTABLISHING AND MAINTAINING A MILK SUPPLY

Step 5 of the Ten Steps to Successful Breastfeeding mandates that hospital staff assist mothers in establishing breastfeeding and educate mothers about how to maintain breastfeeding by establishing an ample milk supply. Even if separated from her baby by prematurity or illness, the mother should be helped to establish a milk supply according to the BFHI Ten Steps model. All maternity staff and mothers are expected to know the importance of feeding frequency to the success of establishing an ample milk supply. Maternity

Table 7-1 How to Share Information With Mothers When You're Not an Expert on Breastfeeding

How should I introduce the topic when it's not what the mother really wanted?

- Distinguish between providing milk and breastfeeding. To begin, if she cannot breastfeed, she will only be providing her milk and she can discontinue this at any time. Avoid value-laden conversation.
- Provide the mother with an explanation as to why the milk is important for her infant. (Hurst [2007] refers to these reasons as "Breast milk as medicine" [p. 234].)
- Leave the mother with the primary message of "Start using the breast pump or expressing manually now and we'll help you sort out how long you want to continue milk expression or breastfeeding later in your baby's hospital stay."

Will I make the mother feel guilty or pressured with this discussion?

- Women want to be able to make an informed decision and want the information with which to do so.
- Women do not feel pressured or coerced when they are merely provided with information and not told "You should ..."

What kinds of questions should I expect from mothers? How do I answer them? I am *not* an expert on breastfeeding.

- Target the two major concerns, which are: (1) lactation involves discomfort or pain; and (2) lifestyle changes that will be required.
- Reassure them that discomfort is "usually preventable, nearly always transient, and can be managed with pain medications or comfort measures" (Rodriguez et al., 2005, p. 114).
- Ensure the correct flange size on the pump kit and demonstrate the correct way to use the pump.
- Reassure that nearly all diets and medications are compatible with milk expression for very-low-birth-weight infants. If uncertain about something, ask the neonatologist or nurse.
- Acknowledge lack of role models and identify potential sources of support, e.g. peer counselors, lactation consultants, other parents in the NICU.
- Establish a group forum where NICU mothers can share their concerns about pumping and milk supplies.

How do I help the mother get started with pumping when she doesn't plan to breastfeed?

- Address the need to establish a milk supply early and stockpile milk in excess of her baby's current needs. Then she can make other choices later as the need arises and know that her baby is still receiving her milk.
- Reassure mothers that they are capable of making enough milk even though they have had a preterm birth. Inform mothers about hormone levels in the first 2 weeks postpartum and how important it is to prime the hormones and structures of the breast in the first few weeks by frequent pumping to assure an adequate supply later.
- Reassure mothers that pumping schedules can be accommodated later to fit school or work schedules or demand from other family members.

What do I say when asked about alternatives to long-term pumping?

- Explain that even small amounts of her milk for short periods of time are important for the best start in life for a very-low-birth-weight infant.

Table 7-1 How to Share Information With Mothers When You're Not an Expert on Breastfeeding (continued)

- Help a mother set short-term goals or milestones that she can accomplish; e.g., milk for the first 2–3 weeks, or milk until the baby's original due date, or American Academy of Pediatrics guidelines of 12 months.
- Praise the mother for pumping.

Source: Adapted from Rodriguez et al., 2005.

staff are expected to know how to help a mother latch a baby on correctly in this step and what the red flags are for an incorrect latch. Nurses are also expected to know how to teach a mother manual expression of milk. For the mother of a preterm or hospitalized infant who is unable to assist in the process of establishing a milk supply, the expectation in all models described in **Table 7-2** is that nurses will help the mother initiate expression and establishment of a milk supply. This does not mean that NICU nurses are the *only* responsible parties, nor does it mean that *only* the postpartum care providers are responsible; *everyone* who has a role in caring for the mother and/or her infant is responsible for knowing and being able to demonstrate basic skills that assist mothers with the establishment of a milk supply. They are responsible for knowing the basic physiology of lactation and practicing skill sets that work with the mother's physiology instead of against it.

Table 7-2 Side-by-Side Comparison of Three Models

Principle	*WHO/UNICEF Ten Steps to Successful Breastfeeding for the Healthy Term Newborn*	*ABI's Ten Steps for the NICU/SCN*	*Nyqvist and Kylberg (2008) Swedish Mothers' 13 Steps*	*Danish Ten Steps to Successful Breastfeeding of Preterm Infants*
Establishing and maintaining milk supply	Step 5. Show mothers how to breastfeed and maintain lactation even if they should be separated from their infants.	Step 5. Enable mothers to begin early milk expression, and provide ongoing education and support to promote adequate milk supply.	Step 6. Inform, encourage, and support mothers in early initiation and establishment of breastmilk expression and maintenance of milk production.	Step 6. The mother is encouraged to establish and maintain milk production by expression.

Term Infants

Establishing a milk supply is dependent on early and frequent stimulation at the breast and the complete delivery of the placenta. In order to achieve high levels of prolactin, the hormone responsible for milk production, ideally, mothers should begin breastfeeding within the first hour of the infant's life. Lactogenesis II, the phase in which milk volume increases dramatically, is triggered by the withdrawal of progesterone caused by delivery of the placenta and usually occurs between 36 and 96 hours postpartum in women with term infants. (According to Czank, Henderson, Kent, Lai, & Hartmann [2007], it takes about 30–40 hours for progesterone to clear the body after delivery of the placenta, and progesterone levels drop tenfold in the first 4 days postpartum.) Prolactin is secreted from the anterior pituitary in response to a sucking stimulus. It binds to specific receptors on the surface of the lactocytes (milk-making cells) in the mammary gland, thus signaling genes for milk production to turn on and start synthesizing milk components. A detailed description of this process may be found in Czank et al. (2007). Prolactin levels are highest in early lactation and decline over the course of lactation. There is also a diurnal rhythm, and prolactin levels are normally higher at night than during the day (Czank et al., 2007).

Prolactin is critical to establishing and maintaining a milk supply in the early weeks and months of lactation. Prolactin levels rise during the time when the infant is actively suckling at the breast and fall when the infant is not suckling, reaching the prefeed serum baseline levels within 3 hours of the beginning of the feeding (Howie, McNeilly, McArdle, Smart, & Houston, 1980). Therefore, to increase prolactin levels and increase the milk-making potential by effectively priming the receptor sites, suckling should occur not only early but frequently—at least 16 times during the first 48 hours of life (usually in the hospital), and then 10–12 times in a 24-hour period thereafter for the first several weeks of life. When fewer feedings per day occur, prolactin levels remain low and prolactin receptor sites are not primed properly, leading to low milk supply. This finding was confirmed by de Carvalho, Robertson, Friedman, and Klaus (1983), who found that the mothers who were told to feed their babies on a 3- to 4-hour schedule, nursing about seven times in a 24-hour period, had lower milk volumes at day 14 than the mothers who were told to feed frequently and who averaged about 10 feedings in a 24-hour period. This also translated into less weight gain for the infants of the scheduled, less frequently feeding mothers.

Glucocorticoids are also essential to the onset of Lactogenesis II and the maintenance of a milk supply. They play a regulatory role in the synthesis of several major components of milk: fat, lactose, and protein. They also regulate the permeability of the alveolus by playing a role in the closure of the paracellular pathway between lactocytes through the formation of tight junctions, and they prevent involution of the lactiferous tissue during established lactation. Glucocorticoids also bind to the same receptor sites as progesterone (Czank et al., 2007).

Effective milk removal from the breast is also an important factor in future milk production and maintenance of a milk supply. If milk is not effectively removed from the breast, milk stasis results. Stasis causes the lactocytes to shut down milk production and involute. The prerequisite of effective and efficient milk removal (milk ejection reflex = letdown reflex) is oxytocin, which is released into the mother's bloodstream from the posterior pituitary in response to nipple stimulation occurring with a correct latch and stretching of the nipple in the infant's mouth. The oxytocin binds with receptor sites on the myoepithelial cells surrounding each alveolus, causing contraction of these cells and forcing milk into the ductal system of the breast and out the nipple. The epithelial cells of the ducts also have oxytocin receptor sites. Oxytocin surges can be observed as changes in the pattern and rate of audible swallowing in the infant. Other stimuli that cause release of oxytocin are the massage-like motion of the infant's hands on the breast (similar to the kneading action of nursing kittens) (Matthiesen, Ransjo-Arvidson, Nissen, & Uvnas-Moberg, 2001), skin-to-skin contact, a conditioned response to the sight, smell, or sounds of the infant (or the thought of the infant), all of which occur during a breastfeeding session (see Prime, Geddes, & Hartmann, 2007 for a review of the roles of oxytocin in the lactating woman).

Factors That Can Delay Lactogenesis II

The factors that can delay Lactogenesis II have to do with disruption of the natural progression of hormonal influence. For example, continued elevated levels of progesterone and lack of decrease would inhibit the attachment of prolactin and glucocorticoids to their respective receptor sites and delay the activation of genes involved with milk production. This may be a reason for the observed delay in Lactogenesis II in obese women, in whom it takes longer for progesterone levels to drop to a critical level. Retained placental fragments may also continue to produce progesterone, tricking the body into thinking it was still pregnant and not time to initiate production of mature milk. Inadequate stimulation of the nipple would also cause less neural stimulation of the pituitary gland, which could result in lower levels of both prolactin and oxytocin. Other factors and possible causes are summarized in Czank et al. (2007, Table 1, p. 105).

Preterm Infants

In the preterm infant, additional risk factors may be present for a delay in Lactogenesis II. The breast itself may not be as fully developed for lactation as if it had undergone the full 40 weeks of gestation. Some speculate that this immaturity may also lead to delay in Lactogenesis II. Additionally, mothers of preterm infants are under a great deal more stress than mothers of healthy, term infants. Women with high salivary cortisol levels (an indicator of stress) during labor and delivery had delayed onset of Lactogenesis II when compared to women with low salivary cortisol levels (Grajeda & Pérez-Escamilla, 2002). Mothers of preterm infants may also have had an emergency (nonelective) cesarean section, which can result in lower prolactin concentrations and fewer oxytocin pulses than those of term vaginal deliveries or elective cesarean sections (see Czank et al., 2007 for a discussion of emergency vs. elective surgical delivery and impact on Lactogenesis II).

Additionally, mothers with impending preterm births are frequently given betamethasone (a corticosteroid) to help the baby's lungs mature more rapidly in utero. Depending on the timing of administration of the betamethasone prior to delivery, onset of Lactogenesis II may be delayed. Betamethasone treatment given within the 2 days prior to delivery to women who deliver between 28 and 34 weeks' gestation "significantly increased milk volume in the first 10 days postpartum compared to women who were treated between 3 and 9 days prior to delivery" (Henderson, Hartmann, Newnham, & Simmer, 2008, p. e92). Delivery at extremely preterm ages delayed onset of Lactogenesis II, and the effect was compounded when betamethasone was not administered in close proximity to the birth (Henderson, et al., 2008).

Cregan, DeMello, Kershaw, McDougall, and Hartmann (2003) measured compositional markers in the milk on day 5 postpartum in women delivering preterm and compared them to the same markers in women delivering term infants. In the preterm mothers, there was a much wider range within the markers, but 82% of the preterm mothers did not have all of the markers present within 3 standard deviations of the mean for term women and they had significantly lower 24-hour milk volumes. The authors concluded that 82% of preterm mothers are at risk for a compromised initiation of lactation.

Establishing and maintaining a milk supply for the mother of a preterm infant is much more difficult. Preterm mothers do not usually have the advantage of a baby with a well-developed suck, swallow, and breathe pattern. Their babies are weak, and if they do go to the breast soon after birth, they may not provide nipple stimulation that is strong enough to evoke a neural response in the pituitary. Separation of mother and baby interferes with not only prolactin production but also oxytocin release. The establishment of a conditioned response to the baby is conditional upon being with the baby and experiencing the sounds, smells, sight, and feel of the infant. Separation therefore leads to inadequate stimulation for release of oxytocin and inefficient milk removal. Milk stasis may be created with inefficient milk removal, and prolactin functioning may be inhibited as a result, leading to lower milk volume.

Establishment and maintenance of a milk supply for a preterm infant must occur without much input from the baby. It is usually entirely mechanical and dependent on a pumping or hand expression regimen. Expressing milk with a mechanical device or manual expression is less effective than having a healthy, breastfeeding term infant remove milk from the breast. It's not uncommon for women to describe a love-hate relationship with the pump. Stress has been shown to be a significant factor in the effectiveness of pumping. Higher salivary cortisol and amylase levels, measures of adrenergic activity, were found in mothers with inadequate milk supplies and correlated with lower prolactin levels in these mothers, leading the authors to conclude that stress suppressed prolactin increases during pumping (Chatterton, Hill, Aldag, Hodges, Belknap, & Zinaman, 2000). How, then, can mothers of preterm infants overcome these difficulties that are already built in? In most cases success rests on the effort that the mother puts into her pumping routine as well as the support she receives from the NICU staff. The goal is to establish an ample milk supply (750–1000 ml/day) in the first week to 10 days postpartum. This type of milk production gives the mother a reserve against diminishing milk volume as the duration of pumping lengthens. According to Meier, Brown, and Hurst (1999), if a mother's milk supply is 1000 ml/day, then her milk supply could decrease by approximately 50% and still be adequate to feed her preterm infant at discharge. The model policy given in **Appendix 7-1** covers many of the practices discussed in the rest of this chapter and will help ensure adequate milk supplies for mothers who are reliant on milk expression.

Initiation and Frequency of Expression

The secret to an adequate milk supply for a preterm infant is to trick the mother's body into thinking that she is nursing a full-term, healthy infant. This means that she must begin expressing/pumping (i.e., feeding) early to prime receptor sites properly. Milk volume and frequency of expression on day 4 were predictive of milk supply at 6 weeks postpartum in preterm mothers. Mothers with the lowest milk production and fewer expressions at day 4 were 9.5 times more likely to have an inadequate milk supply at week 6 than mothers with higher milk production and greater pumping frequency on day 4 (Hill & Aldag, 2005). Research shows that later milk volume is influenced by how soon the mother begins to stimulate her breasts. The optimal window is within the first 6 hours after delivery according to Furman, Minich, and Hack (2002), although imitating what a healthy term infant would do, i.e., initiate expression within the first 2 hours postpartum, might be even more effective. In one study, there was no significant difference in milk weight (as a measure of volume) at 2–5 weeks postpartum between early initiators (< 48 hours after birth) and late initiators (> 48 hours after birth) when initiation alone was analyzed, but when mothers got an early start at pumping but pumped infrequently (< 6 times in a 24-hour period), milk volume was positively influenced (Hill, Aldag, & Chatterton, 2001). Since mothers frequently have difficulty pumping as often as they are instructed, earlier initiation might compensate for lower levels of stimulation later.

In the past, textbook coverage of expression frequency has indicated that expression should occur six times in a 24-hour period. However, this is not what a healthy, term infant would be doing. If a mother was feeding her baby this infrequently, her baby would be at serious risk for failure to thrive and perhaps hypernatremia and dehydration. She would be giving her body messages that she was weaning and her milk supply would decrease. What does work with breastfeeding is nursing 10–12 times in a 24-hour period, for an average feeding interval of 2–2.5 hours. This is a difficult schedule for a pumping mother to maintain around the clock for weeks and months. However, a minimum of eight times in a 24-hour period is the expectation for establishing and maintaining a milk supply when dependent on a pump. In a comparison of mothers of preterm infants who were pumping and term mothers who were both breastfeeding and pumping, Hill, Aldag, Chatterton, and Zinaman (2005) instructed the preterm mothers to pump at least eight times a day. Examination of the mothers' daily logs for pumping and milk volume showed that actual pumping averaged only six times a day, compared to the mothers of term infants who were feeding about nine times a day. The authors also measured milk volume at postpartum day 6 or 7 and found they could predict milk adequacy at 2 and 6 weeks postpartum. Mothers of preterm infants were 2.81 times more at risk for an inadequate milk supply than term mothers were. In a separate study, inadequate milk supply was a predictor for using artificial milk by week 12 postpartum (Hill, Aldag, Zinaman, & Chatterton, 2007). Therefore, establishing an ample supply from the beginning with *early* and *frequent* stimulation prolongs the adequacy of milk supply and lengthens the duration of (breast)feeding for the preterm infant.

There are examples of frequency extending the duration of milk supply. In the case of the Harris sextuplets, the first recorded set of surviving African American sextuplets, their mother, Diamond, pumped for 6 months for them. Born July 27, 2002 at 26 weeks' gestation, the babies had no medical conditions or birth defects. Diamond initially set a goal of pumping for the first month, but decided to continue when she saw how well the four boys and two girls were doing on her milk. She pumped 12 times a day, every 2 hours, with her husband attaching the pumping equipment and caring for the collected milk while she slept. She pumped 50 bottles of milk per day, more milk than she needed (Harris Family Sextuplets Web site, 2007).

In our illustrative case shown in Chapter 1, Bonnie established and maintained a full milk supply by pumping 10 times in a 24-hour period. She had the help of her mother who set her alarm and woke Bonnie to pump in the middle of the night and then made sure that the milk was refrigerated and the kit cleaned for the next time the alarm went off. Bonnie continued to pump after the baby was discharged and was able to supply her infant with pumped milk exclusively for 4 months after discharge. In both these cases, in-person support was a key ingredient to achieving adequate frequency of expression.

Pumping Style: When and How Long

In one study comparing an experimental pump to breastfeeding by term mothers with well established milk supplies, Mitoulas, Lai, Gurrin, Larsson, and Hartmann (2002) found that infants averaged 16.6 minutes to drain the breast. Other protocols that appear as part of research suggest either pumping for 10 minutes on a side or pumping until the milk flow stops (e.g., Groh-Wargo et al., 1995; Jones, Dimmock, & Spencer, 2001). However, one must think of the amount of nipple stimulation that occurs in a breastfeeding and simulate that optimally to increase prolactin levels. A more common recommendation for pump-dependent mothers seen in hospital protocols is that mothers express for a minimum of 15 minutes per side, even if milk flow ceases. In this way mothers can approximate the observation of Mitoulas et al. (2002) for breastfeeding mothers.

The 15-minute session can be done in one continuous time frame or in several shorter clusters that equal 15 minutes (see the Power Pumping section later in this chapter). If only one breast is pumped at a time, the mother needs to spend at least 15 minutes per breast. If she is doing simultaneous pumping she can do both sides in the same 15-minute session. Dairy research demonstrates that pumping more than one teat at a time increases prolactin levels exponentially. Simultaneous pumping therefore has the advantage of saving the mother time as well as spiking her prolactin levels higher and increasing her milk-making potential. In a pilot study, both simultaneous (both breasts) and sequential (single breast) pumping were effective in raising serum levels of prolactin. The difference between the two groups came in the decrease in the amount of prolactin that is observed between 3 and 6 weeks postpartum. The decline was much more rapid in the sequential pumpers, and at day 42 the prolactin levels and milk volume were higher in the simultaneous group than in the sequential group (Hill, Aldag, & Chatterton, 1996).

At least one expression should be in the middle of the night, when the diurnal rhythm of prolactin is naturally highest in the mother's body. Dissenters protest that it is more important for mothers to get their rest at night than to express milk, but this extends at least one of the intervals between pumping sessions too far and does not take advantage of the mother's natural high nighttime hormone levels. It is reasonable to suggest to mothers that they have been getting up in the middle of the night during pregnancy for a reason—to get their bodies used to being up, caring for, and feeding a baby in the middle of the night. In the case of the Harris sextuplets, the nighttime expressions combined with frequency were a large part of her success. More will be said about the importance of support that is ongoing and personal in Chapter 12, which discusses support systems and interventions both prior to and after discharge.

Type of Pump and Kit

Technological developments in the last 25 years or so have influenced thinking about expressing milk and the possibility of women going back to work without having to resort to formula use. It has also influenced thinking about a mother being able to supply her own milk for a preterm infant rather than rely on a donor milk bank. However, much of the research on pumps and pumping that has been done recently (in the last 10 years) is compromised by the close relationships between the researchers and the manufacturers who stand to benefit from sales of their products to hospitals, to the government through the Special Supplemental Nutrition Program for Women, Infants, and Children or Medicaid program, or directly to mothers. When formula companies provide researchers with funds to study breastfeeding, the lactation community is very quick to point the finger and claim that the study is biased. Why do they not suspect the same bias when research is conducted with breast pump manufacturer funding? (See **Box 7-1** for a digression.)

The standard recommendation is that mothers of hospitalized preterm infants use an electric autocycling pump that is not designed for casual use. The most effective types of pumps appear to be rental-grade pumps (frequently incorrectly referred to as "hospital grade," which merely indicates the type of plug that must be present for hospital use).

The size of the pump flange may have a significant impact on a mother's success with expression, and this may make as much difference as the type of pump used. Anecdotal reports exist of mothers who say that no pump ever invented worked for them; these mothers were unable to extract any milk from the breast. However, if the tunnel part of the flange is too small in diameter for the nipple diameter, then the nipple may get stuck and compressed to the point that milk may not be able to exit the nipple pores (Geddes, 2007). If mothers report pain while they are expressing, the diameter of the flange should be examined and the behavior of the nipple in the flange during an actual pumping session should be observed. If the nipple does not stretch or move, turns red, milk flows for a few seconds and then shuts down, or the mother reports pain in the nipple, the mother may need a larger diameter flange. Only observation of the nipple while pumping will give this information; this cannot be seen when the mother is not pumping and just relaxing.

Issues with Gadgets and Devices Such as Breast Pumps

While breast pumps and gadgets definitely have a role to play in assisting some mothers to establish and maintain a milk supply/breastfeeding, the tendency in many cases is to reach for the gadget or device quickly because we

Box 7-1 The Ethics of Breast Pumps—A Digression

For years, Ross Laboratories, a major manufacturer of infant formula, was, by default, the keeper of breastfeeding statistics. They collected marketing data on formula use and breastfeeding for the obvious purpose of expanding market share and then published this data in respected journals such as *Pediatrics* as scientific research. This was clearly a conflict of interest. Today, a less biased government entity, the Centers for Disease Control and Prevention, is the collector and publisher of breastfeeding rates, mining this information from questions on the National Immunization Survey.

Recent research on pumps has similar conflict of interest issues, in this author's opinion. It is conducted exclusively by individuals whose grant funding comes either all or in part from the pump manufacturers themselves, compares different models of pumps from the same manufacturer, is published in reputable breastfeeding journals, and is an advertisement for the pump(s) being researched. While the disclosure of the funding source, now required in all peer-reviewed journals, is more honest and open, it does not lessen or mitigate the effects of the advertising that is going on.

Lepore (2008) writes: "Today, breast pumps are such a ubiquitous personal accessory that they're more like cell phones than like catheters" (p. 2). Pumps show up in movies, where companies pay exorbitantly for product placement, and are subjects of commentary in the popular press, such as the aforementioned Lepore article, which appeared in the *New Yorker*. According to Lepore we have confused pumping with breastfeeding.

> The cynical politics of pump promotion would seem, at first, to be obvious. Breast pumps can be useful, even indispensable and, in some cases, lifesaving. But a thing doesn't have to be underhanded to feel coldblooded.... Pumps put milk into bottles, even though many of breastfeeding's benefits to the baby, and all of its social and emotional benefits, come not from the liquid itself but from the smiling and cuddling ... Breastfeeding involves cradling your baby; pumping involves cupping plastic shields on your breasts and watching your nipples squirt milk down a tube.

What are we telling mothers about their own bodies? Are we telling them that their bodies won't perform unless they have a pump? That's what we seem to have convinced women of in the United States! You need at least one breast pump, maybe several, in order to breastfeed, because your body won't be able to lactate and provide adequate milk without one. It's the same thing as the free sample of formula—both are to be used when the mother has doubts that her body can function properly. Women in developing countries see us using formula/pumps and think this is the modern way and we must know something that they don't about how women's bodies need the gadget/device/formula because they cannot possibly perform adequately (even though our bodies have been doing extremely well in this regard since prehistoric times!).

Of a more dubious ethical nature is the type of research that expands the reach of pump companies to countries where neither the political stability nor the infrastructure would support the widespread use of breast pumps and bottled milk. This research is in the guise of making expressed maternal milk more available to the preterm population. In one study that took place in Kenya and Nigeria, a comparison was made between manual expression and several types of pumps and volume expressed. The pump company donated all the pumps and kits needed for the study. Both pumps, one foot-powered, the other electrically powered,

Box 7-1 The Ethics of Breast Pumps—A Digression (continued)

could extract more milk than hand expression, with only the difference between the electric pump and manual expression being statistically significant (Slusher et al., 2007).

What happens to those mothers when they go home and don't have electricity? That is what the foot-powered pump is for. But what if they also don't have running water and a safe way of cleaning/sterilizing the kit? What if fuel for a fire to boil the water is scarce? What if power or running water is not reliable or clean even when available?

The corollary of providing pumps is that women (and the healthcare providers assisting them to care for a preterm infant) have lost the basic skill of manual expression. Extracting milk from the breast for a preterm infant who is too weak to suck is vital to the survival of the infant. Most women in the world are unable to afford pumps for individual use. Even if the hospital provides the pump for use in the unit, what does the mother do when she goes home? How safe is pump use in resource-poor areas? Boo, Nordiah, Alfizah, Nor-Rohaini, and Lim (2001) tell us that manual expression is the cleanest form of milk expression. Inappropriate marketing of technology is no more ethical than marketing infant formula in resource-challenged areas of the world.

Breast pumps are useful in certain situations and have a role to play in lactation support, just as formula occasionally has a role to play in providing adequate nutrition for babies when breastfeeding is not going well and the infant's well-being is compromised. However, we should not be naïve in our relationship with *any* manufacturer or distributor.

run out of ideas and skills that will help us solve the problem. These gadgets and devices abound and are easily obtained. However, they are costly to the mother in monetary terms (breastfeeding is supposed to be the least expensive way to feed a baby!) and have the added consequence of undermining her confidence level. An example of this is a prospective study by Alexander, Grant, and Campbell (1992), in which the researchers randomly assigned women with truly inverted nipples (nipples that did no protrude at all) to one of four treatment options prenatally. The four options were (1) use of breast shells, (2) use of exercises, (3) use of both breast shells and exercises, and (4) no treatment at all. They then looked at breastfeeding rates at 6 weeks postpartum for each of the groups, finding that the control group (no treatment) was breastfeeding at the highest rate of all the groups. The groups who were assigned the breast shells were breastfeeding at significantly lower rates. Another finding was that some women in the groups assigned shells actually changed their minds about breastfeeding prior to the birth *because of* the shells! They were uncomfortable and caused pain and skin problems; they were conspicuous underneath clothing and caused embarrassment; and they caused sweating and leakage of colostrum. Not only were the shells ineffective in changing the protractility of the nipple, but also they discouraged women from breastfeeding and became a disincentive. Prenatally, they undermined women's confidence in the ability of their body to function normally.

The Special Supplemental Nutrition Program for Women, Infants, and Children that has incentivized breastfeeding initiation by offering free breast pumps to its clients found that in the beginning this had a positive effect on increasing initiation rates. However, over time, the effects of this incentive waned, and the most successful intervention was the one where there was ongoing support and individualized help provided by either a peer counselor of a lactation care provider—services that went beyond standard education strategies (Ahluwahlia, Tessaro, Grummer-Strawn, MacGowan, & Benton-Davis, 2000). Nothing appears to substitute for the personal approach to support for an individual mother.

The question should *not* be what type of pump we offer a mother with a preterm infant, but what type of support do we offer her, and are we doing a good job providing that support? In the case of *this* mother, what does *she* need? Some mothers need more support than others, especially when their confidence levels have been undermined, and, in the case of a preterm infant, this is a mother whose body has not functioned appropriately by carrying the baby to term. She already feels inadequate and is dubious about her ability to establish and maintain a milk supply under difficult circumstances. If her body failed her in carrying her baby, she may have an underlying expectation that she will fail at milk production as well. Individualized support and encouragement that is frequent and easily accessible is crucial. The pump is only helpful.

Manual Expression

In the United States we make the assumption that pumps are needed for most women who have hospitalized infants or are returning to work. Pumps are expensive to rent or purchase, but they are necessary, we think, and make life more convenient. (Although reading Lepore's (2009) description of pumping makes one wonder if perhaps they really are so convenient after all!) What about manual expression? Would mothers of hospitalized infants benefit from more hand expression? Manual expression is the only option available to many mothers of preterm infants in developing countries. Those of us who have been fortunate enough to travel in many of these countries have observed women hand expressing very easily and successfully. In step 5 of the Ten Steps for the BFHI, teaching hand expression is one of the criteria. It is a skill that every new mother should be taught because it is a technique that is always available to the mother, even in a power outage or if she is without clean water to safely care for her equipment. Hand expression is an essential skill, not just because it is a simple technique but also because it helps women become comfortable with touching and handling their breasts and accustoms them to the feel of their breasts. This has the advantage of women becoming knowledgeable about what feels normal and what feels unusual and may be a life-saving technique for the mother when she does breast self-exams. For the mother of a baby in the NICU, an added benefit of hand expression is that breast massage and compression help increase hormone levels and maintain milk supply. Pumps that operate on compression (a tactile component) *and* vacuum together yield higher concentrations of prolactin (Alekseev et al., 1998). The mother can roll her nipple and stretch it to get a milk ejection reflex started. She can manually move milk forward in the breast, including the fat. Should manual expression be included as part of the pumping regimen, i.e., a mix of methods is used, and would this be effective in helping mothers establish and maintain a more ample supply of milk? Would incorporation of such techniques along with mechanical expression help produce larger milk supplies and prevent early dwindling of supply?

Many healthcare providers feel very uncomfortable teaching manual expression to mothers because they don't know how to do it themselves. One method of training involves the use of a medical model where the trainee practices on the anatomical model of the breast. When the hand expression is done correctly, the trainee gets rewarded with a shot of hand lotion; incorrect expression gets no reward.

Many mothers report that they do not like hand expression and don't want to do it as a direct result of the way they were taught to do it; teaching was hands on and invasive. Lang (1997) mentions the following three methods for teaching mothers hand expression: using a breast model, demonstrating on the trainer's body, or demonstrating using the mother's breast. In the latter a hands-on technique is used. The trainer stands behind the mother and places her hand on the mother's breast and demonstrates how to express, then has the mother replace her hand in the same position. "Using the mother's own breast ensures that she sees how simple the skill of hand expression is, and knows how it feels for herself" (Lang, 1997, p. 50). The problem with this type of teaching is that the trainer cannot always evaluate how much pressure she is applying and whether she is causing the mother pain. It also is a type of training and assistance that mothers detest. They feel mauled and violated, even if they have given permission for their breasts to be touched, and this makes them more reluctant to try to hand express. Weimers, Svensson, Dumas, Naver, and Wahlberg (2006) found that mothers who experienced unexpected hands-on assistance with breastfeeding in a NICU regarded the behavior as unpleasant. In-depth interviews were conducted with mothers who had experienced this hands-on approach. Most felt that the hands-on help was an insult to the mother's integrity as well as the baby's when actual feeding at the breast was begun. Mothers described this type of help as slightly brutal, disrespectful, and even unhelpful. They described having their breasts pushed and pulled and shoved into the baby's mouth, often out in the open and exposed to other people in the NICU. Mothers did not understand why the physical help was given, and felt that they grew dependent on this type of help, leaving them with a lack of confidence in their ability to breastfeed when staff were no longer available to help. Some mothers also felt that their breasts had become objects that did not belong to them.

An alternative to this type of teaching model is to sit next to the mother with a doll or a breast model and demonstrate breastfeeding or manual expression on the inanimate object. The mother imitates what she sees without experiencing the invasion of her body space.

TROUBLESHOOTING SUPPLY PROBLEMS

Effects of Smoking on Milk Supply

Smoking during pregnancy is a risk factor for premature delivery and low birth weight. According to the March of Dimes, pregnant women who smoke cigarettes are two times more likely to have a low-birth-weight infant than women who do not smoke (March of Dimes, 2009). Fetuses exposed to cigarette smoking are also more likely to be born with septal and right-sided heart defects (Malik et al., 2008). These babies are nearly certain to be admitted to the NICU. It has also been known from studies conducted in the 1980s that there is an association of early weaning from the breast and cigarette smoking (for example, Woodward & Hand, 1988) and that women who smoke also seem to have lower prolactin levels and perhaps lower milk supplies as a result (Andersen et al., 1982; Vio, Salazar, & Infante, 1991). Hopkinson, Schanler, Fraley, and Garza (1992) conducted a study to determine whether smoking mothers of preterm infants who were totally pump dependent produced less milk or milk of a different composition from women who did not smoke. Over the first 6 weeks postpartum the 24-hour milk production of the smoking mothers did not increase whereas the nonsmoking control group had a significant and continuing increase in milk volume. Fat concentrations were significantly higher in milk from nonsmoking control subjects as well, although concentrations of other components of human milk were similar between the two groups. Finally, cigarette smoking during pregnancy was the strongest risk factor for early cessation of milk expression in a German NICU (Killersreiter, Grimmer, Buhrer, Dudenhausen, & Obladen, 2001).

More recent studies have confirmed that smoking women have shorter breastfeeding durations (Amir & Donath, 2002; Hill & Aldag, 1996). In their systematic review of the epidemiologic evidence, Amir and Donath found that there was an inverse dose–response relationship between the number of cigarettes smoked per day and the duration of breastfeeding, even after correcting for confounding variables. Hill and Aldag included mothers of low-birth-weight infants in their sample and found that smoking mothers of both term and preterm infants reported insufficient milk as a reason for stopping breastfeeding by 8 weeks.

Batstra, Neeleman, and Hadders-Algra (2003) found that "the negative effects of maternal smoking on children's cognitive performance were limited to those who had *not* [italics added] been breastfed" (Batstra et al., 2003, p. 404). Dorea (2007) argues that because smoking women tend to bottle-feed at a higher rate and place their infants at risk for higher morbidity and mortality rates, encouraging women to breastfeed despite associations with earlier weaning protects infants better than if they were exclusively formula fed.

> Therefore, if public health policies cannot stop addicted mothers from smoking during pregnancy it is fundamental not to miss the chance of encouraging and supporting breastfeeding. The food and health inequalities of socially disadvantaged groups demand well crafted public health policies to reduce the incidence of diseases and compress morbidity: these policies need to make it clear that breastfeeding is better and safer. (Dorea, 2007, p. 287)

Given that smoking mothers are at risk for preterm and low-birth-weight deliveries of babies with potential congenital defects, and given that they are at risk for low milk supplies because of their smoking habits, every effort should be made to assist mothers with smoking cessation programs or smoking reduction. Extra attention also needs to be paid to these mothers' pumping routines to ensure that they are pumping frequently enough and to provide support for the mother and reinforcement of the importance of her milk for her infant.

Guided Imagery

Those of us who have been working in the field of lactation for years have frequently suggested to working (pumping) mothers that techniques to remind them of the infant are useful in assisting them with a milk ejection reflex and collection of larger volumes of milk to leave for their infant. We have suggested putting a picture of the baby inside the pump case, and perhaps taking an article of clothing that belongs to the baby to sniff while pumping. Thinking about the baby and visualizing the baby is supposed to help the mother relax and let down to an inanimate object that is not the baby. Sometimes we suggest making a tape recording of the baby's babbling or crying to play while we pump. Many of these suggestions have been transplanted into the NICU over the years, and mothers have found that pumping next to the baby's bed or looking at a photo of the baby and snuggling with a blanket that has covered the baby to be helpful with milk expression. Being able to do KMC immediately before a pumping session has a similar effect of increasing milk supply and the amount of milk the mother is able to collect.

Feher found that a relaxation and imagery audiotape produced similar results in mothers of preterm infants (Feher, Berger, Johnson, & Wilde, 1989). A 20-minute audiocassette tape was developed. The first part of the tape consisted of a progressive relaxation exercise that involved deep rhythmic breathing while alternately tensing and relaxing various muscle groups. The second section of the tape was a guided imagery session in which the mother was to imagine the warmth of the baby's skin against hers or milk flowing from her breasts. The mothers were to play the tapes just prior to a milk expression. Mothers in the study were randomly assigned to receive and listen to the tape or to a no-tape control group. Both groups received information about use of an electric breast pump and protocols for expression. After one week of enrollment in the study, a single expression of milk was obtained in the hospital.

The mothers receiving the tape, despite not having listened to it as often as the study protocol recommended, succeeded in expressing a 63% larger average volume of milk than the control group, a statistically significant difference. The differences in milk volumes were greatest for a subsample of primiparous low-income women, and there was a dose–response relationship of milk volume and the number of times the mother had listened to the tape. In the subset of mothers with seriously ill and ventilated infants, the differences were even greater, with the intervention mothers having a volume increase of 121% over the control group.

The authors point out that producing an audiotape and providing recorders/players may be an expensive proposition and should be compared with other techniques such as personalized psychosocial support. However, it is a valuable adjunct to parent education and counseling and was effective in reducing stress in mothers and getting better results with the pump.

Power Pumping

Another technique that has been successful in increasing milk supplies for women in the workforce has been a technique called "power pumping." The idea behind this technique is to simulate cluster feeding in the baby. Babies who cluster feed (i.e., have several feedings in the space of 2–3 hours and then have a long nap) have much shorter intervals between feedings. As a result, prolactin levels, which normally fall between feedings, do not have a chance to fall as far toward the baseline and instead get bumped up to even higher levels with the potential to produce more milk, particularly in the early weeks and months of milk production. For many healthy, term babies this is a normal pattern of breastfeeding and they may have one or two periods during the day when they practice cluster feeding. Power pumping mimics this by having a mother express in short, frequent segments. She pumps for 5 minutes or so, then gets up and gets herself a glass of water and takes a small break of several minutes. She returns to the pump and expresses for another 5 minutes or so, repeating the minibreak again and pumping for another 5 minutes for a total of 15 minutes or so. At the next opportunity for expression she may repeat this technique. In this way she maintains high prolactin levels and increases her milk volume.

Working mothers frequently report that when they go back to work and the number of times they can pump is limited to two or three times a day, they lose their milk supply by the end of the workweek. Once they can feed the baby at home on the weekend ad lib, they can boost their milk supply back up to normal levels by Monday. However, if they practice a power pumping session each workday, they have a better chance of maintaining their milk supply during the week.

Power pumping is also useful in increasing milk volume in mothers of preterm infants, especially when they find that their supply is decreasing or plateauing just when the baby's needs are increasing. Expressing milk takes energy and an enormous time commitment on the part of the mother, and if the volume of milk that is expressed is small or decreasing, the mother can become discouraged very easily. A decreasing milk supply may contribute to the mother's stress levels. This technique, coupled with support and encouragement and visualization techniques can minimize problems with milk volume and help turn a decreasing milk supply around.

Skin-to-Skin Contact

Practicing skin-to-skin (STS) contact also helps increase faltering milk supply. Hurst, Valentine, Renfro, Burns, and Ferlic (1997) demonstrated a greater milk volume when STS was implemented, compared to a control group that did not initiate STS. Average baseline 24-hour milk volume was 499 ± 139 ml (STS) compared with 218 ± 132 ml (no STS). Milk volumes increased over weeks 2–4 postpartum for the mothers doing STS, but actually decreased slightly in the control group during the same period of time. Increasing milk volume helps to increase duration of breastfeeding, and numerous studies, discussed more in depth in Chapter 9 (Step 7), find that practicing STS/kangaroo mother care (KMC) increases the duration of breastfeeding. Mothers report that they feel more confident about breastfeeding and their ability to produce an adequate milk supply for their infants' needs when they practice KMC (Affonso, Wahlberg, & Persson, 1989).

Galactogogues

Drugs that stimulate milk production, otherwise known as galactogogues, have been used to increase the milk supply in mothers with preterm infants. These include the dopamine antagonists metoclopramide (Reglan) and domperidone (Motilium), which influence prolactin production and therefore have the potential to influence milk supply. There are ongoing questions about the use of these medications and whether they actually work.

Release of prolactin stored in the pituitary is inhibited by dopamine concentrations. When the dopamine receptor sites in the pituitary are blocked by these medications, then prolactin is released in larger amounts. However, this affects only prolactin that has been previously synthesized and stored and does not increase the synthesis of new prolactin. The release of this stored prolactin also blunts the prolactin surge that is seen following nipple stimulation and maintains prolactin levels at an elevated but level state. Whether or not these drugs work also depends on the mother's baseline prolactin levels. In women with low baseline levels, the increase in release from the galactogogue increases milk supply dramatically at relatively low doses, but in women who already have high baseline levels of prolactin, these drugs may not have an impact, and additional milk synthesis may not happen (Hale, 2007).

In the United States, metoclopramide is the most commonly used galactogogue. Use of metoclopramide for this purpose is off label. Studies done in the 1980s found that 10–15 mg doses taken three times a day were effective in increasing prolactin levels and milk supplies in mothers, but also noted that some mothers simply do not respond if they already have elevated prolactin levels (Ehrenkranz & Ackerman, 1986; Kauppila, Kivinen, & Ylikorkola, 1981). In a more recent, randomized, controlled trial where either a placebo or 10-mg tablets were given to mothers of preterm infants prophylactically beginning within 96 hours of birth, there were no significant differences between the two groups in milk volume on day 17 or in the duration of breastfeeding (Hansen, McAndrew, Harris, & Zimmerman, 2005). Of the 14 clinical trials found by Anderson and Valdes (2007), only 4 met the methodological criteria for inclusion in their systematic review, with most of the studies lacking adequate placebo control groups, true randomization, or blinding. To further confound the literature, many of the studies also had poor lactation management practices.

There is also the potential for serious side effects with metoclopramide use. Because it is a dopamine antagonist, many of the side effects are neurological in nature, ranging from depression (seen often), extrapyramidal reactions (seen rarely) such as involuntary movements of limbs, facial grimacing, torticollis, or tardive dyskinesia. Cardiovascular symptoms, gastrointestinal symptoms (diarrhea or cramping), and allergic reactions may also be seen as side effects (RxList, 2009). For this reason, Hale (2007) recommends that this medication be used only over the short term and then discontinued with a careful tapering of the dose so that lactation failure does not occur (see also Protocol No. 9, ABM 2004; Appendices 4-M1 and 4-M2 of the California Perinatal Quality Care Collaborative [CPQCC, 2008b, 2008c]).

Use of domperidone is also an off-label use. In 2004, the FDA issued a warning letter to providers in the United States stating that prescribing or compounding of this medication in the United States violates the Federal Food, Drug, and Cosmetic Act because the drug is not approved for any use in the United States. (For a more thorough discussion of this issue please see Appendix 4-N of the CPQCC [2008a].) In other countries, it is commonly prescribed as an antiemetic. This medication also is used to stimulate milk production and increase prolactin levels. It has the added benefit of not penetrating the blood–brain barrier easily and therefore may not cause the side effects that metoclopramide does. In a randomized, double-blind placebo-controlled trial of 16 mothers, the women assigned the domperidone treatment for 7 days had significantly higher increases in prolactin levels and in milk volume (da Silva, Knoppert, Angelini, & Forret, 2001). In another double-blind, randomized, crossover trial of six mothers, two of the mothers were nonresponders and had no increase in milk supply even though serum prolactin levels increased (Wan et al., 2008).

Fenugreek is used as a spice around the world in cooking and is also used in some places as an herbal galactogogue. In its protocol on galactogogues, the Academy of Breastfeeding Medicine cites two abstracts and an anecdotal report where effectiveness was suggested (ABM, 2004). Fenugreek is known to reduce blood sugar levels and have uterine-stimulating effects. Skidmore-Roth (2006) also notes that fenugreek may interfere with the absorption of all medications that the mother may be taking concurrently. It is therefore very important for the HCP working with a mother with low milk supply to fully evaluate the mother following the steps in ABM's protocol No. 9, which include:

- Evaluate current milk supply and effectiveness of milk transfer. Is her pump working well? Is she really pumping as often as she says she is? What does she mean when she says her milk supply is low? Does the flange of the collecting kit fit her breast properly?
- Inform mothers about evidence (or lack thereof) regarding safety and efficacy of using a therapy to increase milk supply.
- Screen the mother for contraindications to use of a particular therapy. Inform her of potential side effects.
- Ensure adequate follow-up of both the mother and the infant for any side effects and effects on milk supply.
- Be aware that long-term use has not been studied and long-term effects are unknown. Hale (2007) would add to this that if no change in milk supply is seen within a week of starting treatment, then the medication should be discontinued.

Additional caveats from Hale would be:

- There is no evidence that prolactin responds to any of these medications in a dose-dependent manner, so doubling or tripling the dose will not make a difference.
- Discontinuation of the medication should be done in a gradual manner.

Mothers need to understand that in order to establish, maintain, and increase their milk supply, they must be compliant with instructions. Simply popping a pill or drinking more tea will not substitute for putting in the effort of frequent and early pumping and making the hormones of lactation work normally from the beginning. As Anderson and Valdes state, "If mothers are provided education and practice techniques that support lactation physiology, galactogogues appear to have little or no added benefit" (Anderson & Valdes, 2007, p. 240).

COLLECTION OF MILK: GETTING STARTED

Milk storage and handling recommendations can be a contentious issue. There are those who believe that the inherent anti-infective properties are strong enough to protect any baby under any conditions and who assume the best-case scenario when developing recommendations. Then there are those who assume the worst-case scenario when generating guidelines. Having been trained in public health, I fall in the latter camp. When making a public health recommendation it is important to be conservative and assume that many individuals for whom the recommendations are designed are not operating under ideal circumstances. The recommendation therefore covers as many outliers on the bell-shaped curve as possible. Using bench research does not always give us the answers, either, because by definition, bench research is done under tightly controlled (ideal and best case) conditions. We still use it to support some of our recommendations because often it is the only research available. Yet it frequently does not represent the real world in which mothers operate. **Box 7-2** gives an example from the research literature looking at the methodology behind a recommendation for storage durations in the NICU.

Appendix 7-2 delineates recommendations for safe collection, handling and storage of mothers' expressed milk in the hospital setting. These recommendations were originally developed for the Human Milk Banking Association of North America by the author and underwent a peer review process in all three editions. They have been updated here with additional and more recent references. It should be noted that the Human Milk Banking Association of North America currently publishes its own recommendations, which combine protocols for both the NICU and the healthy term infant in the home. Because babies in the NICU are more vulnerable due to their premature and/or sick status, recommendations for milk storage in the NICU will be more conservative than those for the home. To avoid potential confusion

Box 7-2 Methods and Madness: How a Research Finding Became Translated to Policy

In this example from the research literature, analysis of the methodology of a study leads to questions about the appropriateness of the study recommendations. Done in 1994 in a NICU, the study compares durations of storage in the refrigerator or freezer and makes recommendations based on study findings (Pardou, Serruys, Mascart-Lemone, Dramaix, & Vis, 1994). We cannot, however, accept the recommendations from this study (refrigeration for 8 days is preferable to freezing milk) without a critical reading of the entire study and consideration of the application of the study's findings to recommendations for time of storage at certain temperatures. Careful reading of this study with attention to the methodology makes it difficult to develop public health recommendations based on this study. The second arm of the study is the most pertinent for this discussion.

Methods

1. All the mothers in the second arm of the study were mothers of *term* infants who participated in providing samples of milk between days 4 and 7 postpartum. Knowing what we now know about milk composition, is it wise to extrapolate findings from term mothers to preterm mothers?
2. Participants in the study were given instructions to do the following:
   - Wash their hands.
   - Clean the nipple and areola with sterile gauze and sterile water.

Do postpartum mothers who are not participating in a research study clean their breasts before they express milk *every time*?

3. Three methods of expression were used.
   - Hand expression
   - A rubber bulb breast pump (bicycle horn pump)
   - Electric breast pump (no model was specified)

No directions seem to have been given about cleaning or sterilizing the pumps. Was each pump brand new for the purposes of this study? If not, how was it cleaned/sterilized? Bicycle horn pumps are notorious for contamination and mothers' inability to adequately clean/sterilize the bulb. How were the samples distributed categorically? Were there more bicycle horn pump samples in the frozen samples or particular bacterial class than in another? This is an important variable that is not controlled or adjusted for.

4. Samples of expressed milk were drawn into sterile syringes and divided into eight 1-ml aliquots, which were placed in individual screw-cap plastic test tubes. In real life, how many mothers have a new sterile container to store their milk in *every time*? A mother of a NICU baby expressing into new sterile containers each time is probably the most likely scenario, but is probably not standard operating procedure for the mother of a healthy, term infant.
5. Four of the 1-ml samples were placed in the refrigerator (0–4°C) for 8 days and four were put in the freezer (-20°C) for 8 days. At the end of the 8 days the frozen samples were thawed by microwave (cold microwaving). What does this mean? Does it mean that the thawing was so short that the 1-ml sample never got hot? We know, however, that microwaving usually does alter proteins—that's how it works! Will that affect the ability of the antibacterial proteins in the thawed samples to function? A 1-ml sample could have been thawed in a very short time by putting the bottom of the test tube in the palm of the researcher's hand!
6. One sample of the thawed milk and one of the refrigerated milk were immediately analyzed for bacterial contamination, which served as a baseline for bacterial growth. The other samples were held at 26°C (room temperature) for 2, 4, and 6 hours to simulate a tube feeding and the duration of time that milk might be exposed to room temperatures if the baby was being fed continuously.

Box 7-2 Methods and Madness: How a Research Finding Became Translated to Policy (continued)

7. Standard bacteriological techniques were employed to test for bacterial growth. Samples containing < 10^5 CFU/ml (100,000 colony forming units of bacteria per ml) were classified after incubation overnight 37°C. What happened to the samples containing greater than 10^5 CFU/ml? They were actually discarded because this NICU tested all its mothers for bacteria (a practice that can discourage mothers and lead them to believe that they cannot be trusted to supply a safe feeding for their infant) and would never use anything with higher levels for nutritional purposes. But putting a limit on the number of bacteria is not reality. Many mothers of perfectly healthy babies have bacteria levels that are higher than this. This is simply an arbitrary choice. It would have been useful information to examine these discarded samples and see how they behaved and what bacterial growth was like under the same conditions.
8. The samples were categorized into three classes reflecting the type of bacterial growth after the overnight incubation.
   - Class I: milk that had no growth after overnight incubation
   - Class II: milk that contained nonpathogenic bacteria
   - Class III: milk that contained pathogens (*Pseudomonas*, *Staphylococcus aureus*, group B streptococci, enterococci, *Enterobacteriaceae*)

Results

	Class I Samples	*Class II Samples*	*Class III Samples*
0–4°C	• Remained sterile after 8 days in the refrigerator (range 0 CFU/ml) • Still sterile after 6 hrs at 26°C (range 0 CFU/ml)	• Bacteria counts decreased over 8 days in refrigerator (range 0.1–2.8 × 10^3 CFU/ml) • Bacterial load varied over time (range 0–2.4 × 10^3 CFU/ml)	• Bacteria counts decreased over 8 days in refrigerator (range 0–30.0 × 10^3 CFU/ml) • Bacteria counts stable over 6 hrs. (range 0–30.0 × 10^3 CFU/ml)
-20°C	• Small amount of bacteria after 8 days in freezer (range 0–0.2 × 10^3 CFU/ml) • Bacteria increase during hang time. (range 0–5.0 × 10^3 CFU/ml)	• No decrease in bacteria during 8 days in freezer (range 0.10–11.0 × 10^3 CFU/ml) • Insignificant increase in bacteria over 6 hrs at 26°C (range 0–10.0 x 10^3 CFU/ml at 6 hrs)	• Some decrease in bacteria but not significant (range 0.7–65.2 × 10^3 CFU/ml) • Bacteria increased over time and was significant only at 6 hrs, not 2 or 4 hrs. (range 2.6–30.0 × 10^3 CFU/ml at 6 hrs)

No sample exceeded 30.0 × 10^3 bacteria counts (30,000 CFU/ml), the highest bacteria count in the entire study. All milk in the study, therefore, started out as extremely clean milk in comparison to other studies and to real life.

(*continues*)

Box 7-2 Methods and Madness: How a Research Finding Became Translated to Policy (continued)

Discussion

Bacteria have the capability of producing lipases, proteases, and decarboxylases, enzymes that can impact the quality of milk by reducing IgA, lipids, and other components of milk. Bacterial growth also uses milk as a substrate for growth, depleting basic nutrients in milk to support bacterial growth and colonization. Bacteria also have the potential to make individuals ill if concentrations are too high, and it is understood that acceptable limits for certain bacteria in the healthy infant may be too high and unacceptable for the sick, preterm infant. Having bacterial counts as low as the ones in this study is an ideal that is not always achieved in the NICU.

The authors explain the loss of bacterial inhibition in the more contaminated samples (Class III) that have been frozen as being due to the freezing itself, a loss that was not seen in the samples that were only refrigerated. The authors state that they prefer storage in the refrigerator for 8 days rather than freezing because of the lack of suppression of bacterial growth in the frozen samples. While the authors' conclusions may be valid, how they reached these conclusions is questionable because of variables in the methodology. Was it the microwaving that actually was more detrimental than the freezing process itself? Ideally this study should be repeated on mothers of preterm infants and reflect their common everyday practices of expressing milk for their hospitalized infants and eliminate the confounder of microwaving only the frozen milk. The repeat study should also consider the following:

1. Instructions for collection should include hand washing only, as most mothers express without nipple and breast cleansing.
2. Collection methods should be standardized to an electric pump with a kit that has been used numerous times and washed/cleaned by the mother according to her interpretation of instructions.
3. No bacterial limits should be placed on samples in the study. All samples should be analyzed and categorized.
4. Thawing should be done quickly in a constant temperature water bath set at or below body temperature to avoid overheating. Microwaving should not be used.
5. Dividing samples into aliquots should be done under aseptic conditions to avoid contamination from outside sources. No mention of this is in the methodology unless it is assumed to be part of standard bacteriological technique.

Only when studies are done that include real life scenarios can we safely make recommendations for longer storage times and that storage in the refrigerator for 8 days is preferable to freezing regardless of the bacteria counts of the mother, especially as routine bacteria counts on expressed milk have been shown to be ineffective and costly (Law Urias, Lertzman, Robson, & Romance, 1989).

from combining both sets of recommendations in one document, this appendix covers only the hospital setting and is more conservative in its recommendations. More research that is methodologically appropriate and reflects what mothers actually do is needed in this area (see Box 7-2). The following topics, while covered in the recommendations themselves, are those that need a more in-depth discussion because of their controversial nature and new developments that have not been well researched.

Container Types

Appendix 7-2 has a detailed discussion of container types based on the materials from which they are made. Much of this literature is old and needs to be redone since none of it was undertaken before the widespread use of polycarbonate in infant feeding materials.[1]

There are several other issues relating to storage containers for the NICU. Many hospitals have relied/may still be relying on the formula companies for free bottles of sterile water/glucose water, which the hospital then handed out to mothers, telling them to dump the water and reuse the container for the expressed milk. There were/are several problems with this arrangement, including: (1) the caps are not always reusable and may rust if used more than once; (2) the size of the bottles may be large for the amount that the mother is expressing and may cause discouragement and failure of confidence when she sees that she is only getting a small amount (made to appear even smaller by the large size of the bottle in comparison); (3) formula companies may restrict the number of bottles used this way if they deem too many are being given out, leaving mothers with a short supply; (4) this type of advertising raises the cost of everything else related to formula use; and (5) there is an expectation on the part of the formula company that there will be some net benefit derived from the hospital (see also Chapter 11 in this book).

Hospitals have resorted to other types of containers as well, including milk storage bags, which are used once and discarded but which may tear and break at their weakest point, the heat seal on the bottom, especially after freezing (see Appendix 7-2 for a discussion of other hazards and problems with polyethylene bags); sterile urine specimen cups, again used only once (these do not fit on the pump body and are made for body fluids that are waste products (urine, sputum, etc.) and may not be made out of food-grade materials; and volumetric feeders from formula companies (in the past without lids, but now being packaged with screw-cap lids by the formula companies). Pump companies

[1] Bisphenol-A (BPA) is a polymer used in the manufacture of polycarbonate plastics frequently used in infant feeding. It binds to estrogen receptors, and exposure to BPA has been linked to endocrine disruption, recurrent miscarriages, altered mammary gland development, prostate cancer, altered brain development and behavior, and insulin resistance. Environmental exposure occurs over time with leaching of the polymer into the food in the container, especially with heating, pouring hot liquids into the container, repeated washing of containers, and storage of acidic foods. Several manufacturers of baby bottles have now removed BPA from their products. However, BPA is also known to be present in the linings of cans that contain formula (see Alaska Community Action on Toxics 2007; Center for Health, Environment, and Justice [n.d.])

also purvey milk storage bags, and one company has developed a small container specifically for expressing colostrum. It is a shortened volumetric feeder with a rounded bottom, is a little over an ounce in size, and fits onto the pump kit directly. The advantage of the rounded bottom is that colostrum doesn't get caught in the angle between a flat bottom and the straight side of the container; instead it all slides to the same point in the bowl.

A company that makes containers of all sorts that is not related to the formula industry has now started making volumetric containers with snap-cap lids that attach to standard pump bodies. The lid remains attached to the bottle while the mother is pumping, lessening the risk of contamination by putting the cap down on a dirty surface. These containers are approved by the FDA for the collection and storage of human milk and have the added advantage that fat does not adhere to the sides of the container. They are reusable and can be easily cleaned in a dishwasher, making them a more cost-effective option for milk storage than bags with their one-time-only use. Before these snap-cap bottles became available, one physician had mothers in her unit take home sterile water bottles and wash and reuse them. A bucket was provided for each mother and when the milk was used, the bottle was rinsed thoroughly and placed in the bucket so that the mother could take it home and clean it and reuse it. No increase in infection rates in babies was observed as a result of this practice (N. Wight, personal communication, July 2000). However, there is no research to show that mothers can clean such containers adequately over time if they were to take them home from the NICU and reuse them. More research is needed on this practice which could be very cost-effective.

Multiuser Pump Contamination

There are a number of reports in the literature about outbreaks of infection in the NICU caused by pathogens such as *Pseudomonas aeruginosa*, *Klebsiella* sp., and *Serratia marcescens* associated with contaminated breast pumps (Cabasson, Godron, Bordes-Couecou, Hernandorena, & Jouvencal, 2007; Donowitz, Marsik, Fisher, & Wenzel, 1981; Moloney, Quoraishi, Parry, & Hall, 1987; Thom, Cole, & Watrasiewicz, 1970). A neglected area of possible milk contamination is the cleanliness of multiuser pumps. In visits to NICUs around the country, I have observed that pump cleanliness is seldom a priority. In many NICUs, there is no person in charge of making sure that pumps and work surfaces are cleaned between users. In many instances there are not even cleaning products available with which mothers could clean up milk spills and swab the surface of the pump down. Once spilled milk dries on a surface it is very difficult to clean up; being proactive and cleaning spills as they occur is therefore imperative. Frequently this is a question of staff time and location of the pumping area.

When pumps are set up in separate areas that mothers use and share (sometimes with other hospital staff who are expressing) they are out of sight of most personnel who would be responsible for the care and cleaning of the equipment. This means a special effort must be made and a specific individual assigned to check frequently on a schedule and make sure that cleanliness is maintained. Having shared pumps on trolleys that can be used at the baby's bedside would have an advantage in this regard. The nurse who brings the pump to the mother could double-check the cleanliness before the mother begins to use it and then ensure that it is cleaned when the mother finishes. Pumping at the bedside is also advantageous for the mother in helping her to establish and maintain her milk supply. However, privacy may be an issue and mothers could feel uncomfortable pumping next to the baby's bedside, even when a privacy screen is provided. Healthcare providers may feel that they can interrupt her despite the screen, but if the mother is in a separate pumping room she is out of sight and less likely to be interrupted.

Cytomegalovirus

Lawrence (2006) has reviewed the literature on cytomegalovirus (CMV) and its impact on premature infants. Because CMV can cause serious harm and sometimes death to premature infants depending on the timing of exposure, the virus is a concern to neonatologists. CMV can be transmitted in human milk, and in the healthy, term infant, this postnatal mode of transmission may be one method of immunizing the infant without harm. Since the prevalence of the virus in milk tends to be quite high, many attempts have been made to make milk safer and either remove or inactivate the virus by various methods. Pasteurization is one such method; however, the immunologic benefits of human milk are compromised by such treatment. Repeated freezing and thawing also does not appear to be as effective at inactivating the virus as previously thought (Maschmann et al., 2006).

Lawrence (2006) recommends the following practices in NICUs:

- Screen cord blood (or maternal blood) for CMV serostatus of all premature and low-birth-weight infants admitted to the NICU.
- Evaluate each infant for signs of congenital CMV infection and test if warranted.

- Screen all infants of CMV-seropositive mothers for congenital CMV if the infant is to receive his own mother's milk.
- Discuss the risks and benefits of breastfeeding with a CMV-seropositive mother in a balanced manner.
- Evaluate the feasibility, risks, and benefits of various procedures that would inactivate CMV, e.g., pasteurization and freezing.
- Reassess all current policies about breastmilk use in infants of seropositive mothers.
- Examine existing policies for collection, storage, and handling of breastmilk, both for mother-infant-specific and donor milk.
- Continue to monitor and evaluate the frequency and nature of CMV infections in the unit.
- Establish safe practices and guidelines for the prevention of CMV transmission through blood products.
- Continue the use of human milk in the NICU, especially for all well, full-term infants and infants of CMV-seronegative mothers.
- Revise policies as new findings are published.

Fortification and the Potential for Contamination

In term infants clusters of deaths from meningitis caused by *Enterobacter sakazakii* (ES) have occurred in several countries. Normally, a bacterium of this sort would cause diarrhea, so public health officials were surprised to find this bacterium infecting the central nervous system. The common denominator in these clusters of cases was found to be powdered infant formula. Numerous brands were involved, so this could not be blamed on just one company and an oversight. Liquid infant formulas (ready-to-feed and concentrates) are sterilized in the manufacturing process. A powder cannot be sterilized because of the way it is sprayed to form the powder. Groups at greatest risk of infection are infants, particularly those under 2 months of age, premature infants, low-birth-weight infants, and immunocompromised infants (WHO, 2007).

ES is a persistent bacterium, surviving in powdered formula for very long periods of time. According to Hunter, Petrosyan, Ford, and Prasadarao (2008), it was the only organism isolated from powdered infant formula that had been stored for 2.5 years. It is able to survive for at least 12 months in powder and is resistant to routine sterilization methods. Hunter's recommendations include promotion of breastfeeding, limited use of powdered formulas with populations at risk, and reduced hang time (no more than 4 hours) for enteral feedings (see also Chapter 2 of this book and the discussion of fortifiers; Bowen & Braden, 2006; CDC, 2002; FDA, 2002; Stoll, Hansen, Faranoff, & Lemons, 2004).

An expert panel convened by WHO and the Food and Agriculture Organization of the United Nations met in 2004 and reconvened in 2006 to develop guidelines for preparation of powdered infant formulas. These involve mixing powdered infant formula with water that has been heated to greater than 70°C (158°F). For preparing powdered infant formula feedings in the healthcare setting, WHO recommends that "It is best to prepare feeds fresh each time and to feed immediately" (WHO, 2007, p. 10). However, infants could suffer severe burns if formula still at 70°C was fed immediately; quick cooling to temperatures that are safe for feeding is therefore advisable. Feedings not used within 2 hours should be discarded. If feedings cannot be used immediately and must be prepared in advance, then cooled feedings should be placed in a dedicated refrigerator whose temperature is monitored and does not exceed 5°C. If the refrigerated feeding is not used within 24 hours, then it must be discarded (WHO, 2007, p. 11).

How does this relate to fortifiers for human milk? Those manufactured by the formula industry come in two forms, liquid and powdered. The disadvantage of the liquid form is that it displaces volume of human milk that a baby consumes; if a baby is to get only 30 ml of volume at each feeding and 5 ml of that is liquid fortifier, then the baby only gets 25 ml of milk. On the other hand, if the powdered form is used, it is added to the 30 ml of milk. Many neonatologists prefer to use the powdered form for this reason. However, the technology of manufacturing a powdered fortifier is the same as that of manufacturing powdered infant formula, and it is also not a sterile product.

Cases of ES have occurred in NICU settings in the United States when powdered infant formula was being used when breastmilk was unavailable (CDC, 2002). A powdered infant fortifier has been under investigation in Illinois by the Department of Health as a source of ES in cerebral spinal fluid and serum in a neonate (Illinois Department of Health, 2007).

Parents should be made aware of the potential for this infection despite its rarity and be given the option of having a liquid bovine-based fortifier or a fortifier made out of human milk components used. Chan, Lee, and Rechtman (2007) found that use of two different bovine-based fortifiers almost totally inhibited antibacterial activity of human milk against *Escherichia coli, E. sakazakii, Clostridium difficile,* and *Shigella soneii*. Using a human milk-based fortifier maintained the antibacterial activity of human milk against these organisms. As of this writing, the company producing this human milk-based fortifier (made from components extracted from human milk) is currently conducting clinical trials on safety and efficacy of their product for preterm infants. (See Chapter 2 for further discussion of issues related to fortifiers and the need for further research, particularly clinical trials.)

SUMMARY

In this chapter, techniques to help the mother of a hospitalized infant establish and maintain her milk supply have been addressed. Mothers deserve the opportunity to change their minds about whether they want to supply their milk, and then they need to be provided with the support that will enable them to achieve their goals. Besides providing equipment and supplies that are needed, hospital staff need to become a cheering section for the mother, touching base frequently to see how she is doing and offering help and suggestions when they are needed, as in the case of a faltering milk supply. Policies and protocols need to be in place so that every mother gets consistent information from staff, motivating them to continue expressing their milk. Sample policies given in Appendices 7-1 and 7-2 may serve as models for development of NICU policies.

REFERENCES

Academy of Breastfeeding Medicine (ABM). (2004). *Use of galactogogues in initiating and augmenting maternal milk supply*. Retrieved January 7, 2009, from http://www.bfmed.org/Resources/Protocols.aspx

Affonso, D., Wahlberg, V., & Persson, B. (1989). Exploration of mothers' reactions to the kangaroo method of prematurity care. *Neonatal Network, 7*(6), 43–51.

Ahluwahlia, I., Tessaro, I., Grummer-Strawn, L., MacGowan, C., & Benton-Davis, S. (2000). Georgia's breastfeeding promotion program for low-income women. *Pediatrics, 105*(6), e85. Retrieved June 1, 2009 from http://www.pediatrics.aappublications.org/cgi/content/full/105/6/e85

Alaska Community Action on Toxics. (2007). *Bisphenol-A and your health*. Retrieved March 6, 2009, from http://www.chej.org/documents/Bisphenol%20A%20Fact%20sheet.pdf

Alekseev, N., Ilyin, V., Yaroslavski, V., Gaidukov, S., Tikhonova, T., Specivcev, Y., et al. (1998). Compression stimuli increase the efficacy of breast pump function. *European Journal of Obstetrics and Gynecology and Reproductive Biology, 77*(2), 131–139.

Alexander, J., Grant, A., & Campbell, M. (1992). Randomised controlled trial of breast shells and Hoffman's exercises for inverted and non-protractile nipples. *British Medical Journal, 304*(6833), 1030–1032.

Amir, L., & Donath, S. (2002). Does maternal smoking have a negative physiological effect on breastfeeding? The epidemiological evidence. *Birth, 29*(2), 112–123.

Andersen, A., Lund-Andersen, C., Larsen, J., Christensen, N., Legros, J, Louis, F., et al. (1982). Suppressed prolactin but normal neurophysin levels in cigarette smoking breast-feeding women. *Clinical Endocrinology (Oxford), 17*(4), 363–368.

Anderson, P. & Valdes, V. (2007). A critical review of pharmaceutical galactogogues. *Breastfeeding Medicine, 2*(4), 229–242.

Batstra, L., Neeleman, J., & Hadders-Algra, M. (2003). Can breast feeding modify the adverse effects of smoking during pregnancy on the child's cognitive development? *Journal of Epidemiology and Community Health, 57*(6), 403–404.

Boo, N., Nordiah, A., Alfizah, H., Nor-Rohaini, A., & Lim, V. (2001). Contamination of breast milk obtained by manual expression and breast pumps in mothers of very low birthweight infants. *Journal of Hospital Infection, 49*(4), 274–281.

Bowen, A., & Braden, C. (2006). Invasive *Enterobacter sakazakii* disease in infants. *Emerging Infectious Diseases, 12*(8), 1185–1189.

Cabasson, S., Godron, A., Bordes-Couecou, S., Hernandorena, X., & Jouvencal, P. (2007). Infection nosocomiale fatale chez un nouveau-né prématuré liée à une contamination par un tire-lait [Lethal nosocomial infection in a premature newborn due to a breast pump contamination]. *Archives of Pediatrics, 14*(3), 294–295.

California Perinatal Quality Care Collaborative. (2008a). *Domperidone for improving breastmilk production. Appendix 4-N.* Available at: http://www.cpqcc.org/quality_improvement/qi_toolkits/nutritional_support_of_the_vlbw_infant_rev_december_2008

California Perinatal Quality Care Collaborative. (2008b). *Family information sheet: Use of Reglan® (metoclopramide) to increase maternal milk supply. Appendix 4–M2.* Available at: http://www.cpqcc.org/quality_improvement/qi_toolkits/nutritional_support_of_the_vlbw_infant_rev_december_2008

California Perinatal Quality Care Collaborative. (2008c). *Professional information sheet: Use of Reglan® (metoclopramide) to increase maternal milk supply. Appendix 4–M1.* Available at: http://www.cpqcc.org/quality_improvement/qi_toolkits/nutritional_support_of_the_vlbw_infant_rev_december_2008

Center for Health, Environment and Justice. (n.d.). *Baby's toxic bottle: Bisphenol A leaching from popular baby bottles.* Retrieved June 1, 2009, from http://www.chej.org/documents/BabysToxicBottleFinal.pdf

Centers for Disease Control and Prevention (CDC). (2002). Enterobacter sakazakii *infections associated with the use of powdered infant formula—Tennessee, 2001.* Retrieved March 6, 2009, from http://www.cdc.gov/mmwr/preview/mmwrhtml/mm5114a1.htm

Centers for Disease Control and Prevention (CDC). (2008a). *Breastfeeding among U.S. children born 1999–2005, CDC National Immunization Survey.* Retrieved January 25, 2009, from http://www.cdc.gov/breastfeeding/data/NIS_data/index.htm

Centers for Disease Control and Prevention, National Center for Health Statistics (CDC). (2008b). *Breastfeeding in the United States: Findings from the National Health and Nutrition Examination Surveys, 1999–2006. National Center for Health Statistics Data Brief No. 5.* Retrieved January 25, 2009, from http://www.cdc.gov/nchs/data/databriefs/db05.pdf

Chan, G., Lee, M., & Rechtman, D. (2007). Effects of a human milk-derived human milk fortifier on the antibacterial actions of human milk. *Breastfeeding Medicine, 2*(4), 205–208.

Chatterton, R., Hill, P., Aldag, H., Hodges, K., Belknap, S., & Zinaman, M. (2000). Relation of plasma oxytocin and prolactin concentrations to milk production in mothers of preterm infants: Influence of stress. *Journal of Clinical Endocrinology and Metabolism, 85*(10), 3661–3668.

Cregan, M., DeMello, T., Kershaw, D., McDougall, K., & Hartmann, P. (2002). Initiation of lactation in women after preterm delivery. *Acta Obstetricia et Gynecologica Scandinavica, 81*(9), 870–877.

Czank, C., Henderson, J., Kent, J., Lai, C., & Hartmann, P. (2007). Hormonal control of the lactation cycle. In T. Hale & P. Hartmann (Eds.), *Textbook of human lactation* (pp. 89–111). Amarillo, TX: Hale Publishing, L.P.

da Silva, O., Knoppert, D., Angelini, M., & Forret, P. (2001). Effect of domperidone on milk production in mothers of premature newborns: A randomized, double-blind, placebo-controlled trial. *Canadian Medical Association Journal, 164*(1), 17–21.

de Carvalho, M., Robertson, S., Friedman, A., & Klaus, M. (1983). Effect of frequent breast-feeding on early milk production and infant weight gain. *Pediatrics, 72*(3), 307–311.

Donowitz, L., Marsik, F., Fisher, K., & Wenzel, R. (1981). Contaminated breast milk: A source of Klebsiella bacteremia in a newborn intensive care unit. *Reviews of Infectious Diseases, 3*(4), 716–720.

Dorea, J. (2007). Maternal smoking and infant feeding: Breastfeeding is better and safer. *Maternal Child Health Journal, 11*(3), 287–291.

Ehrenkranz, R., & Ackerman, B. (1986). Metoclopramide effect on faltering milk production by mothers of premature infants. *Pediatrics, 78*(4), 614–620.

Feher, S., Berger, L., Johnson, J., & Wilde, J. (1989). Increasing breast milk production for premature infants with a relaxation/imagery audiotape. *Pediatrics, 83*(1), 57–60.

Food and Drug Administration, Center for Food Safety and Applied Nutrition. (2002). *Health professionals letter on* Enterobacter sakazakii *infections associated with use of powdered (dry) infant formulas in neonatal intensive care units.* Retrieved March 6, 2009, from http://www.cfsan.fda.gov/~dms/inf-ltr3.html

Furman, L., Minich, N., & Hack, M. (1998). Breastfeeding of very low birth weight infants. *Journal of Human Lactation, 14*(1), 29–34.

Furman, L., Minich, N., & Hack, M. (2002). Correlates of lactation in mothers of very low birth weight infants. *Pediatrics, 109*(4), e57.

Geddes, D. (2007). Gross anatomy of the lactating breast. In T. Hale & P. Hartmann (Eds.), *Textbook of human lactation* (pp. 19–34). Amarillo, TX: Hale Publishing, L.P.

Grajeda, R., & Pérez-Escamilla, R. (2002). Stress during labor and delivery is associated with delayed onset of lactation among urban Guatemalan women. *Journal of Nutrition, 132*(10), 3055–3060.

Groh-Wargo, S., Toth, A., Mahoney, K., Simonian, S., Wasser, T., & Rose, S. (1995). The utility of a bilateral breast pumping system for mothers of premature infants. *Neonatal Network, 14*(8), 31–36.

Hale, T. (2007). Medications that alter milk production. In T. Hale & P. Hartmann (Eds.), *Textbook of human lactation* (pp.479–489). Amarillo, TX: Hale Publishing, L.P.

Hansen, W., McAndrew, S., Harris, K., & Zimmerman, M. (2005). Metoclopramide effect on breastfeeding the preterm infant: A randomized trial. *Obstetrics and Gynecology, 105*(2), 383–389.

Harris Family Sextuplets Web site. (2007). *The Harris family sextuplets: America's first surviving African-American sextuplets.* Retrieved March 6, 2009, from www.harrissextuplets.net/background.shtml

Henderson, J. J., Hartmann, P. E., Newnham, J. P., & Simmer, K. (2008). Effect of preterm birth and antenatal corticosteroid treatment on lactogenesis II in women. *Pediatrics, 121*(1), e92–e100.

Hill, P., & Aldag, J. (1996). Smoking and breastfeeding status. *Research in Nursing and Health, 19*(2), 125–132.

Hill, P., & Aldag, J. (2005). Milk volume on day 4 and income predictive of lactation adequacy at 6 weeks of mothers of nonnursing preterm infants. *Journal of Perinatal and Neonatal Nursing, 19*(3), 273–282.

Hill, P., Aldag, J., & Chatterton, R. (1996). The effect of sequential and simultaneous breast pumping on milk volume and prolactin levels: A pilot study. *Journal of Human Lactation, 12*(3), 193–199.

Hill, P., Aldag, J. & Chatterton, R. (2001). Initiation and frequency of pumping and milk production in mothers of non-nursing preterm infants. *Journal of Human Lactation, 17*(1), 9–13.

Hill, P., Aldag, J. Chatterton, R., & Zinaman, M. (2005). Comparison of milk output between mothers of preterm and term infants: The first 6 weeks after birth. *Journal of Human Lactation, 21*(1), 22–30.

Hill, P., Aldag, J., Zinaman, M., & Chatterton, R. (2007). Predictors of preterm infant feeding methods and perceived insufficient milk supply at week 12 postpartum. *Journal of Human Lactation, 23*(1), 32–38.

Hopkinson, J., Schanler, R., Fraley, K., & Garza, C. (1992). Milk production by mothers of premature infants: Influence of cigarette smoking. *Pediatrics, 90*(6), 934–938.

Howie, P. W., McNeilly A. S., McArdle, T., Smart, L., & Houston, M. (1980). The relationship between suckling-induced prolactin response and lactogenesis. *Journal of Clinical Endocrinology and Metabolism. 50*(4), 670–673.

Hunter, C., Petrosyan, M., Ford, H., & Prasadarao, N. (2008). *Enterobacter sakazakii*: An emerging pathogen in infants and neonates. *Surgical Infections, 9*(5), 533–539.

Hurst, N. (2007). The 3 M's of breast-feeding the preterm infant. *Journal of Perinatal and Neonatal Nursing, 21*(3), 234–239.

Hurst, N., Valentine, C., Renfro, L., Burns, P., & Ferlic, L. (1997). Skin-to-skin holding in the neonatal intensive care unit influences maternal milk volume. *Journal of Perinatology, 17*(3), 213–217.

Illinois Department of Health. (2007). Memorandum to all local health departments, hospital infection control practitioners and hospital laboratories on *Enterobacter sakazakii* investigation. December 4, 2007.

Jones, E., Dimmock, P., & Spencer, S. (2001). A randomized controlled trial to compare methods of milk expression after preterm delivery. *Archives of Disease in Childhood, Fetal and Neonatal Edition, 85*(2), F91–F95.

Kauppila, A., Kivinen, S., & Ylikorkola, O. (1981). A dose response relation between improved lactation and metoclopramide. *The Lancet, 1*(8231), 1175–1177.

Kavanaugh, K., Meier, P., Zimmerman, B., & Mead, L. (1997). The rewards outweigh the efforts: Breastfeeding outcomes for mothers of preterm infants. *Journal of Human Lactation, 13*(1), 15–21.

Killersreiter, B., Grimmer, I., Buhrer, C., Dudenhausen, J., & Obladen, M. (2001). Early cessation of breast milk feeding in very low birthweight infants. *Early Human Development, 60*(3), 193–205.

Lang, S. (1997). *Breastfeeding special care babies*. London: Bailliere Tindall.

Law, B. J., Urias, B. A., Lertzman, J., Robson, D., & Romance, L. (1989). Is ingestion of milk-associated bacteria by premature infants fed raw human milk controlled by routine bacteriologic screening? *Journal of Clinical Microbiology, 27*(7), 1560–1566.

Lawrence, R. M. (2006). Cytomegalovirus in human breast milk: Risk to the premature infant. *Breastfeeding Medicine, 1*(2), 99–107.

Lepore, J. (2009, January 19). *Maternity department: Baby food—if breast is best, why are women bottling their milk?* Retrieved January 17, 2009, from http://www.newyorker.com/reporting/2009/01/19/090119fa_fact_lepore?printable=true

Lu, M., Lange, L., Slusser, W., Hamilton, J., & Halfon, N. (2001). Provider encouragement of breastfeeding: Evidence from a national survey. *Obstetrics and Gynecology, 97*(2), 290–295.

Lucas, A., Cole. T., Morley, R., Lucas, P., Davis, J., Bamford, M., et al. (1988). Factors associated with maternal choice to provide breast milk for low birth weight infants. *Archives of Disease in Childhood, 63*(1), 48–52.

Malik, S., Cleves, M., Honein, M., Romitti, P., Botto, L., Yang, S., et al. (2008). Maternal smoking and congenital heart defects. *Pediatrics, 121*(4), e810–e816.

March of Dimes. (2008). *Nation gets a "D" as March of Dimes releases premature birth report card*. Retrieved December 1, 2008, from http://www.marchofdimes.com/printableArticles/22684_42538.asp

March of Dimes. (2009). *Why are babies born with low birthweight?* Retrieved January 19, 2009, from http://search.marchofdimes.com/cgi-bin/MsmGo.exe?grab_id=6&page_id=611328&query=smoking&hiword=smoking

Marinelli, K., & Hamelin, K. (2005). Breastfeeding and the use of human milk in the neonatal intensive care unit. In M. MacDonald, M. Mullet, & M. Seshia (Eds.), *Avery's neonatology: Pathophysiology and management of the newborn* (6th ed., pp. 413–444). Philadelphia: Lippincott Williams & Wilkins.

Maschmann, J., Hamprecht, K., Weissbrih, B., Dietz, K., Jahn, G., & Speer, C. (2006). Freeze-thawing of breast milk does not prevent cytomegalovirus transmission to a preterm infant. *Archives of Disease in Childhood, Fetal and Neonatal Edition, 91*(4), F288–F290.

Matthiesen, A., Ransjo-Arvidson, A., Nissen, E, & Uvnas-Moberg, K. (2001). Postpartum maternal oxytocin release by newborns: Effects of infant hand massage and sucking. *Birth, 28*(1), 13–19.

Meier, P. (2001). Breastfeeding in the special care nursery. Prematures and infants with medical problems. *Pediatric Clinics of North America, 48*(2), 425–442.

Meier, P., Brown, L., & Hurst, N. (1999). Breastfeeding the preterm infant. In J. Riordan & K. Auerbach (Eds.), *Breastfeeding and human lactation* (2nd ed., pp. 449–481). Sudbury, MA: Jones and Bartlett.

Miracle, D., Meier, P., & Bennett, P. (2004a). Making my baby healthy: Changing the decision from formula to human milk feedings for very-low-birth-weight infants. *Advances in Experimental Medicine and Biology, 554*, 317–319.

Miracle, D., Meier, P., & Bennett, P. (2004b). Mothers' decisions to change from formula to mothers' milk for very-low-birth-weight infants. *Journal of Obstetric, Gynecologic, and Neonatal Nursing, 33*(6), 692–703.

Mitoulas, L., Lai C., Gurrin, L., Larsson, M., & Hartmann, P. (2002). Efficacy of breast milk expression using an electric breast pump. *Journal of Human Lactation, 18*(4), 344–352.

Moloney, A., Quoraishi, A., Parry, P., & Hall, V. (1987). A bacteriological examination of breast pumps. *Journal of Hospital Infection, 9*(2), 169–174.

Pardou, A., Serruys, E., Mascart-Lemone, F., Dramaix, M., & Vis, H. (1994). Human milk banking: Influence of storage processes and of bacterial contamination on some milk constituents. *Biology of the Neonate, 65*(5), 302–309.

Prime, D., Geddes, D., & Hartmann, P. (2007). Oxytocin: Milk ejections and maternal-infant well-being. In T. Hale & P. Hartmann (Eds.), *Textbook of human lactation* (pp. 141–155). Amarillo, TX: Hale Publishing, L.P.

Rodriguez, N., Miracle, D., & Meier, P. (2005). Sharing the science on human milk feedings with mothers of very-low-birth-weight infants. *Journal of Obstetric, Gynecologic, and Neonatal Nursing, 34*(1), 109–119.

Ryan, A., Wenjun, Z., & Acosta, A. (2002). Breastfeeding continues to increase into the new millennium. *Pediatrics, 110*(6), 1103–1109.

RxList. (2009). *Reglan*. Retrieved January 7, 2009, from http://www.rxlist.com/reglan-drug/htm

Sisk, P., Lovelady, C., & Dillard, R. (2004). Effect of education and lactation support on maternal decision to provide human milk for very-low-birth-weight infants. *Advances in Experimental Medicine and Biology, 554*, 307–311.

Skidmore-Roth, L. (2006). *Mosby's handbook of herbs and natural supplements* (3rd ed.). St. Louis, MO: Mosby/Elsevier.

Slusher, T., Slusher, I., Biomdo, M., Bode-Thomas, F., Curtis, B., & Meier, P. (2007). Electric breast pump use increases maternal milk volume in African nurseries. *Journal of Tropical Pediatrics, 53*(2), 125–130.

Stoll, B., Hansen, N., Fanaroff, A., & Lemons, J. for the National Institute of Child Health and Human Development Neonatal Research Network. (2004). *Enterobacter sakazakii* is a rare cause of neonatal septicemia or meningitis in VLBW infants. *Journal of Pediatrics, 144*(6), 821–823.

Thom, A., Cole, A., & Watrasiewicz, K. (1970, March 14). Pseudomonas aeruginosa infection in a neonatal nursery, possibly transmitted by a breast-milk pump. *The Lancet, 1*(7646), 560–561.

Vio, F., Salazar, G., & Infante, C. (1991). Smoking during pregnancy and lactation and its effect on breast-milk volume. *American Journal of Clinical Nutrition, 54*(6), 1011–1016.

Wan, E., Davey, K., Page-Sharp, M., Hartmann, P., Simmer, K., & Ilett, K. (2008). Dose-effect study of domperidone as a galactogogue in preterm mothers with insufficient milk supply, and its transfer into milk. *British Journal of Clinical Pharmacology, 66*(2), 283–289.

Weimers, L., Svensson, K., Dumas, L., Naver, L., & Wahlberg, V. (2006). Hands-on approach during breastfeeding support in a neonatal intensive care unit: A qualitative study of Swedish mothers' experiences. *International Breastfeeding Journal, 1*. Retrieved January 25, 2009, from http://internationalbreastfeedingjournal.com/content/1/1/20

Wight, N., & Morton, J. (2007). Human milk, breastfeeding, and the preterm infant. In T. Hale & P. Hartmann (Eds.), *Textbook of human lactation* (pp. 215–253). Amarillo, TX: Hale Publishing, L.P.

Woodward, A., & Hand, K. (1988). Smoking and reduced duration of breastfeeding. *Medical Journal of Australia, 148*(9), 477–478.

World Health Organization (WHO). (2007). *Safe preparation, storage and handling of powdered infant formula: Guidelines*. Retrieved March 6, 2009, from http://www.who.int/foodsafety/publications/micro/pif_guidelines.pdf

Appendix 7-1

STEP 5

Enable mothers to begin early milk expression, and provide ongoing education and support, to promote adequate milk supply.

Policies 5.1–5.7

Title

Assisting mothers to establish and maintain an optimal milk supply.

Purpose

To provide support and education to promote a full and ongoing maternal milk supply. Success at establishing and maintaining an ample milk supply is an essential ingredient in the health and well-being of both the hospitalized infant and its mother. When babies cannot assist in the process of establishing and maintaining a milk supply directly through breastfeeding, proper education, support, and equipment should be provided.

Supportive Data

Human milk feeding is important for the health and normal development of the hospitalized infant (Marinelli & Hamelin, 2005; Wight & Morton, 2007). Establishment and maintenance of a milk supply under stressful circumstances requires a great deal of effort and motivation as well as patience on the part of the mother, above and beyond learning how to breastfeed.

Rationale

Early proactive support works best for all new mothers. Anticipating periods for the NICU/SCN mother when problems may arise or questions may be raised and addressing them in a proactive and anticipatory manner will (1) help instill confidence in the NICU mother that she can meet her infant's needs, (2) avoid common pitfalls that compromise milk supply, and (3) prolong breastfeeding duration.

Mothers of NICU/SCN babies are less likely to breastfeed than mothers of healthy, term infants (Furman, Minich, & Hack, 2002). Frequently, healthcare professionals and/or family members discourage these mothers from initiating lactation because they believe that providing milk will be too stressful in an already stress-filled situation (Meier, 2001). Mothers may be erroneously advised that their own high-risk health conditions may interfere with adequate volumes or composition of milk. Mothers of NICU/SCN infants feel a loss of their role as a mother and a loss of control over their lives and their babies' lives when mothering cannot occur naturally because of separation. Several studies show that providing milk for their infants helps mothers cope with the emotional stresses surrounding the NICU/SCN experience and gives them a tangible claim on their babies. Providing breastmilk is something only the mother can do (Kavanaugh, Meier, Zimmerman, & Mead, 1997).

A full milk supply must be established for the preterm or sick infant, just as it is for a full-term, healthy infant. If a mother is just keeping up with the infant's current needs, which may be quite small depending on the gestational age and level of illness, she will be unable to develop a larger milk supply when the infant's nutritional needs increase according to normal lactation physiology. Therefore, the key to success is early and frequent breast stimulation, which has the added advantage of providing colostrum for the infant.

Scope

The policies apply to all NICU/SCN personnel, including the medical director, nursing director, nursing supervisors, licensed staff, ancillary staff, and volunteers.

Policy 5.1

All postpartum and NICU/SCN staff should be trained to implement Step 5 as per Step 2.

Policy 5.2

Mothers should receive written information about milk expression and the use of a breast pump in order to establish and maintain a full milk supply for the nonsuckling or partially suckling infant.

Policy 5.3

Mothers should be assisted in beginning milk expression as soon as possible within 6 hours of delivery.

Procedure 5.3.1
Instructions on hand expression should be given to all mothers including a demonstration and return demonstration and documented in the medical record.

Procedure 5.3.2
If hand expression will not be the sole method of expression used, a mother should be provided with a rental-grade electric pump for in-hospital use. A double collecting kit for personal use should be provided each mother in hospital for the most efficient establishment of a full milk supply. Collecting kits should fit the pump the mother will be using and should also fit the mother's breasts.

Procedure 5.3.3
Mothers should be shown how to use the pump and disassemble and assemble the collecting kit. A return demonstration should be documented in the medical record. The pump and collecting kit should be used according to the manufacturer's instructions.

Procedure 5.3.4
If a mother is physically incapable of expressing milk herself, either because of a temporary medical condition or due to a long-term physical disability, staff should ensure that expression is initiated by either staff or other support persons, such as the father, within 6 hours of the delivery. As the mother recovers she may assume responsibility for expression.

Procedure 5.3.5
Upon her hospital discharge, the mother should be assisted in locating a rental grade pump for home use, similar to the one she has been using in the hospital.

Policy 5.4

All mothers should receive collection and storage guidelines for expressed milk. Instructions are provided per the NICU/SCN protocols, and a return demonstration should be given. Guidelines should include (but not be limited to) information on:

- Hand washing prior to expression
- Use of nipple products and creams
- Frequency and duration of pumping sessions
- Packaging instructions for feedings

- Labeling instructions
- Cleaning of pump kits and accessories
- Storage durations for refrigerators and freezers

Policy 5.5

An ample supply of clean collecting containers should be provided on a continuous basis by the NICU/SCN, along with personalized, waterproof labels containing the infant's identifying name and hospital medical record number.

Procedure 5.5.1
Preferred containers are hard-sided plastic, with airtight lids, calibrated, and of small portion size. Use of polyethylene bags for milk collection and storage during the hospitalization is strongly discouraged due to risk of contamination, loss of milk, and loss of valuable components in the milk, such as fat.

Procedure 5.5.2
Any colostrum or milk expressed should be saved for the infant. Small drops of colostrum expressed into the flange of the pump kit should be drawn into and stored in syringes until needed. Alternatively, small containers specifically designed for direct expression of colostrum without loss may also be used.

Policy 5.6

Protocols for storage of expressed milk should be developed according to the following basic guidelines:

- Freshly expressed milk must be refrigerated within 1 hour of expression if the milk will be used fresh within 48 hours. If milk will not be used within 48 hours, it should be frozen as soon as possible after expression.
- Milk can be refrigerated for up to 24 hours before freezing.
- Frozen expressed milk should be used within 3 months.
- Thawed milk should be used within 24 hours.

Procedure 5.6.1
Each NICU should have locked refrigerators and freezers with alarms dedicated solely for the storage of a mother's expressed milk.

Procedure 5.6.2
Mothers should be instructed on how to transport their frozen or refrigerated milk to the NICU/SCN and how to place it in the freezer/refrigerator for use.

Policy 5.7

The NICU/SCN and/or lactation staff should encourage mothers to express their feelings and concerns about adequate milk supply and transfer, beginning with the first NICU/SCN visit and continuing until the baby's discharge in an ongoing fashion.

Procedure 5.7.1
Mothers should be requested to keep a daily log of expressed milk volumes.

Procedure 5.7.2
NICU/SCN staff should access and evaluate mothers' daily logs a minimum of twice weekly.

Procedure 5.7.3
Mothers should be informed on a daily basis of current infant feeding volumes, so that packaging in feeding-sized portions can be adjusted as needed.

Procedure 5.7.4
Mothers who are pumping a minimum of eight times in a 24-hour period but whose volumes of expressed milk do not/cannot increase (e.g., insufficient glandular tissue, hormonal imbalances, breast surgery/injury) and are unable to meet the nutritional needs of their infants should be offered support and be provided opportunities to discuss their feelings and concerns in an ongoing manner.

Procedure 5.7.5
A NICU/SCN lactation support group that meets a minimum of once a week, facilitated by medical and or nursing and /or lactation staff, should be established to allow mothers to air their frustrations, ask for help, and realize that they are not alone. (See Step 10.)

REFERENCES

Furman, L., Minich, N., & Hack, M. (1998). Breastfeeding of very low birth weight infants. *Journal of Human Lactation, 14*(1), 29–34.

Kavanaugh, K., Meier, P., Zimmerman, B., & Mead, L. (1997). The rewards outweigh the efforts: Breastfeeding outcomes for mothers of preterm infants. *Journal of Human Lactation, 13*(1), 15–21.

Marinelli, K., & Hamelin, K. (2005). Breastfeeding and the use of human milk in the neonatal intensive care unit. In M. MacDonald, M. Mullet, & M. Seshia (Eds.), *Avery's neonatology: Pathophysiology and management of the newborn* (6th ed., pp. 413–444). Philadelphia: Lippincott Williams & Wilkins.

Meier, P. (2001). Breastfeeding in the special care nursery. Prematures and infants with medical problems. *Pediatric Clinics of North America, 48*(2), 425–442.

Wight, N., & Morton, J. (2007). Human milk, breastfeeding, and the preterm infant. In T. Hale & P. Hartmann (Eds.), *Textbook of human lactation* (pp. 215–253). Amarillo, TX: Hale Publishing, L.P.

Appendix 7-2

Recommendations for Collection, Storage, and Handling of a Mother's Own Milk for Her Infant in the Hospital Setting, 4th Edition

PREFACE

With the growing body of published evidence about the importance of feeding human milk to premature infants, it is now even more important that hospitals have protocols in place that assist mothers in expressing and storing their milk safely. Hospital protocols and policies should minimize barriers for the mother as well as minimize damage to the milk itself. Keeping expressed milk clean and safe is paramount; therefore recommendations of a public health nature must be conservative to cover as many outliers as possible and protect as many individuals as possible without placing undue burdens on them.

The importance of minimizing barriers to mothers cannot be overemphasized. Overloading mothers with rules and restrictions related to breastfeeding discourages mothers and leads them to choose formula feeding instead (Gabriel, Gabriel, & Lawrence, 1986). Similarly, if there are too many rules and restrictions for the expression of human milk, overwhelmed mothers may choose not to undertake this task despite knowing the benefits to the infant. Hospital staff should be knowledgeable about the physiology of lactation so that they may provide appropriate information and support to mothers who express their milk for hospitalized infants (Pantazi, Jaeger, & Lawson, 1998). Hospital staff also should know how to assist mothers with milk expression and storage in order to keep the process as simple as possible yet safe for the milk and for the infant. This should be the job of everyone who comes in contact with a mother in the NICU who is expressing milk, not just the role of the lactation specialist.

Since 1999, several articles have been published questioning whether it is safe for infants in NICUs to be fed milk that is collected at home (Rozolen, Goulart, & Kopelman, 2006; Ng, Lee, Leung, Wong, & Ho, 2004). However, these reports come from developing countries (Brazil, China) where it is probable that many mothers do not have access to clean water sources or a means of carefully cleaning containers for milk in the home. Cultural practices may also encourage higher than normal bacterial growth—in China it is traditional for many women to avoid bathing for one month postpartum (Ng, Lee, et al., 2004). In the United States, this is rarely a problem; more often the problem of milk contamination relates to lack of appropriate teaching and support for the mother. Reports such as these should not deter us in providing mothers' expressed milk as a rule, rather than as the exception, with as few restrictions placed on its use as possible.

These recommendations are intended to help hospitals establish evidence-based protocols and policies. Where research is lacking, the clinical experience of neonatologists and lactation care providers and common sense are used. These recommendations are specifically designed for the sick and hospitalized infant, not for the healthy, term infant whose mother will be returning to the workplace. Much of the research available is older research. Opportunities for future research abound.

Recommendations	Rationales
Section I: Parent Education and Support	
A. Written and verbal and/or video instructions should be supplied to each mother. Written instructions should be clear, easy to read (at no more than a sixth-grade reading level), translated into appropriate languages for the hospital population, and should include instructions for: 1. Proper hand-washing techniques 2. Washing and cleaning of pump parts 3. Storage, handling, and transport of milk 4. Labeling 5. Timing and length of pumping sessions to assure optimal milk supply 6. A phone number and a person to contact when concerns or questions arise	A. Research shows that mothers of hospitalized infants have many questions about expressing and storing their milk and keeping it as clean as possible (Forte, Mayberry, & Ferketich, 1987; Hopkinson, Schanler, & Garza, 1988). Verbal and video instructions are valuable, but written instructions for use at home are also essential for quality control. Translating of materials into appropriate languages for the hospital population enables clearer comprehension of instructions and better compliance with them. D'Amico, DiNardo, and Krystofiak (2003) stress the importance of repetitive education as well as face-to-face education between the nurse and the mother.

Recommendations	Rationales
Section II: Technology of Expression—Pumps and Accessory Kits for Expression	
A. Electric breast pumps that meet hospital electrical and biomedical requirements should be used to establish and maintain an adequate milk supply for a hospitalized infant.	A. In older studies, regular and frequent use of an electric breast pump with automatic cycling that met hospital electrical and biomedical standards established and maintained a milk supply that was higher in fat content than other forms of expression (Garza, Johnson, Harrist, & Nichols, 1982; Green, Moye, Schreiner, & Lemons, 1982). Most mothers find these pumps easier to use when frequent expression is required.
B. Manual expression should be taught to mothers as an adjunct to pumping mechanically.	B. Manual expression has been found to be the cleanest form of expression (Boo, Nordiah, Alfizah, Nor-Rohaini, & Lim, 2001; Liebhaber, Lewiston, Asquith, & Sunshine, 1978). An additional advantage of manual expression is the skin-to-skin contact that the mother has during massage and expression that helps maintain prolactin levels and milk supply.
C. Hand pumps of the bicycle horn variety should never be used to collect milk that will be fed to an infant.	C. There is no way of sterilizing the rubber bulbs of these older models of hand pumps. The bulbs themselves can become a major source of contamination (Lawrence & Lawrence, 2005; Liebhaber et al., 1978).
D. Each mother should be supplied with her own personal pumping kit with flanges that fit each breast and nipple.	D. Sharing of pump kits may be a source of cross-contamination. Tight nipple compression during expression may impede milk flow, causing long-term problems with milk supply and the potential for clogs and mastitis. The diameter of the flange tunnel should be large enough so that the nipple slides easily in and out of the tunnel without compression (Geddes, 2007).
E. Accessory kits (or manual pumps) should be cleaned after each use with hot soapy water and thoroughly rinsed. Washing in a dishwasher is also acceptable. F. Parts of accessory kits that do not actually touch the milk, e.g. tubing, should be cleaned or replaced according to the manufacturer's instructions. Tubing that has been washed may	E.–H. Manufacturer's instructions for cleaning accessory kits (and manual pumps) should be followed. There is no research to support the need for sterilization of pump kits after every use (Asquith, Sharp, & Stevenson, 1984). D'Amico et al. (2003) report that pumps and pump kits can be a significant vector for

Recommendations	Rationales
Section II: Technology of Expression—Pumps and Accessory Kits for Expression	
be dried by pouring rubbing alcohol through the tubing and allowing it to air dry. G. Bottled/boiled water should be used for cleaning pump kits in areas with contaminated water supplies. H. Washed pump parts and accessory kits can be placed, upside down, on a clean towel, covered with another clean paper or cloth towel, and allowed to air dry at home or at the baby's bedside on the counter or in a drawer.	bacterial infections in the NICU. Mothers should be advised not to touch the barrier filter membrane used in some pump setups because contamination of this membrane could lead to contamination of the milk. Collection bottles for the kit should be turned upside down and allowed to air dry or dried with a clean paper towel before being placed in other storage receptacles. Bacteria may multiply in the small droplets of moisture left behind.
Section III: Collection of Expressed Human Milk	
A. Mothers should wash their hands thoroughly before expression. Special care should be taken to clean nails and nail beds.	
1. If using an antimicrobial soap and water, wet hands with warm or cool water, apply soap and rub hands together vigorously for *at least* 15 seconds. Rinse hands with water; dry thoroughly with a clean paper towel. Use the towel to turn off the faucet.	1. Thorough hand washing is important as it reduces the potential for and degree of contamination of expressed milk (Barger & Bull, 1987; Larson, Zuill, Zier, & Berg, 1984; Sosa & Barness, 1987). According to the CDC, washing with regular soap suspends microorganisms and allows them to be rinsed off; washing with antimicrobial soap actually kills pathogens (CDC, 2002). When washing with soap and water, hands should be rubbed together for at least 15 seconds before rinsing and drying with a disposable paper towel.
2. If using an alcohol-based hand rub, follow manufacturer's instructions. Apply recommended amount to palm of hand and rub hands together, covering all surfaces. Rub until hands are dry. If hands are dry in less than 15 seconds, inadequate amounts of the hand-rub preparation have been used.	2. Alcohol-based hand cleaners are preferred by the CDC because of their excellent in vitro germicidal activity against both gram-positive and gram-negative bacteria as well as various fungi and enveloped viruses (CDC, 2002). They are more effective than antimicrobial soaps for standard handwashing and reducing the number of multidrug-resistant pathogens on the hands of healthcare workers.
3. Mothers should be instructed that long fingernails, artificial fingernails, and rings are sources of bacterial contamination, and that short fingernails are best.	3. Artificial nails are more likely to harbor gram-negative bacteria even after hand washing and have been implicated in outbreaks of infection in hospital settings. The concentration of

Recommendations	Rationales
Section III: Collection of Expressed Human Milk	
	gram-negative bacteria and *Staphylococcus aureus* rises with the number of rings worn (Kennedy, Elward, & Fraser, 2004). Artificial nails and extenders are not recommended for individuals in contact with patients in intensive care settings and natural nail tips should be kept at less than 0.25 inch in length. No recommendations about rings were made (CDC, 2002).
B. Breast cleansing routines are unnecessary and can be damaging to nipple skin. Routine daily hygiene is sufficient.	B. Routine daily hygiene is gentle on the breast and nipple tissue. Two protocols in past literature suggested the use of an antibacterial soap (Costa, 1989; Meier & Wilks, 1987) and one suggested the use of isopropanol (Minder, Roten, Zurbrugg, Gehriger, Lebek, & Nagel, 1982) to wash the breasts. The use of isopropanol and other breast cleansing protocols appear to be unnecessarily harsh on the nipple skin and may be a source of nipple pain. In some climates, extreme cleaning procedures (harsh soaps, drying agents, very hot water) may lead to chapping, flaking, and breakdown of skin and may result in cracks, which provide sites for infections. Studies that relied on daily hygiene rather than breast cleansing techniques (Barger & Bull, 1987; Sosa & Barness, 1987) or rinsing the breasts with sterile water prior to expression (Larson et al., 1984; Nwankwo, Offor, Okolo, & Omene, 1988; Pittard, Anderson, Cerutti, & Boxerbaum, 1985) showed no increase in contamination of milk.
C. Routine use of nipple lubricants is unnecessary. Where use is warranted, a product that can be safely ingested by the baby should be chosen.	C. Many commonly used nipple lubricants are not intended for internal use. If consumed while breastfeeding or in expressed milk they may be harmful to the infant (Lawrence & Lawrence, 2005, p. 284).

Recommendations	Rationales
Section III: Collection of Expressed Human Milk	
D. Mothers of hospitalized infants should be assisted with expressing their milk on a regular basis within the first 6 hours postpartum. 1. Delivery room, recovery room, postpartum, and NICU staff should know how to help a mother establish a milk supply through pumping. 2. When physically capable, mothers should begin expression within the first 6 hours postdelivery. 3. When a mother is physically incapable of expressing milk herself, staff should ensure that expression is initiated by either staff or other support persons within 12 hours of the mother's recovery (optimally sooner). Sufficient numbers of electric pumps should be available in delivery rooms and postpartum units as well as special pumping rooms. Electric pumps that meet hospital, electrical, and biomedical standards should be available to mothers for use during visits to the infant.	D. Delay of initiation in expression may result in lower prolactin levels and lower milk production (Hill, Brown, & Harker, 1995; Hopkinson et al., 1988; Lawrence & Lawrence, 2005). Helping a mother to express within the first 6 hours postdelivery resulted in higher milk volumes later (Furman, Minich, & Hack, 2002; Hill & Aldag, 2005; Hill, Aldag, & Chatterton, 2001). Delayed expression of milk is also associated with higher bacteria counts in the early milk of mothers of hospitalized infants (Asquith, Pedrotti, Harrod, Stevenson, & Sunshine, 1984). This is most likely due to stasis of the milk. Bacterial counts dropped dramatically with the establishment of the free flow of milk.
E. It is unnecessary to express and discard the first few ccs of milk prior to expressing and saving milk for a feeding.	E. While discarding the first several ccs of milk has been suggested by some for the collection of *banked donor* milk (Asquith & Harrod, 1979), this practice may seriously affect the amount of expressed milk that is available to a mother's own baby, since many mothers are not able to express large amounts of milk, especially in the colostral phase (Lawrence & Lawrence, 2005, p. 768). Although some early literature suggested that bacteria counts in early milk could be lowered by discarding the first few ccs of an expression (West, Hewett, & Murphy, 1979), other studies and clinical practice in many settings have shown it to be unnecessary (Carroll, Osman, & Davies, 1980; Pittard et al., 1985; Pittard, Geddes, Brown, Mintz, & Hulsey, 1991).

Recommendations	Rationales
Section III: Collection of Expressed Human Milk	
F. Each expression of milk should be collected in its own separate container. Expressions should not be layered. Even small drops of colostrum should be drawn into a syringe and saved to be used for either feeding or oral care.	F. Layering milk from several expressions requires opening the container several times to add fresh milk to what has already been expressed. Each time the container is opened the opportunity for milk contamination increases. Small samples chill more rapidly than large ones in the refrigerator.
G. Mothers should be encouraged to store expressed milk in feeding-sized portions. 1. Mothers should receive frequent updates on feeding volumes so that feeding portions can be adjusted appropriately.	G. Storing expressed milk in feeding-sized portions will minimize waste and decrease the risk of contamination from frequent entry into the container (Larson et al., 1984).
H. Individualized labels for each container should be provided. These should include the infant's name and hospital ID number. Mothers should add the date and time of expression with a waterproof marker. Any illnesses or use of medications can also be clearly indicated on the label.	H. Clear labeling will help prevent feeding errors and assure that each infant receives his/her own mother's milk.
I. Milk that is only partially thawed and not previously fed to the infant (e.g., milk that partially thaws while being transported from home; less than 50% of volume thawed) may be refrozen in the interest of maximizing the volume of milk available to the infant and preventing waste.	I. There is no research to indicate that milk that has been partially thawed is unsafe, and intrinsic anti-infective properties of the milk may still be active although at a reduced level. Neville (1995) reports that repeated freezing and thawing may break down the milk fat globule membrane and expose the inner surface to binding by ions and other milk components. Frequent partial thawing should therefore be avoided. Other researchers report that lipases remain active during refrigeration and freezing (Berkow et al., 1984; Lavine & Clark, 1987). Breakdown of the fats during lipolysis may actually increase the antiviral, antibacterial, and antiparasitic activity of the milk (Hamosh, 1994; Hamosh et al., 1996; Isaacs & Thormar, 1990).
Section IV: Types of Containers	
A. Mothers should have access to an ample supply of suitable food-grade aseptic containers. Containers should be free of bisphenol A (BPA).	A. Although most hospital policies recommend the use of sterile containers for collection of a mother's own milk, aseptic or clean containers used for storage of human milk show no increase in bacterial contamination when compared to sterile containers (Pittard et al., 1991).

Recommendations	Rationales
Section IV: Types of Containers	
B. Containers should attach directly to standard pump kits to avoid transfer of milk and potential contamination during transfer.	B. Any time milk is transferred from one container to another, the potential for external contamination increases.
C. Aseptic containers should have caps that will provide an airtight seal.	C. Container lids that will provide an airtight seal are preferred over nipple units for human milk storage. Tight caps reduce the risk of contamination of the expressed milk as well as the exposure of nutrients in the milk to oxidation.
D. Storage containers for expressed human milk should be hard sided, either plastic or glass.	D. Several manufacturers now make containers with tight-fitting lids that are FDA approved, attach directly to pump bodies, are BPA-free, and have zero fat adhesion. However, the types of materials containers are made from have drawbacks (Hurst, Myatt, & Schanler, 1998). Hard plastic or glass containers show the smallest loss of immunologic factors during storage compared to milk storage bags. Fat is lost to a greater extent in many plastic containers because of adherence to the sides of the containers and the inability to mix the fat back into the milk with gentle shaking (Hamosh, 1994). Forceful shaking breaks the milk fat globule membrane. In an early study that looked at brief milk storage duration, white blood cells present in the milk appeared to adhere more to glass than plastic (Paxson & Cress, 1979). Later studies that looked at different types of blood cells as well as the duration of milk storage found that white cells actually detach more rapidly from glass than plastic over time (Goldblum et al., 1981; Hamosh, 1994; Pittard & Bill, 1981). Lysozyme, lactoferrin, sIgA, and other immunologic components of human milk may also be affected by the type of storage container, with storage in glass appearing to maintain concentrations better than plastic (Goldblum et al., 1981; Lawrence, 1999, 2001). Some vitamins are also lost when plastic containers are used for storage, although these losses may not be statistically significant (Van Zoeren-Grobben, Schrijver, Van den Berg, & Berger, 1987). Heat is the most significant cause of vitamin content being altered.

Recommendations	Rationales
Section IV: Types of Containers	
E. Use of polyethylene bags for milk storage is strongly discouraged.	E. Loss of fat is considerably higher when milk is stored in polyethylene bags. Coupled with the later loss of fat when feeding tubes are used, this loss may be significant to a premature infant who needs to maximize caloric intake for improved growth and weight gain (Mehta et al., 1988). Fat-soluble vitamins may also be lost as a result of storage in bags (Hamosh, 1994). Early research indicated that 60% of sIgA specific for *Escherichia coli* polysaccharides was lost when milk was stored in polyethylene bags (Goldblum, Garza, Johnson, Harrist, Nichols, & Goldman, 1981; Garza & Nichols, 1984). However, newer research using enzyme-linked immunosorbent assay (ELISA) testing was not able to confirm this finding (Beezhold, 1998). Bags puncture and split easily, even the thicker ones, and the risk of milk contamination and loss of milk is much greater than with hard-sided containers. The heat-sealed seam is the weakest point. Drawing feedings into syringes from bags is extremely difficult to do without increasing contamination of the milk and breaking fat globule membranes (Garza & Nichols, 1984; Garza et al., 1986). Bags are difficult to seal. They are not airtight, and milk components may become oxidized and lost.
Section V: Storage	
A. Definitions of types of storage include the following: 1. **Fresh milk**: Milk held at room temperature (less than 25°C [77°F]) or milk held in a refrigerator at approximately 4°C (39°F). 2. **Frozen milk**: Milk held at approximately -20°C (-4°F) or -70°C (-94°F). 3. **Thawed milk**: Milk that has been previously frozen.	
B. Freezers that maintain -20°C (-4°F) should be used. Manual defrost freezers are preferable because (1) they do not warm up every 24 hrs to remove the collected frost (as in frost free); and (2) the cooling element may actually be in the shelf itself.	B. Freezers should maintain -20°C within a narrow range of variation. This can be done best when freezers are opened infrequently. Since NICU freezers are opened frequently, having the cooling element in the shelf will help maintain lower temperatures more consistently.

Recommendations	Rationales
Section V: Storage	
	Freezers that hold -70°C (-94°F) are usually intended for research purposes, but storage at this temperature or -20°C has minimal effect on milk components. As long as the milk fat globule membrane is intact, milk lipases remain relatively inactive (Berkow et al., 1984). Most home refrigerator freezers and some freezers in hospitals do not approach -20°C (-4°F) because of frequent door opening, and milk composition may change more rapidly in these cases. Hospital staff should ascertain the adequacy of home freezer space and help the family problem-solve if they do not have room at home for overflow from NICU freezers.
C. Dedicated freezers and refrigerators should be provided for human milk storage. They should be tilted slightly backward at installation so that doors close automatically.	C. Providing storage space for human milk that is separate from other food items, specimens, or drugs is a hospital code requirement. Tilting freezers slightly backwards will prevent accidental thawing of freezer contents if the door does not get closed properly.
D. Freezers and refrigerators that store human milk should be plugged into the emergency power supply (red plugs in hospitals). Alarms should be installed on freezers to alert hospital staff if the temperature rises above acceptable levels.	D. It is important to prevent thawing of the milk during a power failure or accidental failure to close the freezer door completely.
E. Freezers or refrigerators in hospitals that are placed in areas accessible to the public should have locks.	E. Locks on freezers and refrigerators will protect milk against sabotage. There should be a written policy on access to freezers and refrigerators used for human milk storage.
F. Policies should be developed for periodic cleaning and sanitizing of freezers and refrigerators used for the storage of human milk.	F. Refrigerators used for human milk storage should be cleaned with a bacteriocidal/viricidal solution on a regular basis and whenever there are spills of thawed or fresh milk so that other storage containers are not exposed to contaminants from the spills. Freezers also need to be defrosted and thoroughly cleaned on a regular basis, particularly if they are manual defrost types of freezers (for example, when the frost builds up to a specified thickness.) Frost-free freezers need periodic cleaning with a bacteriocidal/viricidal solution to ensure cleanliness, especially the door handles.
G. It is inappropriate to label freezers used for human milk with biohazard stickers.	G. Besides the inappropriate message that may be conveyed to mothers and hospital staff, human milk does not constitute a biohazard and does

Recommendations	Rationales
Section V: Storage	
	not require universal precautions when handled for feeding. "Although universal precautions do not apply to human breast milk, gloves may be worn by health care workers in situations where exposures to breast milk might be frequent, e.g., in breast [donor] milk banking." (CDC, 1999; see also OSHA, 1992).
H. Storage durations	
1. Expressed milk should be refrigerated immediately or placed in a cooler with blue ice within 1 hour of expressing.	1. For the preterm or sick infant, caution is appropriate, and it is safest to refrigerate milk right after pumping. Numerous studies have looked at the effects of storage time and temperature on bacterial counts in human milk (Barger & Bull, 1987; Larson et al., 1984; Olowe et al., 1987; Pardou et al., 1994; Pittard et al., 1985; Sosa & Barness, 1987). Some researchers studying milk held at room temperature report a variety of safe storage times (Nwankwo et al., 1988; Ajusi, Onyango, Mutanda, & Wamola, 1989; Hamosh, Ellis, Pollock, Henderson, & Hamosh, 1996). However, study designs vary considerably, definitions of room temperature may be different, and results may be inappropriate for the preterm or ill infant.
2. Milk that will not be used completely by 48 hours after expression should be frozen.	2. Several studies looking at the effects of refrigeration on storage for varying periods from 24 hours to 8 days found no appreciable bacterial growth over these storage times (Larson et al., 1984; Olowe, Ahmed, Lawal, & Ransome-Kuti, 1987; Pardou et al., 1994; Pittard et al., 1985; Sosa & Barness, 1987). In a majority of samples, colony counts decreased or remained the same over time, with refrigeration having a greater inhibitory effect on bacterial growth than freezing. The recommended 48 hours of refrigerated storage is within a bacteriologically safe range and is conservative enough to cover variables in home refrigeration, time and temperature,

Recommendations	Rationales
Section V: Storage	
	collection techniques, hospital transport, and hospital exposure to multiple caregivers. Schanler, Slutzah, Codipilly, and Potak (2008) recommend that storage in the refrigerator beyond 48 hours be considered based on a small pilot study of milk held in the refrigerator for 96 hours. There were no significant differences in osmolality, white blood cell count, gram-negative colony count, or concentrations of sIgA and lactoferrin, but pH and total and gram-positive bacteria counts decreased significantly. Hanna et al. (2004) found that antioxidant activity of human milk was better preserved with refrigeration for up to 48 hours. Longer durations of storage in either the refrigerator or the freezer resulted in greater loss of antioxidant activity. (See also Ankrah, Appiah-Opong, & Dzokoto, 2000.)
3. Frozen milk should be used by oldest date first. Milk should be used within 3 months of expression for the hospitalized, premature infant. However, use of older milk is preferable to no human milk, and older milk should not be discarded. As feedings are begun, colostrum and transitional milk, even if frozen, should be used first before fresh milk.	3. The milk enzymes, lipoprotein lipase, and bile salt stimulated lipase remain active during storage at -20°C (-4°F). As the temperature declines there is a reduction in the rate of chemical reactions. At -70°C (-94°F) enzymatic reactions that denature fat do not occur. At -20°C (-4°F) milk fat continues to be hydrolyzed and triglyceride concentrations decrease, resulting in smells ranging from a slightly soapy smell to a rancid smell. Infants may or may not reject this flavor change (Lawrence, 1999). Three months of freezing was found to cause minimal loss of biologic activity in human milk (Friend, Shahani, Long, & Vaughn, 1983). However, Berkow, Freed, Hamosh, Bitman, Wood, Happ, et al. (1984) found that lipase activity was minimal as long as the milk fat globule membrane stayed intact (see I. later in this table).

Recommendations	Rationales
Section V: Storage	
4. Colostrum, either fresh or frozen, should always be used first for feeding purposes before mature milk. Fresh, mature milk that the mother has brought in should be used preferentially over frozen milk, despite its being out of order of expression dates.	4. A hierarchy of enteral feeding order exists. Colostrum, whether it is frozen or fresh, should always be used first when enteral feedings are initiated, before any mature milk is used. This will help protect the gut and prime it. The next choice is fresh milk because fewer components have been compromised in the freezing process and live white blood cells in the milk may also be protective of the infant. Finally, frozen milk should be used.
Section VI: Bacteriological Quality Control	
A. Bacteriological screening of a mother's milk	
1. Withholding a mother's milk from her infant while waiting for routine bacteriological screening of the milk is unnecessary and not medically indicated in most circumstances. 2. If an infant becomes ill, bacteriological screening of the milk may be beneficial and should be considered as part of standard techniques for determining the origin of infection.	1. Mothers should never be made to feel that their milk is dirty. Routine screening programs often preclude feeding fresh breastmilk to an infant. Frequently it takes longer than 48 hours to get laboratory culture results. In a large study (Law, Urias, Lertzman, Robson, & Romance, 1989) routine screening was ineffective in limiting the bacterial content for less prevalent and potentially pathogenic organisms. Furthermore, those infants receiving milk that contained these organisms appeared to suffer no ill effects. Other studies also report no ill effects in infants from being fed potential pathogens in human milk (Narayanan, Prakash, & Gujral, 1983).
B. Hospital pumps	
1. Hospital staff should be responsible for monitoring electric breast pumps used by multiple mothers, such as pumps placed in lactation rooms. Pumps should be cleaned daily, checked for milk backup, and regularly monitored for suction levels with pressure gauges according to the manufacturers' instructions. Pumps contaminated internally with milk or that have been used by someone with an infectious disease should be removed from use and serviced completely according to protocols for hospital equipment.	1. Hospital pumps can malfunction, be misused, and may be overlooked as a possible source of contamination. Pumps that malfunction or do not function optimally may inhibit establishment of a good milk supply. Pumps are patient equipment and should be treated similarly to other hospital equipment.

Recommendations	Rationales
Section VI: Bacteriological Quality Control	
2. To avoid the possibility of cross-contamination, accessory kits should exclude the possibility of milk backup into the pump and backflow of aerosols into the milk. Mothers should be instructed carefully in the proper configuration of the kit.	2. Instructions from pump companies for use of the kit should be followed. a. Accessory kits used incorrectly may easily cause milk backup in a pump, necessitating the pump's removal from service for thorough cleaning. b. Just as with other patient equipment, if a mother or baby has a communicable disease, the mother should not share a pump with other mothers. The pump kit may be likened to a piece of personal hygiene equipment.
Section VII: Transporting Milk	
A. For short-distance transport, milk should be packed tightly in a cooler *without* ice during transport to the hospital. A clean towel or Styrofoam beads can be used to fill extra space. Blue ice or freezer gel packs may be used.	A. Milk should be maintained in a frozen state during transport to reduce the risk of warming of the milk that could encourage bacterial growth. *Note*: Milk freezes at a lower temperature than water; therefore, ice is warmer than frozen milk and actually may thaw milk somewhat. Freezer gel packs are acceptable because they have a lower freezing point than water.
B. Frozen milk that must be shipped requiring more than 18 hours' removal from the freezer should be packed in dry ice and shipped in a sturdy insulated container. Ambient weather temperatures should be considered when packing milk for shipping. Bottles should be individually wrapped and well cushioned to prevent breakage and to provide better insulation. *Note*: Not all shippers will allow dry ice as part of the shipment. Check with shipping companies for allowable weight limits for dry ice. Some shippers only allow 5.0 pounds per package.	B. Frozen milk will remain frozen for several hours if well packed in a cooler. Dry ice for longer shipping distances will help prevent milk from partially thawing and prevent bacterial growth and deterioration of nutrient quality.

(*continues*)

Recommendations	Rationales
Section VIII: Feeding Expressed Milk to the Infant	
A. Staff should always practice good hand-washing techniques prior to handling, preparing feedings, or during actual feeding.	A. Careful hand cleansing by staff when handling human milk decreases the risk of contamination or disease transmission from the care provider or milk handler to the milk during the preparation process. Use of an alcohol-based hand rub and gloves in one NICU setting reduced the incidence of methicillin-resistant *Staphylococcus aureus* (MRSA) septicemia as well as the incidence of late onset systemic infection (including NEC) significantly (Ng, Wong, Lyon, So, Liu, Lam, et al., 2004).
B. Thawing procedures:	
1. Rapid thawing may be done either by holding the bottle of milk under cool or *lukewarm* running tap water or by allowing milk containers to stand in warm water until thawed. The water level should not touch the bottle cap.	1.–4. Rapid thawing has the advantage over slower thawing of causing less damage to milk fat globule membranes (Berkow et al., 1984). Thawing under running tap water may introduce contamination if the container lid becomes wet. Thawing in running water should never be unattended.
2. Basins of warming or thawing milk should never be left in the sink, where they may become contaminated.	
3. Bottle warmers using dry heat may be used according to hospital protocols. Settings should not overheat the milk.	
4. To avoid using the wrong milk, milk for each infant should be thawed and warmed separately from milk for another infant.	
5. Thawing should never be done in a microwave oven.	5. Microwave thawing significantly decreases the activity of many anti-infective factors, including lysozyme, total IgA, and secretory IgA specific to several forms of *E. coli*, allowing for greater *E. coli* growth (Quan, Yang, Rubenstein, Lewiston, Sunshine, Stevenson, et al., 1992; Sigman, Burke, Swarner, & Shavlik, 1989). Vitamin C appears to be negatively affected by microwaving as well and can be reduced by as much as 40% (Lawrence, 1999). Other components may be affected because of the excessive heat rather than the microwaves themselves. There is an increased potential for hot spots with uneven heating in the microwave, and safety becomes an issue (Nemethy & Clore, 1990).

Recommendations	Rationales
Section VIII: Feeding Expressed Milk to the Infant	
C. Warming milk	
1. Human milk should only be warmed to approximately body temperature (37°C [98.6°F]) and not be subjected to excessive heat. Warming milk for feeding can be done rapidly by holding the container under warm running tap water prior to use. Gentle swirling is also recommended to resuspend fats.	1. Milk needs to be warmed very little. Excessive heat destroys components that are beneficial to the premature and sick infant. For example, bile salt-dependent lipase is very sensitive to heat. (Bjørkstén, Burman, De Château, Fredrikzon, Gothefors, & Hernell, 1980; Garza, Hopkinson, & Schanler, 1986; Wardell, Wright, Bardsley, & D'Souza, 1984). Bile salt-dependent lipase activity is reduced by 15–20% when milk is kept at 38°C (100.4°F) for several hours, only slightly above body temperature. (Hamosh, Henderson, Ellis, Mao, & Hamosh, 1997). *Note*: Controlled temperature hot air incubators can be advantageous for warming milk for a particular baby. Individual characteristics need to be determined, and each hospital needs to establish its own quality control conditions for warming milk.
2. Only the amount of milk needed for a feeding should be warmed. Milk that has been warmed for a feeding but not used should be discarded.	2. Warming can initiate bacterial proliferation.
3. Pasteurizing of mothers' own milk is not recommended except under rare medical circumstances.	3. Pasteurizing a mother's own milk for her infant is unnecessary and may destroy not only her sense of competence as a mother but also her milk's unique immunological protection for her infant.
D. Tube (gavage) feeding 1. Short feeding tubes and single syringe infusion pumps should be used. 2. The syringe pump apparatus should be placed below the isolette and oriented with the tip pointing upward. 3. All syringes should be emptied completely and flushed following hospital protocols.	1.–3. When tube feeding human milk to infants, a major concern is loss of fat due to its separation and adherence to the walls of feeding tubes (Mehta, Hamosh, Bitman, & Wood, 1988; Narayanan, Singh, & Harvey, 1984; Stocks, Davies, Allen, & Sewell, 1985; Tacken, Vogelsang, van Lingen, Slootstra, Dikkeschel, & Van Zoeren-Grobben, 2009). Reduction of available surface area by shortening feeding tubes and orienting the syringe so that fat will rise and be pushed through the tube first will minimize these losses. Larger bore tubing also reduces the fat loss (Brennan-Behm, Carlson, Meier, &

(*continues*)

Recommendations	Rationales
Section VIII: Feeding Expressed Milk to the Infant	
	Engstrom, 1994). Lavine and Clark (1989) found that refrigeration of milk for three days (4°C) increased delivery of lipids during an 8-hour continuous infusion.
4. With continuous feedings, syringe systems should be changed every 4 hours.	4. Continuous tube feedings of human milk require holding milk at room temperature for long periods of time, which could allow small numbers of bacteria to increase substantially, particularly if the milk has been warmed (Botsford, Weinstein, Boyer, Nathan, Carman, & Paton, 1986). Hamosh et al. (1996) showed that storage of freshly expressed milk at room temperature (25°C; 77°F) is safe for 4 hours and does not result in an increase in bacteria. Similar results were found in a study of tube feeding on previously frozen milk although no ambient temperature was given (Dodd & Froman, 1991). Changing the syringe every 4 hours also reduces breakdown of milk components that are light sensitive (Bates, Liu, Fuller, & Lucas, 1985; Jocson, Mason, & Schanler, 1997; Lemons, Miller, Eitzen, Strodtbeck, & Lemons, 1983; Santiago, Codipilly, Potak, & Schanler, 2005).
E. Preparation of feedings	
1. Fortifiers and other additives should be added by experienced personnel in separate preparation areas using specific protocols that assure clean techniques.	1. Mixing of feedings in designated areas by trained personnel: a. promotes appropriate supplementation b. prevents contamination c. reduces the risk of errors (see Dumm, Peel, Jones, Lore, Hunter, Kendall-Harris, et al., 2007)
2. Human milk to which fortifiers have been added should be used within 24 hours of fortification.	2. Total bacterial colony counts were significantly higher in fortified human milk than in unfortified human milk held in the refrigerator and increased over time. Bacterial counts did not change significantly during the first 20 hours of refrigeration but increased during a 4-hour simulation of warming and feeding (Jocson et al., 1997; Schanler, 1996).

Recommendations	Rationales
Section VIII: Feeding Expressed Milk to the Infant	
3. Labels on milk must state the time and date when additives were placed in the milk so that any left at the end of 24 hours may be discarded.	
F. Duration of usage	
1. Milk left in the feeding container after a feeding should be discarded and not reused.	1. There is no research to suggest that refeeding partially fed bottles is safe.
2. Thawed milk that has not been warmed for use or fed to the infant should be stored in the refrigerator and used within 24 hours.	
G. Charting of feedings	
1. The type of feeding (e.g., fresh, refrigerated, thawed), the method of feeding (e.g., gavage, bottle, cup), and the amount fed should be recorded in the baby's chart.	1. All feedings should be charted in detail.
2. Fortifiers and other additives should also be documented in the infant's chart.	
H. Protocols for accidental feedings	
1. Hospitals should have policies and procedures in place in order to prevent and deal with any accidental feeding of a mother's milk to the wrong infant.	1. While this situation appears to occur infrequently, it is a significant error and may be extremely traumatic for the parents of the infant who was fed incorrectly, for the mother who became the inadvertent donor, and for the staff involved in the feeding error. Hospitals may address this issue in a variety of ways, e.g., double checking by another staff person before feeding an infant to ensure that labels match, similar to check-off procedures before blood transfusions are given; preparing the feeding at the infant's bedside rather than in a common work space, etc. One tertiary care center in the United States implemented six sigma quality improvement methodologies and reduced the risk of breast milk administration errors to fewer than 3.4 mistakes per 1 million opportunities (Drenckpohl, Bowers, & Cooper, 2007).
2. When administration errors are made, and the wrong milk is fed to an infant, the exposure should be treated in the same manner as an accidental exposure to other body fluids would be treated. The hospital should bear the cost of any testing for both the donor and recipient.	2. The CDC has a protocol available for what to do in the case of an administration error (CDC, 2007).

REFERENCES

Ajusi, J. D., Onyango, F. E., Mutanda, L. N., & Wamola, I. A. (1989). Bacteriology of unheated expressed breast milk stored at room temperature. *East African Medical Journal, 66*(6), 381–387.

Ankrah, N., Appiah-Opong, R., & Dzokoto, C. (2000). Human breastmilk storage and the glutathione content. *Journal of Tropical Pediatrics, 46*(2), 111–113.

Asquith, M. T., & Harrod, J. (1979). Reduction of bacterial contamination in banked human milk. *Journal of Pediatics, 95*(6), 993–994.

Asquith, M. T., Pedrotti, P. W., Harrod, J. R., Stevenson, D. K., & Sunshine, P. (1984). The bacterial content of breast milk after the early initiation of expression using a standard technique. *Journal of Pediatric Gastroenterology and Nutrition, 3*(1), 104–107.

Asquith, M. T., Sharp, R., & Stevenson, D. K. (1984). Decreased bacterial contamination of human milk expressed with an electric breast pump. *Journal of the California Perinatal Association, 4*(22), 45–47.

Barger, J., & Bull, P. (1987, August). A comparison of the bacterial composition of breast milk stored at room temperature and stored in the refrigerator. *International Journal of Childbirth Education, 2*(3), 29–30.

Bates, C., Liu, D., Fuller, N., & Lucas, A. (1985). Susceptibility of riboflavin and vitamin A in breast milk to photodegradation and its implications for the use of banked breast milk in infant feeding. *Acta Paediatrica Scandinavica, 74*(1), 40–44.

Beezhold, D. H. (1998). Polyethylene storage containers do not affect secretory IgA levels in human breast milk. *Canadian Journal of Allergy and Clinical Immunology, 3*(4), 177–180.

Berkow, S., Freed, L., Hamosh, M., Bitman, J., Wood, D., Happ, B., et al. (1984). Lipases and lipids in human milk: Effect of freeze-thawing and storage. *Pediatric Research, 18*(12), 1257–1262.

Bjørkstén, B., Burman, L. G., De Château, P., Fredrikzon, B., Gothefors, L., & Hernell, O. (1980). Collecting and banking human milk: To heat or not to heat? *British Medical Journal, 281*(6243), 765–769.

Boo, N., Nordiah, A., Alfizah, H., Nor-Rohaini, A., & Lim, V. (2001). Contamination of breast milk obtained by manual expression and breast pumps in mothers of very low birthweight infants. *Journal of Hospital Infection, 49*(4), 274–281.

Botsford, K. B., Weinstein, R. A., Boyer, K. M., Nathan, C., Carman, M., & Paton, J. B. (1986). Gram-negative bacilli in human milk feedings: Quantitation and clinical consequences for premature infants. *Journal of Pediatrics, 109*(4), 707–710.

Brennan-Behm, M., Carlson, G. E., Meier, P., & Engstrom, J. (1994). Caloric loss from expressed mother's milk during continuous gavage infusion. *Neonatal Network, 13*(2), 27–32.

Carroll, L., Osman, M., & Davies, D. P. (1980). Does discarding the first few millilitres of breast milk improve the bacteriological quality of bank breast milk? *Archives of Disease in Childhood, 55*(11), 898–899.

Centers for Disease Control and Prevention, Hospital Infections Program, National Center for Infectious Diseases (CDC). (1999). *Universal precautions for prevention of transmission of HIV and other bloodborne infections.* Retrieved March 5, 2009, from http://www.cdc.gov/ncidod/dhqp/bp_universal_precautions.html

Centers for Disease Control and Prevention (CDC). (2002). Guideline for hand hygiene in health-care settings. Recommendations of the Healthcare Infection Control Practices Advisory Committee and the HICPAC/SHEA/APIC/IDSA Hand Hygiene Task Force. In J. Boyce & D. Pittet (Eds.), *Morbidity and Mortality Weekly Report, 51*(RR-16), 1–44. Retrieved March 5, 2009, from http://www.cdc.gov/mmwr/preview/mmwrhtml/rr5116a1.htm

Centers for Disease Control and Prevention (CDC). (2007). *What to do if an infant is mistakenly fed another woman's expressed breast milk*. Retrieved March 5, 2009, from http://www.cdc.gov/breastfeeding/recommendations/other_mothers_milk.htm

Costa, K. M. (1989). A comparison of colony counts of breast milk using two methods of breast cleansing. *Journal of Obstetric, Gynecologic, and Neonatal Nursing, 18*(3), 231–236.

D'Amico, C. J., DiNardo, C. A., & Krystofiak, S. (2003). Preventing contamination of breast pump kit attachments in the NICU. *Journal of Perinatal and Neonatal Nursing, 17*(2), 150–157.

Dodd, V., & Froman, R. (1991). A field study of bacterial growth in continuous feedings in a neonatal intensive care unit. *Neonatal Network, 9*(6), 17–21.

Drenckpohl, D., Bowers, L., & Cooper H. (2007). Use of the six sigma methodology to reduce incidence of breast milk administration errors in the NICU. *Neonatal Network, 26*(3), 161–166.

Dumm, M., Peel, L., Jones, A., Lore, P., Hunter, C., Kendall-Harris, M., et al. (2007). Certified formula room technician program improves safety and quality of product delivered to infants in neonatal intensive care. *Journal of the American Dietetic Association, 107*(8), A49.

Forte, A., Mayberry, L. J., & Ferketich, S. (1987). Breast milk collection and storage practices among mothers of hospitalized neonates. *Journal of Perinatology, 7*(1), 35–39.

Friend, B. A., Shahani, K. M., Long, C. A., & Vaughn, L. A. (1983). The effect of processing and storage on key enzymes, B vitamins, and lipids of mature human milk. I. Evaluation of fresh samples and effects of freezing and frozen storage. *Pediatric Research, 17*(1), 61–64.

Furman, L., Minich, N., & Hack, M. (2002). Correlates of lactation in mothers of very low birth weight infants. *Pediatrics, 109*(4), e57.

Gabriel, A., Gabriel, K. R., & Lawrence, R. A. (1986). Cultural values and biomedical knowledge: Choices in infant feeding: analysis of a survey. *Social Science and Medicine, 23*(5), 501–509.

Garza, C., Hopkinson, J., & Schanler, R. J. (1986). Human milk banking. In R. R. Howell, F. H. Morriss, & L. K. Pickering (Eds.), *Human milk in infant nutrition and health* (pp. 225–255). Springfield, IL: Charles C. Thomas Publisher.

Garza, C., Johnson, C. A., Harrist, R., & Nichols, B. L. (1982). Effects of methods of collection and storage on nutrients in human milk. *Early Human Development, 6*(3), 295–303.

Garza, C., & Nichols, B. L. (1984). Studies of human milk relevant to milk banking. *Journal of the American College of Nutrition, 3*(2), 123–129.

Geddes, D. (2007). Gross anatomy of the lactating breast. In T. Hale & P. Hartmann (Eds.), *Textbook of human lactation* (pp. 19–34). Amarillo, TX: Hale Publishing, L.P.

Goldblum, R. M., Garza, C., Johnson, C. A., Harrist, R., Nichols, B. L., & Goldman, A. S. (1981). Human milk banking. I. Effects of container upon immunologic factors in mature milk. *Nutrition Research, 1*(5), 449–459.

Green, D., Moye, L., Schreiner, R. L., & Lemons, J. A. (1982). The relative efficacy of four methods of human milk expression. *Early Human Development, 6*(2), 153–159.

Hamosh, M. (1994). *Breast milk storage: Review of the literature and recommendations for research needs*. San Diego, CA: Wellstart International.

Hamosh, M., Ellis, L. A., Pollock, D. R., Henderson, T. R., & Hamosh, P. (1996). Breastfeeding and the working mother: Effect of time and temperature of short-term storage on proteolysis, lipolysis, and bacterial growth in milk. *Pediatrics, 97*(4), 492–498.

Hamosh, M., Henderson, T. R., Ellis, L. A., Mao, J. I., & Hamosh, P. (1997). Digestive enzymes in human milk: Stability at suboptimal storage temperatures. *Journal of Pediatric Gastroenterology and Nutrition, 24*(1), 38–43.

Hanna, N., Ahmend, K., Anwar, M., Petrova, A., Hiatt, M., & Hegyi, T. (2004). Effect of storage on breast milk antioxidant activity. *Archives of Disease in Childhood, Fetal and Neonatal Edition, 89*(6), F518–F520.

Hill, P., & Aldag, J. (2005). Milk volume on day 4 and income predictive of lactation adequacy at 5 weeks of mothers of nonnursing preterm infants. *Journal of Perinatal and Neonatal Nursing, 19*(3), 273–282.

Hill, P., Aldag, J., & Chatterton, R. (2001). Initiation and frequency of pumping and milk production in mothers of non-nursing preterm infants. *Journal of Human Lactation, 17*(1), 9–13.

Hill, P. D., Brown, L. P., & Harker, T. L. (1995). Initiation and frequency of breast expression in breastfeeding mothers of LBW and VLBW infants. *Nursing Research, 44*(6), 352–355.

Hopkinson, J., Schanler, R., & Garza, C. (1988). Milk production by mothers of premature infants. *Pediatrics, 81*(6), 815–820.

Hurst, N. M., Myatt, A., & Schanler, R. J. (1998). Growth and development of a hospital-based lactation program and mother's own milk bank. *Journal of Obstetric, Gynecologic, and Neonatal Nursing, 27*(5), 503–510.

Isaacs, C. E., & Thormar, H. (1990). Human milk lipids inactivate enveloped viruses. In S. A. Atkinson, L. A. Hanson, & R. K. Chandra (Eds.), *Breastfeeding, nutrition, infection and infant growth in developed and emerging countries* (pp. 161–174). St. John's, Newfoundland, Canada: ARTS Biomedical Publishers and Distributors.

Jocson, M., Mason, E. O., & Schanler, R. J. (1997). The effects of nutrient fortification and varying storage conditions on host defense properties of human milk. *Pediatrics, 100*(2 Pt. 1), 240–243.

Kennedy, A., Elward, A., & Fraser, V. (2004). Survey of knowledge, beliefs, and practices of neonatal intensive care unit healthcare workers regarding nosocomial infections, central venous catheter care, and hand hygiene. *Infection Control and Hospital Epidemiology, 25*(9), 747–752.

Larson, E., Zuill, R., Zier, V., & Berg, B. (1984). Storage of human breast milk. *Infection Control, 5*(3), 127–130.

Lavine, M., & Clark, R. M. (1987). Changing patterns of free fatty acids in breast milk during storage. *Journal of Pediatric Gastroenterology and Nutrition, 6*(5), 769–774.

Lavine, M., & Clark, R. M. (1989). The effect of short-term refrigeration of milk and addition of breast milk fortifier on the delivery of lipids during tube feeding. *Journal of Pediatric Gastroenterology and Nutrition, 8*(4), 496–499.

Law, B. J., Urias, B. A., Lertzman, J., Robson, D., & Romance, L. (1989). Is ingestion of milk-associated bacteria by premature infants fed raw human milk controlled by routine bacteriologic screening? *Journal of Clinical Microbiology, 27*(7), 1560–1566.

Lawrence, R. A. (1999). Storage of human milk and the influence of procedures on immunological components of human milk. *Acta Paediatrica, 88*(430), 14–18.

Lawrence, R. A. (2001). Milk banking: The influence of storage procedures and subsequent processing on immunologic components of human milk. *Advances in Nutritional Research, 10*, 389–404.

Lawrence, R. A., & Lawrence, R. M. (2005). *Breastfeeding: A guide for the medical profession* (6th ed.). Philadelphia: Elsevier Mosby.

Lemons, P., Miller, K., Eitzen, H., Strodtbeck, F., & Lemons, J. (1983). Bacterial growth in human milk during continuous feeding. *American Journal of Perinatology, 1*(1), 76–80.

Liebhaber, M., Lewiston, N. J., Asquith, M. T., & Sunshine, P. (1978). Comparison of bacterial contamination with two methods of human milk collection. *Journal of Pediatrics, 92*(2), 236–237.

Mehta, N., Hamosh, M., Bitman, J., & Wood, D. L. (1988). Adherence of medium-chain fatty acids to feeding tubes during gavage feeding of human milk fortified with medium-chain triglycerides. *Journal of Pediatrics, 112*(3), 474–476.

Meier, P., & Wilks, S. (1987). The bacteria in expressed mothers' milk. *Maternal Child Nursing, 12*(6), 420–423.

Minder, W., Roten, H., Zurbrugg, R. P., Gehriger, G., Lebek, G., & Nagel, G. (1982). Quality of breast milk: Its control and preservation. *Helvetica Paediatrica Acta, 37*(2), 115–137.

Narayanan, I., Prakash, K, & Gujral, V. V. (1983). Bacteriological analysis of expressed human milk and its relation to the outcome of high risk low birth weight infants. *Indian Pediatrics, 20*(12), 915–920.

Narayanan, I., Singh, B., & Harvey, D. (1984). Fat loss during feeding of human milk. *Archives of Disease in Childhood, 59*(5), 475-477.

Nemethy, M., & Clore, E. R. (1990). Microwave heating of infant formula and breast milk. *Journal of Pediatric Health Care, 4*(3), 131–135.

Neville, M. C. (1995). Sampling and storage of human milk. In R. G. Jensen (Ed.), *Handbook of milk composition* (pp. 63–79). San Diego, CA: Academic Press.

Ng, D., Lee, S., Leung, L., Wong, S., & Ho, J. (2004). Bacteriological screening of expressed breast milk revealed a high rate of bacterial contamination in Chinese women. *Journal of Hospital Infection, 58*(2), 146–150.

Ng, P. C., Wong, H. L., Lyon, D. J., So, K., Liu, F., Lam, R., et al. (2004). Combined use of alcohol hand rub and gloves reduces the incidence of late onset infection in very low birthweight infants. *Archives of Disease in Childhood, Fetal Neonatal Edition, 89*(4), F336–F340.

Nwankwo, M. U., Offor, E., Okolo, A. A., & Omene, J. A. (1988). Bacterial growth in expressed breast-milk. *Annals of Tropical Paediatrics, 8*(2), 92–95.

Occupational Safety and Health Administration (OSHA). (1992). Breast milk does not constitute occupational exposure as defined by standard. Standard No. 1910.1030. *Interpretation and compliance letters.* Retrieved June 16, 2009, from http://www.osha.gov/pls/oshaweb/owadisp.show_document?p_table=INTERPRETATIONS&p_id=20952

Olowe, S. A., Ahmed, I., Lawal, S. F., & Ransome-Kuti, S. (1987). Bacteriological quality of raw human milk: Effect of storage in a refrigerator. *Annals of Tropical Paediatrics, 7*(4), 233–237.

Pantazi, M., Jaeger, M. C., & Lawson, M. (1998). Staff support for mothers to provide breast milk in pediatric hospitals and neonatal units. *Journal of Human Lactation, 14*(4), 291–296.

Pardou, A., Serruys, E., Mascart-Lemone, F., Dramaix, M., & Vis, H. (1994). Human milk banking: Influence of storage processes and of bacterial contamination on some milk constituents. *Biology of the Neonate, 65*(5), 302–309.

Paxson, C. L., & Cress, C. C. (1979). Survival of human milk leukocytes. *Journal of Pediatrics, 94*(1), 61–64.

Pittard, W. B., III, Anderson, D. M., Cerutti, E. R., & Boxerbaum, B. (1985). Bacteriostatic qualities of human milk. *Journal of Pediatrics, 107*(2), 240–243.

Pittard, W. B., III, & Bill, K. (1981). Human milk banking: Effect of refrigeration on cellular components. *Clinical Pediatrics, 20*(1), 31–33.

Pittard, W. B., III, Geddes, K. M., Brown, S., Mintz, S., & Hulsey, T. C. (1991). Bacterial contamination of human milk: Container type and method of expression. *American Journal of Perinatology, 8*(1), 25–27.

Quan, R., Yang, C., Rubenstein, S., Lewiston, N. J., Sunshine, P., Stevenson, D. K., et al. (1992). Effects of microwave radiation on anti-infective factors in human milk. *Pediatrics, 89*(4 Pt. 1), 667–669.

Rozolen, C., Goulart, A., & Kopelman, B. (2006). Is breast milk collected at home suitable for raw consumption by neonates in Brazilian public neonatal intensive care units? *Journal of Human Lactation, 22*(4), 418–425.

Santiago, M., Codipilly, C., Potak, D., & Schanler, R. (2005). Effect of human milk fortifiers on bacterial growth in human milk. *Journal of Perinatology, 25*(10), 647–649.

Schanler, R. J. (1996). Human milk fortification for premature infants. *American Journal of Clinical Nutrition, 64*, 249–250.

Schanler, R., Slutzah, M., Codipilly, C., & Potak, D. (2008). Can human milk be stored at refrigerator temperature for more than 48 hours in the neonatal intensive care unit? [Platform Abstract No. 4]. *Breastfeeding Medicine, 3*, 191.

Sigman, M., Burke, K. I., Swarner, O. W., & Shavlik, G. W. (1989). Effects of microwaving human milk: Changes in IgA content and bacterial count. *Journal of the American Dietetic Association, 89*(5), 690–692.

Sosa, R., & Barness, L. (1987). Bacterial growth in refrigerated human milk. *American Journal of Disease in Childhood, 141*(1), 111–112.

Stocks, R. J., Davies, D. P., Allen, F., & Sewell, D. (1985). Loss of breast milk nutrients during tube feeding. *Archives of Disease in Childhood, 60*(2), 164–166.

Tacken, K. J., Vogelsang, A., van Lingen, R. A., Slootstra, J., Dikkeschei, B. D., & Van Zoeren-Grobben, D. (2009, May 4). Loss of triglycerides and carotenoids in human milk after processing. *Archives of Disease in Childhood, Fetal and Neonatal Edition* [Epub ahead of print].

Van Zoeren-Grobben, D., Schrijver, J., Van den Berg, H., & Berger, H. M. (1987). Human milk vitamin content after pasteurisation, storage, or tube feeding. *Archives of Disease in Childhood, 62*(2), 161–165.

Wardell, J. M., Wright, A. J., Bardsley, W. G., & D'Souza, S. W. (1984). Bile salt-stimulated lipase and esterase activity in human milk after collection, storage, and heating: Nutritional implications. *Pediatric Research, 18*(4), 382–386.

West, P. A., Hewitt, J. H., & Murphy, O. M. (1979). The influence of methods of collection and storage on the bacteriology of human milk. *Journal of Applied Bacteriology, 46*(2), 269–277.

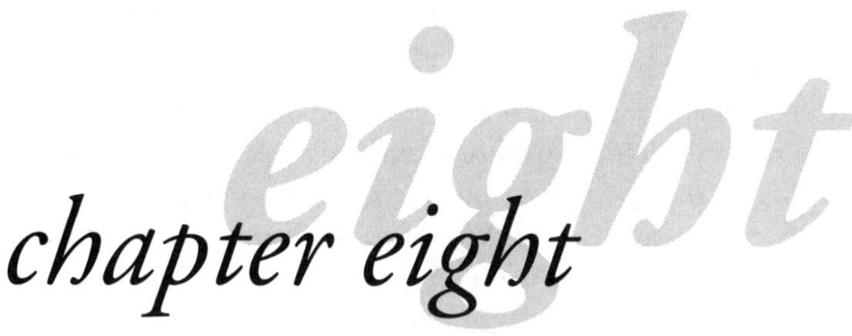

chapter eight

Step 6: Give Preterm and/or Compromised Infants Only Human Milk Unless Medically Contraindicated

EXCLUSIVE BREASTFEEDING FOR HEALTHY, TERM INFANTS

Definition

One of the goals of step 6 of the Ten Steps to Successful Breastfeeding is that the healthy, term infant be exclusively breastfed and supplemented only when there is a medical indication of infant need. Exclusive breastfeeding means that the infant gets nothing to eat except human milk (Labbok & Krasovec, 1990, reporting for the Interagency Group for Action on Breastfeeding). Nearly exclusive breastfeeding includes vitamins and mineral supplements or medications added into the diet for medical reasons. Together these two constitute full breastfeeding.

Benefits of Exclusive Breastfeeding

The benefits of breastfeeding have been discussed elsewhere in this book (see Chapter 5). However, it is recognized that exclusive breastfeeding conveys the greatest health benefits. In developing countries, it has been recognized since the 1930s that there is a dose–response relationship between the amount of breastfeeding and human milk an infant receives and the protection the baby has against disease. An exclusively breastfed baby receives nutritional, immunological, and developmental benefits that mixed-fed babies do not. Among other protective mechanisms, exclusive breastfeeding eliminates exposure to oral pathogens—they simply do not reach the baby's mouth because he is being exclusively breastfed. When complementary foods (culturally appropriate teas and paps) are introduced too early, the baby is exposed to pathogens that he would not normally be exposed to if the mother were exclusively breastfeeding. When breastfeeding is not exclusive, the protective elements of human milk do not work as well, perhaps because of a change in gut pH or dilution of the protective milk components.

In developed countries, this dose–response relationship is also seen (Raisler, Alexander, & Campo, 1999). Using data from the National Maternal and Infant Health Survey in 7092 infants with birth weights greater than 1500 g, the study outcome measures were the number of sick baby medical visits and months of illness related to diarrhea, cough or wheeze, ear infection, runny nose or cold, fever, vomiting, or pneumonia. Five feeding doses were created based on the Interagency Group for Action on Breastfeeding definitions and applied to the baby's feeding methods for each month of the study (see **Table 8-1** for the definitions). The study controlled for demographic characteristics such as race, education, and poverty status, to mention a few, and also controlled for maternal and household smoking, infant birth weight, siblings in the household, day care use, household crowding, and maternal recall interval. Generalized estimating equations regression, a sophisticated longitudinal data analysis, was used to estimate the relationship of breastfeeding doses to the outcome measures over a 6-month period. The summary of results concludes:

> . . . the study results suggested that full breast-feeding has a significant protective effect against common infant illnesses but minimal breast-feeding does not. These findings were consistent among all income groups, even in the United States' environment of clean water, good sanitation, and readily available hygienic infant formula. (Raisler et al., p. 29)

Duration of Exclusive Breastfeeding

Current recommendations for the duration of exclusive breastfeeding in the healthy, term infant are based on a systematic review of the literature conducted by Kramer and Kakuma (2004). This review compared exclusive breastfeeding for 6 months to exclusive breastfeeding for 3–4 months followed by appropriate complementary feeding to 6 months of age. The health

Table 8-1 Definitions of Breastfeeding

Full = 100% breastfeeding
Most = 51–99% breastfeeding
Equal = 50% breastfeeding
Less = 1–49% breastfeeding
None = 0% breastfeeding

Source: Adapted from Raisler et al., 1999.

effects for both mother and infant, infant growth, and infant development were examined. No deficits in either weight or length were found in either group. The authors underscore that each infant must be managed individually so that insufficient growth or other adverse events are not ignored and managed appropriately, but conclude that " . . . the available evidence demonstrates no apparent risks in recommending, as a general policy, exclusive breastfeeding for the first 6 months of life in both developing and developed country settings." (p. 74)

WHO and the World Health Assembly revised their infant feeding recommendations in 2001 to recommend exclusive breastfeeding for the first 6 months of life as the norm (WHO, 2001). Other organizations supporting 6 months of exclusive breastfeeding followed by appropriate complementary feeding include the American Academy of Pediatrics Section on Breastfeeding (2005), the American Academy of Family Physicians (2009), the Academy of Breastfeeding Medicine (2008), the United States Breastfeeding Committee (2000), and UNICEF (WHO/UNICEF, 2003).

CONTRAINDICATIONS FOR USE OF MOTHER'S OWN MILK/BREASTFEEDING

Occasionally there are compelling health reasons why an infant should not be breastfed. They are few in number. The only infant contraindication to breastfeeding according to the CDC (2007) is if the infant has been diagnosed on the newborn screening panel as having galactosemia, a rare metabolic disorder that occurs in 1 in every 30,000 to 60,000 births. The gene for galactosemia is an autosomal recessive gene. In order to show symptoms, the baby must have both recessive genes, one from each parent. The recessive gene is a mutation of the gene that forms the enzyme that metabolizes the simple sugar galactose, one of the two simple sugars that form lactose, the predominant sugar in human milk. When lactose is broken down in the digestive process, glucose and galactose are formed. The galactose can quickly build up in the infant's body and cause damage to the liver, the central nervous system, and other body systems. Individuals with galactosemia cannot tolerate any form of milk, either human or other mammal, because lactose is the defining characteristic of milk (National Library of Medicine, 2009).

WHO and UNICEF (2007) list an additional contraindication to being breastfed—maple syrup urine disease. Babies diagnosed with maple syrup urine disease require a special formula that is free of the amino acids leucine, isoleucine, and valine (all of which appear in human milk). Phenylketonuria is also listed under contraindications in the WHO/UNICEF document along with the acknowledgment that some breastfeeding is possible (with very close monitoring of the infant) in combination with a phenylalanine-free formula.

Other contraindications to breastfeeding relate to the condition of the mother according to the CDC (2007). If the mother meets any of the following conditions, breastfeeding is contraindicated:

- Has been infected with the human immunodeficiency virus (HIV)
- Is taking antiretroviral medications
- Has untreated, active tuberculosis
- Is infected with human T-cell lymphotrophic virus (HTLV) Type I or Type II
- Is using or dependent on an illicit drug
- Is taking prescribed cancer chemotherapy agents, such as antimetabolites that interfere with DNA replication and cell division
- Is undergoing radiation therapy (nuclear medicine therapies and diagnostics require only a temporary interruption of breastfeeding)

Marijuana use falls into this category as it is still illegal and illicit under federal law, despite some states being more willing to consider and legalize the use of marijuana for medical reasons.

ACCEPTABLE MEDICAL REASONS FOR SUPPLEMENTATION (UNICEF/WHO)

According to WHO and UNICEF, there are acceptable medical reasons for the use of breastmilk substitutes in a breastfeeding baby. **Table 8-2** lists these reasons within their categories of providing supplemental nutrition for a limited period of time. Use of breastmilk substitutes when the mother is HIV positive is only recommended if "replacement feeding is acceptable, feasible, affordable, sustainable, and safe" (p. 5). According to the U.S. Committee

Table 8-2 Acceptable Reasons for Using Breastmilk Substitutes

Infants who need supplemental nutrition in addition to breastmilk for a limited period of time
• Very-low-birth-weight infants (birth weight less than 1500g) • Very preterm infants (born at less than 32 weeks' gestation) • Newborns at risk for hypoglycemia "by virtue of impaired metabolic adaptation or increased glucose demand (such as those who are preterm, small for gestational age or who have experienced significant intrapartum hypoxic/ischaemic stress, those who are ill and those whose mothers are diabetic if their blood sugar fails to respond to optimal breastfeeding or breastmilk feeding.)" (p. 4)
Mothers who may need to avoid breastfeeding temporarily
• Mothers with severe illness that prevents them from taking care of their infants (e.g., sepsis) • Herpes simplex virus type 1 (HSV-1) on the breast—direct contact between the infant's mouth and the lesions on the mother's breasts should be avoided until the lesions resolve. • Certain maternal medications, *especially when there are no safer alternatives available*. The list includes sedating psychotherapeutic drugs, antiepileptic drugs, and opioids (which can sedate the infant and cause respiratory depression), radioactive iodine-131 (use a safer alternative if available; mother may resume breastfeeding after 2 months of cessation), and topical iodine and iodophors on open wounds and mucous membranes (these can cause thyroid suppression and electrolyte abnormalities in the breastfed infant).

Source: WHO/UNICEF, 2007.

for UNICEF (1996), acceptable medical reasons in the United States for supplementation of the breastfed baby are:

- Severe dysmaturity
- Very low birth weight
- Inborn errors of metabolism
- Acute water loss
- Mothers who are severely ill
- Mothers who require a medication that is contraindicated

EXCLUSIVE BREASTFEEDING FOR THE PRETERM INFANT

Supplementation of the Breastmilk-Fed Premature Infant

The circumstances of the preterm, low-birth-weight and hospitalized infants who are the subject of this book are included in the list of acceptable reasons for supplementation. Supplementation assumes that other appropriate foods are offered *in addition to* breastfeeding/breastmilk. These babies have severe dysmaturity problems due to their early gestational age at birth, and they have low birth weights. Some may be older gestationally at birth but have metabolic needs in excess of exclusive breastfeeding. According to most U.S. neonatologists, babies born with these conditions require fortification of breastmilk.

I would like to suggest, however, that if we were to feed preterm infants differently, there might not be a need for fortification using other animal or plant products. Research is needed in order to examine whether or not increasing the volume of intake in selected cases would decrease the need for fortification. This means that in the strictest sense, preterm infants are very unlikely to be exclusively breastmilk fed, unless the fortifier is actually made out of human milk components. Again, there is no published research on the safety or efficacy of such products in development. This topic has been extensively discussed in previous chapters (see Chapters 2 and 7). All of the previous discussion simply points to the need for further research using a breastfeeding model rather than a formula-feeding model.

When modifying step 6 of the Ten Steps to Successful Breastfeeding for the healthy, term infant to make it more appropriate for the preterm infant, the emphasis is placed on supplying as much human milk to these babies as possible. (See **Table 8-3** for a side-by-side comparison of the step models.) In the American Breastfeeding Institute (ABI) version of step 6, this means that human milk stands as the standard of care for *all* infants in the NICU, premature or otherwise (see **Appendix 8-1**). Use of premature formulas would become rare and usually unnecessary if human milk is considered as the first choice. On the rare occasions of a metabolic contraindication to human milk for a preterm infant, specialty formulas should, of course, be used.

Gastrointestinal Development and Deficits in the Preterm Infant

Neu (2007) has reviewed issues related to gastrointestinal development of the premature infant. The intestine serves not only as an organ of digestion and absorption but also as an immune organ of the body. It also has exocrine and endocrine functions and a vast amount of neural tissue "equivalent to that of the entire spinal cord" (p. 629S). During the last trimester of pregnancy, the length of the fetal intestine nearly doubles; the increase in intestinal surface area available for absorption is even greater during the same period of time. Gestational age of 34 weeks appears to be critical, since gut motility is impaired and limited largely to infants born at < 34 weeks' gestation. Dysmotility leads to delayed gastric emptying and

Table 8-3 Side-by-Side Comparison of Three Models

Principle	*WHO/UNICEF Ten Steps to Successful Breastfeeding for the Healthy Term Newborn*	*ABI's Ten Steps for the NICU/SCN*	*Nyqvist and Kylberg (2008) Swedish Mothers' 13 Steps*	*Danish Ten Steps to Successful Breastfeeding of Preterm Infants*
Exclusive use of human milk	Step 6. Give (breastfed) newborn infants no food or drink other than breast milk, unless medically indicated.	Step 6: Give preterm and compromised babies only human milk unless *medically* contraindicated.	Step 8. Give the infant the mother's own milk as first choice, and pasteurized donor milk as second choice, fortified when indicated.	

poorer tolerance of enteral feedings. Motility of the small intestine is also more disorganized due to immaturity of the enteric nervous system. This contributes further to delayed transit of food through the intestinal tract. The combination of incomplete innervation and poor motility as well as an immature mucosal barrier and immune response can lead to stasis of food in the GI tract, providing a substrate for subsequent bacterial overgrowth. Because of the immaturity of the infant's immune system, the premature gut also has low levels of secretory IgA and protective mucus, decreased regenerative capacities, and increased permeability, all of which increase the potential for greater tissue damage in the infant who is enterally fed. Low levels of acid output by the GI tract, as well as low levels of digestive enzymes, foster bacterial overgrowth by potential pathogens and damage from their toxins (Neu, 2007).

The Importance of Minimal Enteral Nutrition

In many NICUs, enteral feeding of the critically ill and very premature low-birth-weight infant is replaced by total parenteral nutrition through a line directly into the infant's bloodstream. Parenteral nutrition, especially if used long term, may create problems for the preterm infant such as sepsis caused by infection in the line and liver damage (cholestasis, fatty liver, etc.). The use of minimal enteral nutrition (also known as trophic feedings, minimal enteral feedings, GI priming, gut stimulation, and hypocaloric enteral feedings) begins while parenteral feeding is continued until enteral feeding tolerance is established (Smith, 2005). Parenteral feeding is gradually discontinued as the infant handles larger enteral feedings and the need for additional nutrition decreases. Ideally, parenteral nutrition is discontinued as soon as possible.

In the third trimester of gestation, infants swallow amniotic fluid, up to 450 ml per day, according to Neu (2007). It is therefore abnormal to have an interruption, as occurs with a preterm birth, of fluid traveling through the lumen of the GI tract. Lack of nutrients in the lumen can result in:

- Mucosal atrophy
- Lack of stimulation of trophic hormones
- Sepsis, either from infection of the parenteral line or through bacterial overgrowth of a nonmotile gut
- Increased signs of inflammation
- Poorer feeding tolerance (Neu, 2007; Smith, 2005)

Neu (2007) asks the question, "Is it possible to decrease the use of parenteral nutrition by increasing the use of the immature gastrointestinal tract?" (p. 632S). Can we avoid the issue of growth restriction from undernutrition and the subsequent deficits that occur because of this undernutrition at critical stages of development (e.g., long-term short stature, organ growth failure, and deficits in number of neurons and in dendritic connections resulting in poorer behavioral and cognitive outcomes at later ages) (Hay, 2008)?

The practice of feeding small amounts in order to stimulate development of the intestinal tract is termed *minimal enteral nutrition (MEN)* or *trophic feeding*. MEN improves gastrointestinal blood flow, enzyme activity, hormone release, and motility (Mishra, Agarwal, Jeevasankar, Deorari, & Paul, 2008). Clinical benefits also include improved feeding tolerance, reduced systemic sepsis, shorter hospital stays, and greater postnatal growth. Mishra et al. (2008) observed no ill effects from starting MEN for neonates on total parenteral nutrition or ventilation. Benefits of feeding small amounts within 48 hours of life in extremely low-birth-weight infants (compared to later initiations of feeds) include:

- Significantly earlier achievement of full enteral feedings (12.7 days vs. 45.8 days; $p < 0.01$)
- Earlier regaining of birth weight (13.3 days vs. 15.4 days; $p < 0.05$)

- Trend toward greater overall weight gain in weeks 3–4 of life
- Decreased incidence of low blood glucose levels (Donovan, Puppala, Angst, & Coyle, 2006)

Others report earlier discharge in infants fed MEN (Tyson & Kennedy, 2005).

Some of the challenges with MEN are the weight and maturity of the infant when MEN is begun. Different recommendations are made depending on the size of the infant at birth. The speed with which feedings are advanced is also an issue for many neonatologists, but a current systematic review (McGuire & Bombell, 2008) states that "currently available data do not provide evidence that slow advancement of enteral feed volumes reduces the risk of necrotizing enterocolitis in very low birth weight infants." Tyson and Kennedy (2005), in their systematic review, point out that study methodology continues to be a stumbling block in drawing accurate conclusions; studies are unblinded, have varying outcomes measures, and sample sizes are small. In selecting the studies for their systematic review, Tyson and Kennedy themselves are remiss in not specifying what is in the feeding.

> Trials were included if they enrolled high risk infants randomly assigned to receive trophic feedings (defined as dilute or full strength feedings providing ≤ 25 kcal/kg/d for ≥ 5 d) compared to either 1) no enteral nutrient intake (no feedings or water only) or 2) a specific feeding regimen involving a greater enteral intake of formula or human milk than with trophic feedings. (Tyson & Kennedy, 2005)

Minimal enteral feeding will achieve different results depending on whether the feeding is human milk or formula. When the research design makes no distinction between the two types of feedings, results will be ambiguous, and advantages of trophic feedings or MEN may be diluted. However, if one studies the effects of (1) human milk as MEN compared to (2) formula alone as MEN compared to (3) no MEN, answers may be more obvious and clinicians more willing to use MEN with expressed milk. For example, van Elburg., van den Berg, Bunkers, van Lingen, Smink, van Eyck, et al. (2004) looked at the effects of MEN in infants with intrauterine growth retardation to see if it had an effect on intestinal permeability after birth. The MEN group was fed either 12 feedings of 0.5 ml breastmilk or preterm formula if less than 1000 g at birth; if greater than 1000 g, they received 12 feedings of 1 ml breastmilk or preterm formula. The authors stated that MEN did not reduce intestinal permeability. But if they had done the study comparing three groups based on what was in the feeding, would the results have been different, and would the human milk-fed infants have had a decrease in permeability? Taylor, Basile, Ebeling, and Wagner (2009) asked the same question concerning 62 healthy, preterm infants who were less than 32 weeks' gestation. They defined the infant groupings by the amount of human milk (HM) they received (majority = HM > 75%; partial = 25–75% HM; minimal = < 25% HM). A second type of classification system was defined as either any human milk or formula only, and data were analyzed both ways. Their results are less ambiguous than van Elburg and colleagues' and demonstrate a dose–response relationship; e.g., the less human milk the infant received, the greater the degree of remaining permeability at the end of the first month of life. "Infants who received the majority of feeding as human milk (> 75%) demonstrated significantly lower intestinal permeability when compared to infants receiving minimal (< 25% or none) . . ." (Taylor et al., 2009, p. 11). They conclude that "Human milk promotes intestinal closure earlier and more consistently than formula in the first postnatal month" (p. 15).

Preterm infants are born with high levels of plasma somatostatin, a gut peptide that inhibits various gastrointestinal functions such as gut motility and growth. Somatostatin levels are higher also in sick infants, both term and preterm, and Marchini, Lagercrantz, Feuerberg, Winberg, and Uvnas-Moberg (1988) suggest that gastrointestinal symptoms experienced by sick infants may be related to elevated levels of this inhibitory gut peptide. Increased plasma somatostatin levels are inversely related to gestational age, birth weight, and birth length, and were also higher in infants with respiratory distress syndrome or birth asphyxia (Tornhage, Serenius, Uvnas-Moberg, & Lindberg, 1997) and higher in the first hours of life in 23–36-weeks'-gestation infants (Tornhage, Serenius, Uvnas-Moberg, & Lindberg, 1996). However, somatostatin levels can be down-regulated by feeding the preterm neonate with breastmilk by gavage (Sann, Chayvialle, & Descos, 1982), a desirable outcome since inhibition of gut motility is reduced, and better gastrointestinal development is fostered by the counterbalancing gut hormones, gastrin, cholecystokinin (CCK), enteroglucagon, motilin, and neurotensin (Lucas, Bloom, & Aynsley-Green, 1986). Multiple surges of plasma concentrations of these gut hormones were observed when preterm infants were enterally fed small quantities of human milk—even infants with hyaline membrane disease. Similar surges were not seen with parenteral nutrition only (Lucas et al., 1986). Breastfeeding/breastmilk feeding enhanced the release of CCK in preterm infants and could thus be considered clinically therapeutic, especially for infants who are also being fed parenterally (Lucas et al., 1986; Tornhage, Serenius, Uvnas-Moberg, & Lindberg, 1998b).

The gut hormones produced when the parasympathetic nervous system is activated (gastrin, CCK) cause growth in the infant and increased insulin production. Since growth is a prime objective in the NICU, it is imperative to improve growth and foster it, and we can do this by helping preterm infants to shift the levels of gut peptides, lowering the catabolic ones (somatostatin) and raising the anabolic ones (e.g., gastrin and CCK). Besides the use of species-specific milk (Lucas et al., 1980), peripheral nerve stimulation such as that received during skin-to-skin contact and sucking stimuli increases CCK and affects the release of other gastrointestinal hormones (Holst, Lund, Petersson, & Uvnas-Moberg, 2005; Marchini, et al., 1987; Tornhage, Serenius, Uvnas-Moberg, & Lindberg, 1998a; Uvnas-Moberg, Marchini, & Winberg, 1993). Sucking also increases CCK and gastrin and positively influences the secretory and motor functions of the GI tract. It is therefore important for preterm infants who are being fed by gavage to have the opportunity to simultaneously suck on a pacifier to stimulate gastric hormones. Widstrom et al. (1988) found that the time for tube feeding significantly decreased when the infant sucked on a pacifier during the feeding, and gastric retention was decreased also, indicating better gut motility. Use of a pacifier during tube feeding also stimulated insulin release (Marchini et al., 1987).

Another benefit of the use of human milk rather than formula for MEN relates to the immaturity of the gut and the low acidity of the gut that creates a more basic environment that fosters the growth of pathogens. Human milk helps to maintain the acidity of the gut by fostering colonization of the gut with *Lactobacillus bifidus*, a commensal bacteria in the human gut that actually helps to maintain acidity by producing an acetic acid buffer (Bullen, Tearle, & Stewart, 1977; see discussion Chapter 2 in this book). This is the rationale behind the use of probiotic bacteria in the management of preterm infants. However, the species of *Lactobacillus* used as probiotics (live microorganisms) and mentioned by Neu (2007) are different and may have the potential to cause problems, especially since correct dosages and mechanisms of action have not been determined. Studies of safety of different bacteria used as probiotics and their potential for overgrowth and harm in immature preterm infants have not been done, and according to Neu, case reports do exist of sepsis in infants caused by probiotics. Neu states that "we are permitting the use of these agents without the same standards that we would apply to safety testing for pharmacologic or nutraceutical agents" (p. 631S).

Premji, Paes, Jacobson, and Chessell (2002) and Smith (2005) developed research-based guidelines for early enteral feeding of the very-low-birth-weight infant. In both guidelines, human milk is used preferentially to provide MEN. In the first guideline, MEN is begun at 48 hours for infants weighing less than 1000 g at birth, with nutritional feedings beginning on day 5–6. For infants between 1000 and 1500 g at birth, nutritional feedings are started at 48 hours and advanced at a rate of less than 30 ml/kg/day. In Smith's guideline, feeding regimens were broken out even further into the following four birth-weight classifications: < 750 g, 751–1000 g, 1001–1250 g, and 1251–1500 g. The goals in Smith's guideline were to begin feedings on day 2–3 *when possible*, but if the mother's milk was unavailable, initiation of feedings was supposed to be held off until her milk was available. In Smith's comparative study of preimplementation and postimplementation practice, all of the infants whose feedings were delayed due to lack of mother's milk all received their first feeding by day 3, which was within the goal of the guideline. (See **Box 8-1** for a discussion of the process of guideline development.)

Use of Banked Donor Human Milk

Delay of MEN due to lack of mother's own milk could be avoided if banked donor milk were on hand and prescribed for this use. In Scandinavian countries, banked donor milk is used preferentially (in the absence of the mother's own milk) to begin MEN as early as the first day of life (see Arnold, 1999). Then as the mother's own milk is collected, her milk is substituted and merely supplemented with donor milk. A review and discussion of donor milk banking practices are presented in Chapters 13–16 in this book. Ziegler, Thureen, and Carlson (2002) state that delayed introduction of enteral feedings has no beneficial effects, including a reduction in the incidence of NEC, and actually has negative effects on the overall development and maturation of the gut. Ziegler advocates for aggressive feeding to stimulate gut maturation, including release of gut hormones and to improve gut motility, with the preferred feeding being human milk.

> . . . Feedings should be started on the day of birth. A frequently encountered practical limitation is that breast milk takes at least 2 days to come in and often does not come in for three, four, or five

Box 8-1 Developing an Evidence-Based Guideline

The process of developing a research-based guideline for MEN in very-low-birth-weight infants in Smith's level 3 NICU (2005) was very well planned and implemented and is a good model for an effective process that other institutions could utilize. First, a multidisciplinary nutrition committee was formed to establish goals for development of the guideline—development of a usable research-based guideline that could be individualized as necessary but still provide for consistency of care among many clinicians. The goal was to achieve better growth and nutrition in very-low-birth-weight infants and to establish full enteral nutrition by the 3rd week of life. The process involved members of the committee being assigned to review various topics in the literature, meeting weekly to develop the guidelines. Because human milk was identified as the preferred feeding choice, increasing lactation services and breastfeeding initiation rates for NICU families became a secondary goal, and a dietitian experienced in nutritional needs of preterm infants and a lactation consultant were included in the committee. The committee then established a plan to educate the staff nurses, nurse practitioners, physicians, and NICU families about the guidelines.

Implementation began with education prior to adoption of the guideline. Members of the multidisciplinary team each educated members of their own departments, beginning 2 weeks prior to implementation and then continuing 1 month after implementation. Education was done both formally and informally to facilitate buy-in by the various departments and disciplines.

Evaluation, a key component of assessing the effectiveness and success of any program, was also undertaken in two phases 6 months after the feeding guideline was implemented. Feeding practices of 49 very-low-birth-weight infants were followed prospectively to see if outcomes measures were met. Findings were that consistency of care improved, the incidence of NEC decreased after implementation of standardized feeding schedules, and breastfeeding initiation rates increased significantly due to an increase in the availability of proactive breastfeeding support. Other outcomes need further research.

Source: Smith, 2005.

days. During that time only small amounts of colostrum are available, which is very valuable and must be fed. To supplement colostrum, greater use should be made of donated breast milk, which is available from milk banks. Gastric residuals should not be allowed to interfere with feeding. Infants with cardiovascular instability should be fed. Feeding volumes should be kept low (1–2 ml/feed), and frequency of feedings every 6 hours or less, preferably every 3 hours . . . (Ziegler et al., 2002, p. 240).

Every NICU does not need to start a milk bank of its own, but every NICU should have a supply of frozen donor milk from a donor milk bank for this purpose. When the mother's own milk is unavailable in the volumes the baby requires, donor milk becomes a temporary solution. When mothers cannot supply their own milk long term for any reason, sole use of donor milk should be considered until full enteral feedings are established, and the advantages of optimal gut maturation conferred upon the infant.

WHEN FORMULA MUST BE FED

When neither the mother's own milk nor donor milk is available, it is incumbent on the NICU to ensure that the mother knows how to prepare formula, especially powdered formulas, and how to store it safely. She should be offered the opportunity to prepare the formula in the NICU under supervision so that she is comfortable with the technique prior to the baby's discharge. In Chapter 7 the problem of *Enterobacter sakazakii* in formula and the potential for its presence in powdered bovine-based human milk fortifiers was discussed at length. When infants are discharged while still small and before due dates, they are very vulnerable to infection, and if the mother does not understand the health risks of the powdered formula she may not be as careful in preparation and storage of the liquid as she should be, believing that it is safe. Discharge orders should ensure that mothers preferentially use the liquid formulas, ready-to-feed or concentrate, or be thoroughly informed on safe preparation techniques for powdered infant formulas. A special section on formula preparation has been added to the model policy in Appendix 8-1 despite the fact that this chapter and model policy is about feeding human milk exclusively as much as possible.

SUMMARY

Preterm infants, because of their immature and fragile status, deserve as close to exclusive human milk feeding/breastfeeding as possible. Their fragile gut requires that we not subject it to nonphysiologic fluids (like formula) but ensure that the many bioactive substances present in human milk be allowed to work to foster appropriate gastrointestinal development. While mainstream neonatology agrees on the need for fortification, new methods of accomplishing this without introducing foreign proteins is desirable. The use of human milk should be extended to the use of donor human milk from a milk bank when mother's own milk is absent or inadequate temporarily. Step

6 delineates a policy that can be used or adapted to every level of special care and includes the use of banked donor milk. Formula feeding is associated with significant long-term and short-term problems and/or deficits in the preterm infant. In the best-case scenario, it does not provide the preterm infant with optimal outcomes, even if it does no harm. Policies should reflect the optimal use of human milk for these fragile and compromised infants. In addition, adequate lactation services must be assured for families of preterm infants.

REFERENCES

Academy of Breastfeeding Medicine (ABM). (2008). Position on breastfeeding. *Breastfeeding Medicine, 3*(4), 267–270.

American Academy of Family Physicians. (2009). *Family physicians supporting breastfeeding* [position paper]. Retrieved March 11, 2009, from http://www.aafp.org/online/en/home/policy/policies/b/breastfeedingpositionpaper.printerview.html

American Academy of Pediatrics, Section on Breastfeeding. (2005). Breastfeeding and the use of human milk. *Pediatrics, 115*(2), 496–506.

Arnold, L. D. W. (1999). Donor milk banking in Scandinavia. *Journal of Human Lactation, 15*(1), 55–59.

Bullen, C., Tearle, P., & Stewart, M. (1977). The effect of "humanized" milks and supplemented breast feeding on the faecal flora of infants. *Journal of Medical Microbiology, 10*(4), 403–413.

Centers for Disease Control and Prevention (CDC). (2007). *When should a mother avoid breastfeeding?* Retrieved March 11, 2009, from http://www.cdc.gov/breastfeeding/disease/contraindicators.htm

Donovan, R., Puppala, B., Angst, D., & Coyle, B. (2006). Outcomes of early nutrition support in extremely low-birth-weight infants. *Nutrition in Clinical Practice, 21*(4), 395–400.

Hay, W. (2008). Strategies for feeding the preterm infants. *Neonatology, 94*(4), 245–254.

Holst, S., Lund, I., Petersson, M., & Uvnas-Moberg, K. (2005). Massage-like stroking influences plasma levels of gastrointestinal hormones, including insulin, and increases weight gain in male rats. *Autonomic Neuroscience: Basic & Clinical, 120*(1–2), 73–79.

Kramer, M., & Kakuma, R. (2004). The optimal duration of exclusive breastfeeding: A systematic review. *Advances in Experimental Medicine and Biology, 554*, 63–77.

Labbok, M., & Krasovec, K. (1990). Toward consistency in breastfeeding definitions. *Studies in Family Planning, 21*(4), 226–230.

Labiner-Wolfe, J., Fein, S., & Shealy, K. (2008). Infant formula-handling education and safety. *Pediatrics, 122*(Suppl. 2), S85–S90.

Lucas, A., Bloom, S., & Aynsley-Green, A. (1986). Gut hormones and 'minimal enteral feeding.' *Acta Paediatrica Scandinavica, 75*(5), 719–723.

Lucas, A., Sarson, D., Blackburn, A., Adrian, T., Aynsley-Green, A., & Bloom, S. (1980). Breast vs. bottle: Endocrine responses are different with formula feeding. *The Lancet, 1*(8181), 1267–1269.

Marchini, G., Lagercrantz, H., Feuerberg, Y., Winberg, J., & Uvnas-Moberg, K. (1987). The effect of non-nutritive sucking on plasma insulin, gastrin, and somatostatin levels in infants. *Acta Paediatrica Scandinavica, 76*(4), 573–578.

Marchini, G., Lagercrantz, H., Milerad, J., Winberg, J., & Uvnas-Moberg, K. (1988). Plasma levels of somatostatin and gastrin in sick infants and small for gestational age infants. *Journal of Pediatric Gastroenterology and Nutrition, 7*(5), 641–644.

McGuire, W., & Bombell, S. (2008). Slow advancement of enteral feed volumes to prevent necrotizing enterocolitis in very low birth weight infants. *Cochrane Database Systematic Reviews, 16*, CD001241.

Mishra, S., Agarwal, R., Jeevasankar, M., Deorari, A., & Paul, V. (2008). Minimal enteral nutrition. *Indian Journal of Pediatrics, 75*(3), 267–269.

National Library of Medicine, National Institutes of Health. (2009). *Medical encyclopedia entry: Galactosemia*. Retrieved March 11, 2009 from http://www.nlm.nih.gov/medlineplus/ency/article/000366.htm

Neu, J. (2007). Gastrointestinal development and meeting the nutritional needs of premature infants. *American Journal of Clinical Nutrition, 85*(2), 629S–634S.

Premji, S., Paes, B., Jacobson, K., & Chessell, L. (2002). Evidence-based feeding guidelines for very low-birth-weight infants. *Advances in Neonatal Care, 2*(1), 5–18.

Raisler, J., Alexander, C., & O'Campo, P. (1999). Breast-feeding and infant illness: A dose–response relationship? *American Journal of Public Health, 89*(1), 25–30.

Sann, L., Chayvialle, J., & Descos, F. (1982). Plasma somatostatin concentration in the preterm neonate. *European Journal of Pediatrics, 139*(2), 148–150.

Smith, J. (2005). Early enteral feeding for the very low birth weight infant: The development and impact of a research-based guideline. *Neonatal Network, 24*(4), 9–19.

Taylor, S., Basile, L., Ebeling, M., & Wagner, C. (2009). Intestinal permeability in preterm infants by feeding type: Mother's milk versus formula. *Breastfeeding Medicine, 4*(1), 11–15.

Tornhage, C., Serenius, F., Uvnas-Moberg, K., & Lindberg, T. (1996). Plasma somatostatin and cholecystokinin levels in preterm infants during the first day of life. *Biology of the Neonate, 70*(6), 311–321.

Tornhage, C., Serenius, F., Uvnas-Moberg, K., & Lindberg, T. (1997). Plasma somatostatin and cholecystokinin levels in sick preterm infants during their first six weeks of life. *Acta Paediatrica, 86*(8), 847–850.

Tornhage, C., Serenius, F., Uvnas-Moberg, K., & Lindberg, T. (1998a). Plasma somatostatin and cholecystokinin levels in preterm infants during kangaroo care with and without nasogastric tube-feeding. *Journal of Pediatric Endocrinology and Metabolism, 11*(5), 645–651.

Tornhage, C., Serenius, F., Uvnas-Moberg, K., & Lindberg, T. (1998b). Plasma somatostatin and cholecystokinin levels in response to feeding in preterm infants. *Journal of Pediatric Gastroenterology and Nutrition, 27*(2), 199–205.

Tyson, J., & Kennedy, K. (2005). Trophic feedings for parenterally fed infants. *Cochrane Database Systematic Reviews, 20*, CD000504.

United States Breastfeeding Committee. (2000). *Statement on exclusive breastfeeding*. Raleigh, NC: Author. Retrieved June 18, 2009, from http://www.usbreastfeeding.org/LinkClick.aspx?link=Position-Statements%2fEBF-Statement-2000-08-05-USBC.pdf&tabid=70&mid=393

United States Committee for UNICEF, Wellstart International. (1996). *Guidelines and evaluation criteria for hospital/birthing center level implementation*. New York: Author.

Uvnas-Moberg, K., Lundeberg, T., Bruzelius, G., & Alster, P. (1992). Vagally mediated release of gastrin and cholecystokinin following sensory stimulation. *Acta Physiologica Scandinavica, 146*(3), 349–356.

Uvnas-Moberg, K., Marchini, G., & Winberg, J. (1993). Plasma cholecystokinin concentrations after breast feeding in healthy 4 day old infants. *Archives of Disease in Childhood, 68*(1 Spec No), 46–48.

van Elburg, R., van den Berg, A., Bunkers, C., van Lingen, R., Smink, E., van Eyck, J., et al. (2004). Minimal enteral feeding, fetal blood flow pulsatility, and postnatal intestinal permeability in preterm infants with intrauterine growth retardation. *Archives of Disease in Childhood, Fetal and Neonatal Edition, 89*(4), F293–F296.

Widstrom, A., Marchini, G., Matthiesen, A., Werner, S., Winberg, J., & Uvnas-Moberg, K. (1988). Nonnutritive sucking in tube-fed preterm infants: Effects on gastric motility and gastric contents of somatostatin. *Journal of Pediatric Gastroenterology and Nutrition, 7*(4), 517–523.

World Health Organization (WHO). (2001). *Infant and young child nutrition.* Fifty-fourth World Health Assembly 54.2. Geneva, Switzerland: Author.

World Health Organization (WHO)/UNICEF. (2003). *Global strategy on infant and young child feeding.* Retrieved March 11, 2009, from http://whqlibdoc.who.int/publications/2003/9241562218.pdf

World Health Organization (WHO)/UNICEF. (2007). *Acceptable medical reasons for use of breast-milk substitutes.* Retrieved March 11, 2009, from http://www.who.int/nutrition/publications/infantfeeding/WHO_NMH_NHD_09.01_eng.pdf

World Health Organization (WHO), Food and Agriculture Organization. (2007). *Safe preparation, storage and handling of powdered infant formula: Guidelines.* Retrieved May 2, 2009, from http://www.who.int/foodsafety/publications/micro/pif_guidelines.pdf

Ziegler, E., Thureen, P., & Carlson, S. (2002). Aggressive nutrition of the very low birthweight infant. *Clinics in Perinatology, 29*(2), 225–244.

APPENDIX 8-1

STEP 6

Give preterm and/or compromised infants only human milk unless medically contraindicated.

Policies 6.1–6.7

Title

Use of human milk for all NICU/SCN babies

Purpose

To provide premature and/or compromised NICU/SCN infants with (1) mother's own breastmilk or (2) banked donor human milk when a mother refuses or is unable to provide her milk, use of her milk is contraindicated, her supply falters, and/or she cannot provide adequate amounts of her milk.

Rationale

To ensure that all premature and/or compromised NICU/SCN babies receive only human milk (unless medically contraindicated for the infant) to achieve a standard of short-term growth, prevent feeding-related morbidities, and optimize long-term outcome.

Supportive Data

Nutrition during critical periods in early life may permanently affect the structure and/or function of organs and tissues (Lucas, 1994). It has been shown that early diet can influence long-term health (e.g., brain development, obesity, bone mineralization, blood pressure) and the risk of certain adult diseases (e.g., cardiovascular disease, diabetes, chronic digestive diseases, cancers, bone health) (Koletzko, 2005; Lucas, 1994, 2005; Schack-Nielsen, Larnkjær, & Fleischer Michaelsen, 2005). While there are occasional medical contraindications to the use of a mother's breastmilk, the majority of preterm infants should be fed human milk from their own mothers or from a donor human milk bank.

Scope

These policies apply to all NICU/SCN personnel including the medical director, nursing director, nursing supervisors, licensed staff, ancillary staff, and volunteers.

Policy 6.1

Human milk is the standard of care for preterm nutrition as well as term infant nutrition.

Policy 6.2

All infants should receive their own mother's milk preferentially unless there is a contraindication (e.g., mother being HIV positive in developed countries, mother using illegal drugs, having an infant with galactosemia, etc. [CDC, 2007]).

Procedure 6.2.1

Routine bacteriological screening of a mother's milk prior to feeding is unnecessary, does not prevent exposure to bacteria, gives negative messages to the mother, and should be avoided. (See Appendix 7-2.)

Procedure 6.2.2

Mother's milk being prepared for feeding should not be warmed above body temperature or subjected to excessive heat in any way.

Procedure 6.2.3

Milk that has separated during freezing and thawing can be swirled gently to resuspend fat particulates. It should never be shaken vigorously.

Procedure 6.2.4

If delivered by a single syringe infusion pump, feedings of mother's milk should be managed to ensure as complete delivery of nutrients (particularly fats) as possible.

a. The syringe pump is placed below the isolette.
b. The syringe is oriented with the tip pointing upward.
c. Tubing is kept short to minimize surface area available for loss of milk components.

Procedure 6.2.5
All feedings, including fortifiers and additives, are logged in the baby's medical record.

Policy 6.3

The NICU/SCN should have policies and procedures in place to prevent milk from one mother being accidentally fed to another mother's infant. (See Appendix 7-2.)

Policy 6.4

Members of the multidisciplinary healthcare team should identify infants who may be candidates for receiving banked donor milk. Use of banked donor milk is preferential to the use of formula and should be routine for all NICUs/SCNs.

Procedure 6.4.1
In the absence of a mother's own milk, for whatever reason, donor milk from a milk bank should be used preferentially over formula.

Procedure 6.4.2
Donor milk may be prescribed for the treatment of various medical conditions, *including, but not limited to:*

- Prematurity
- Malabsorption
- Other gastrointestinal disorders
- Feeding intolerance
- Renal failure
- Inborn errors of metabolism
- Cardiac diseases
- Failure to thrive
- Short-gut syndrome
- Treatment of infectious diseases (diarrhea, botulism, pneumonia)
- Immunological deficiencies
- Congenital anomalies
- Supplementation of hypoglycemia
- Postoperative nutrition and healing
- Maternal lactation failure
- Adoption

- Supplementation of inadequate maternal milk supply
- Illness of mother requiring temporary cessation of breastfeeding
- Health risk to the infant from the biological mother's milk
- Death of the mother

Procedure 6.4.3

Informed consent from the potential recipient's mother (or father, if the mother is not available) for use of donor milk should be obtained per institutional policy.

Procedure 6.4.4

A prescription, from the physician, Neonatal Nurse Practitioner (NNP), or Physician's Assistant (PA) (someone licensed to prescribe), is faxed to an approved milk bank. Milk may be ordered for a specific individual or may be ordered in bulk for use by many infants in the NICU/SCN simultaneously.

Procedure 6.4.5

The amount of the next week's needs for donor milk is determined and ordered weekly or biweekly, according to the individual milk bank's policies in order to have a sufficient supply on hand.

Procedure 6.4.6

Processed banked donor milk is shipped frozen overnight to the hospital and transported to the NICU/SCN within the hospital chain of custody procedures. For example, upon arriving in the receiving department, the employee in receiving immediately pages the responsible person caring for the recipient. Milk is transferred to that individual, who transports it to the freezer in the NICU/SCN.

Procedure 6.4.7

Processed banked donor milk is checked against the shipping forms for accuracy, damage, and maintenance of frozen state.

Procedure 6.4.8

Batch numbers of each container of processed banked donor milk are logged in appropriately with the date received.

Procedure 6.4.9

Processed banked donor milk designated for a specific recipient is transferred to the freezer into a bin designated for that specific individual.

Procedure 6.4.10
Frozen milk or milk containing ice crystals is immediately placed in the freezer. Defrosted milk must be used within the next 24 hours or discarded. If milk arrives defrosted, the facility initiating the shipment must be notified.

Procedure 6.4.11
Follow the instructions for thawing processed banked donor milk that accompany the milk or the hospital protocol for thawing frozen human milk.

Procedure 6.4.12
Document the milk bank batch identification number in the baby's medical record with each feeding.

Policy 6.5

If the medical condition of the infant warrants the use of formula, a written medical order is required in the baby's chart documenting the medical indication(s) for its use.

Policy 6.6

Formula and feeding supplies for NICU/SCN use should be purchased at a fair market price to avoid conflicts of interest. Negotiated prices should be similar to the percentage of retail price that the hospital pays for other supplies (e.g., if the hospital pays 40% of retail for aspirin and 20% of retail for gauze bandages, then it would be reasonable to pay between 20 and 40% of retail for formula). (See Chapter 11 in this book.)

Policy 6.7

Recognizing that not all NICU mothers will be discharged breastfeeding, staff should develop a procedure and protocol that specifically addresses the safe preparation of formula and baby-led formula-feeding practices, and teach formula-feeding mothers appropriately in a manner free of commercial bias (Labiner-Wolfe et al., 2008).

Procedure 6.7.1
Instructions should be developed utilizing the World Health Organization's recommendations for safe preparation, storage, and handling (WHO, 2008). Information should include, but not be limited to:

- Handwashing prior to formula preparation;

- Special precautions for preparation of powdered formula to eliminate or reduce contamination with *Enterobacter sakazakii* and prevent infant illness and disease;
- Adequate cleaning techniques for feeding implements, particularly nipples;
- Appropriate mixing procedures for powdered and concentrate formulas, such as whether to add water to premeasured powder or powder to premeasured water;
- Appropriate and safe warming procedures;
- Durations of storage of prepared formula at room temperature and in the refrigerator.

Procedure 6.7.2

Instructions should be developed on baby-led and safe formula feeding practices to prevent over-feeding and reduce the risk of choking and aspiration from feedings that are rushed.

Procedure 6.7.3

Parents who have opted to feed formula to their infants should be educated in safe formula feeding practices as well as proper mixing techniques prior to discharge from the hospital. Education should be given in writing as well as verbally. A return demonstration of formula preparation should be required.

REFERENCES

Centers for Disease Control and Prevention (CDC). (2007). *When should a mother avoid breastfeeding?* Retrieved March 11, 2009, from http://www.cdc.gov/breastfeeding/disease/contraindicators.htm

Koletzko, B. (2005). Early nutrition and its later consequences: New opportunities. Perinatal nutrition programmes adult health. *Advances in Experimental Medicine and Biology, 569*, 1–12.

Lucas, A. (1994). Role of nutritional programming in determining adult morbidity. *Archives of Disease in Childhood, 71*(4), 288–290.

Lucas, A. (2005). The developmental origins of adult health and well-being. *Advances in Experimental Medicine and Biology, 569*, 13–15.

Schack-Nielsen, L., Larnkjær, A., & Fleischer Michaelsen, K. (2005). Long-term effects of breastfeeding on the infant and mother. *Advances in Experimental Medicine and Biology, 569*, 16–23.

chapter nine

Step 7: Implementing Kangaroo Mother Care and Skin-to-Skin Contact in the NICU as Routine Care

> Since attachment among primates is a process, any time an infant spends away from its mother breaks the normal flow of interaction. Although there may not be a "critical period" for bonding, the time after birth is clearly sensitive to the development of a new relationship. Parents are getting to know their babies and they are primed by the excitement of the moment to see, smell and hear everything they can about their child. . . . All these scientific and medical advisors, counselors and researchers seem to miss the fact that culture, in the form of the medical establishment, has intervened in human biology. For millions of years the human female animal gave birth and held that baby to her chest. She carried the baby close and helped it find the nipple. The timing of the bond, the intensity of the attachment, and the need for hooking up physically and emotionally was never in question because the closeness was a given. In all cultures except Western culture, the process is the same today. (Small, 1998, p. 26)

In the Ten Steps to Successful Breastfeeding for the healthy, term infant, fulfilling the criteria of step 7 means that the mother and infant should room in continuously during the hospital stay, with separations only for medical reasons. Should separation be necessary, reinstatement of continuous rooming in is expected as soon as the medical condition is resolved or a medical procedure, such as circumcision, complete. When mothers and babies room in and continue to do skin-to-skin bonding as they did in the delivery room, they learn together and begin to establish mutual attachment that keeps babies safe and healthy. Mothers learn their babies' feeding cues and satiety cues, and mothers and babies learn how to breastfeed together. Each has a learning curve that can be facilitated and shortened if mothers and babies are together and can feed on cue. Breastfeeding outcomes are improved when rooming in with no supplements is instituted as routine. Breastfeeding mothers who room in have larger milk supplies and produce mature milk earlier than mothers who do not room in. Higher rates of exclusive breastfeeding and longer durations of breastfeeding have also been observed when rooming in is instituted, and less physiologic jaundice due to poor feeding is seen in babies who room in. (See Cadwell & Turner-Maffei [2009] for a discussion of this step for healthy, term infants.)

This step does not translate well into the NICU setting unless the facility has individual NICU rooms or one considers it to be a step that allows mothers and their preterm or hospitalized babies as much contact as possible. Increasing contact means not only that the mother must have unrestricted visitation access to her infant, but also that she be allowed to hold her infant as much as possible in skin-to-skin (STS) care or kangaroo mother care (KMC). Step 7 has therefore been modified in the three different step models for the NICU/SCN presented earlier to mean the implementation of routine STS care or KMC. (See **Table 9-1** for a side-by-side comparison of the models.)

In evolutionary terms, it is normal behavior for primate mothers to carry their young and to feed them whenever the infant indicates (see Small, 1998). All primates do this, and as they practice these carrying and feeding behaviors, they teach the next generation by example. A number of years ago, a zoo in the United States was having a problem with one of its gorillas that became pregnant. As soon as the baby was born the mother clearly did not know what to do with it and began playing with it and throwing it around the enclosure, eventually killing it. This mother could not bond with her baby because she had most likely been separated at birth from her own mother and had never bonded as an infant (Small, 1998, p. 18). Having been separated from her group, she had never learned this behavior by observation. The second time the gorilla became pregnant, the zookeepers decided on a different tactic, asking La Leche League for volunteer nursing mothers who sat in front of the gorilla exhibit and breastfed their babies, changed and cleaned them, stroked them (groomed them), talked to them and carried them around in slings and in arms. The gorilla mother observed all this

Table 9-1 Side-by-Side Comparison of Three Models

Principle	*WHO/UNICEF Ten Steps to Successful Breastfeeding for the Healthy Term Newborn*	*ABI's Ten Steps for the NICU/SCN*	*Nyqvist and Kylberg (2008) Swedish Mothers' 13 Steps*	*Danish Ten Steps to Successful Breastfeeding of Preterm Infants*
Mother–infant contact	Step 7. Practice rooming in—allow mothers and infants to remain together 24 hours a day.	Step 7. Promote early and continued skin-to-skin contact for mothers and their premature or compromised infants with full mechanical breastmilk expression.	Step 5. Encourage early, continuous, and prolonged skin-to-skin care (kangaroo mother care) without unwarranted restrictions and offer opportunities for mothers to remain together with their infants 24 hours a day.	Step 4. Parents are encouraged to have skin-to-skin contact with their infants.

behavior day after day during most of her pregnancy, and when her next baby was born she modeled the same behavior, nursing her infant, grooming it, and carrying it around.

If we want mothers of sick and separated babies to bond well with their infants and keep their infants safe, we must provide the model of KMC as often as possible for lengthy durations. When doing so, we provide parents with opportunities to learn about and from their infants; these opportunities have lasting benefits for both mother and baby. We are continuing a chain of learning in mothers that they, in turn, will teach their own children. However, barriers exist to practicing KMC, including fears of safety for certain categories of premature infants and reluctance on the part of nurses, physicians, and families to initiate or participate in KMC (Engler et al., 2002). This chapter provides the evidence for instituting KMC in a NICU setting as a standard of care.

BENEFITS OF KMC FOR THE MOTHER/BABY DYAD

The maternal benefits of STS contact as soon after birth as possible were discussed in Chapter 6. These included better bonding between mother and baby, which lasts long term and results in different mother–infant interactions as the baby grows and matures and is discharged from the hospital. Mothers who socialize with their babies elicit more responses from their babies. Being able to hold their infants skin to skin and touch their infants also impacts mothers' moods and helps to mitigate and resolve depressive symptoms.

Frequent KMC in the NICU over the entire NICU stay also continues to have benefits for the mother/infant dyad. When mothers are encouraged to be with their babies and hold them, they spend more time observing their infant's behavior. Mothers can learn their baby's responses to the environment and their infant's approach and avoidance behaviors. As the babies develop more mature signals, mothers can also begin to recognize feeding cues. (See **Table 9-2** for behavioral signs of distress and for signs of happiness.)

Milk Supply

One of the most beneficial aspects of continuing frequent and lengthy KMC in the NICU is better success in establishing a milk supply and in transitioning the infant to the breast. A small study by Hurst, Valentine, Renfro, Burns, and Ferlic (1997) demonstrated an increase in milk volume when STS was implemented compared to a control group that did not initiate STS. Average baseline 24-hour milk volume was 499 ± 139 ml (STS) compared with 218 ± 132 ml (no STS). Milk volumes increased over weeks 2–4 postpartum for the mothers doing STS care, but actually decreased slightly in the control group during the same period of time. Similar to an earlier study by Affonso, Wahlberg, and Persson (1989), mothers experiencing STS contact in this study reported that they felt more confident about breastfeeding and their ability to produce an adequate milk supply for the infants' needs. Control mothers expressed feelings of insecurity about their milk supply and abandoned breastfeeding earlier because of reported insufficient supply.

Breastfeeding Rates

KMC dyads breastfeed for longer durations of time compared to non-KMC dyads. Hake-Brooks and Anderson (2008) documented feeding method at hospital discharge and at 1.5, 3, 6, 12, and 18 months of age. They report that the difference in durations between the STS group and the standard contact group was statistically significant (KMC = 5.08 months versus no-KMC = 2.05 months; p = 0.003). Bier et al. (1996) had similar significant findings in their study, documenting longer durations of breastfeeding in STS out to 6 months postdischarge, even though breastfeeding rates decreased for both control and STS groups.

Table 9-2 Signs of Distress and Happiness

Signs of Distress
White knuckle syndrome Babies greater than 32 weeks are able to flex their hands and make a fist. Fisting is a common behavior in babies, but clenching the fist so tightly that the knuckles turn white is an indicator of distress.
Finger splay Fingers stretched out are a sign of tension and distress.
Sagging cheeks and chin Sagging cheeks and chin are a sign of fatigue and indication that the baby doesn't have enough energy.
Spitting up Spitting up as a sign of distress needs to be distinguished from normal spitting up that occurs immediately after the feeding due to immature sphincters.
Furrowed brow A furrowed brow is an indication of worry and stress, similar to that in adults.
Ear tuck Babies older than 32 weeks' gestation can flatten their ears back against their head when stressed, as opposed to ears sticking out away from the head in unstressful situations.
Stop sign One of the baby's arms comes up with the hand splayed in an obvious signal to *stop*.
Air sitting In air sitting, the legs lift into the air—the leg version of the stop sign.
Arching back The baby who arches his or her back is trying to pull away from the source of distress.
Hyperalertness Hyperalertness involves staring alertly at something or someone with a look of concern or fear on the baby's face.
Gaze aversion The baby tries to shift her gaze from what she has been looking at and shifts her gaze back and forth without focusing on anything.
Head turning When gaze aversion is not adequate to decrease stress, then the baby turns her head, sometimes in a back-and-forth "no" motion.
Yawning or hiccupping Yawning or hiccupping usually accompanies fatigue or stress.
Tactile reinforcement The baby touches himself and distracts himself from the unpleasant event. Fingers and thumbs touch, hands touch each other, or hands touch the mouth in extreme distress, sometimes sucking on fingers to self-console or calm down.

(continues)

Table 9-2 Signs of Distress and Happiness

Signs of Happiness
Relaxed brow—no worry signs here
Uplifted cheeks and chin indicating good muscle tone and energy
Gently flexed hands in a relaxed position
Flexed posture
Smiling

Source: Adapted from Ludington-Hoe & Golant, 1993, pp. 53–66.

Exclusivity rates for breastfeeding were also higher in the groups that experienced KMC in two studies from India on low-birth-weight babies. At 6 weeks, the number of KMC mothers exclusively breastfeeding their babies was double that of the control group (Ramanathan, Paul, Deorari, Taneja, & George, 2001), and 98% of the KMC group were exclusively breastfeeding at the end of the second study compared to 76% in the control group (Suman, Udani, & Nanavati, 2008). KMC was found to be one of the correlates of successful breastfeeding by Furman, Minich, and Hack (2002).

BENEFITS OF KMC FOR THE BABY

Cardiorespiratory Stability

Bergman, Linley, and Fawcus (2004) compared cardiorespiratory stability in low-birth-weight infants (1200–2199 grams at birth) who were randomized to routine incubator care or KMC for the first 6 hours postdelivery. At the end of 6 hours, 56% of the KMC group had perfect scores for cardiorespiratory stability compared with only 11% of the standard care group. In a subanalysis of those infants weighing less than 1800 grams at birth, 44% of the KMC group had perfect scores compared to none in the standard care group. In a case study, heart rate variability was high when the infant was fussing in the incubator, but when he was placed in STS contact with his mother, his heart rate variability decreased as he fell asleep. The parasympathetic component of heart rate variability was the most volatile and sensitive to the decreasing stress as the infant settled into KMC (McCain, Ludington-Hoe, Swinth, & Hadeed, 2005).

In another study of preterm infants born at older gestational ages (34–36 weeks), KMC was used to assist with recovery from the fatigue of birth. Infants were placed on their mothers' chests skin to skin immediately after the birth in the delivery room and were left there for the first 6 hours post-birth. Heart rates, respiratory rates, and oxygen saturations remained within normal limits, and the grunting respirations of two of the infants disappeared with continuous STS contact. Sleep predominated as the infant state. The infants stayed with their mothers and were discharged within 48 hours fully breastfeeding (Ludington-Hoe et al., 1999). Another case report of a 33-weeks' gestation infant with mild respiratory distress at birth suggests that KMC used in conjunction with ventilatory care may assist with recovery (Swinth, Anderson, & Hadeed, 2003).

Respiratory rates of preterm infants also become more regular when being held in KMC (Anderson, 1991; Bergman et al., 2004). While in the incubator, respiration fluctuated with periodic breathing and apnea. This fluctuation was more pronounced in babies under 1800 grams birth weight, presumably because of lower gestational age. However, the fluctuations became less frequent and less pronounced in the KMC infants of all weights (Bergman et al., 2004). Apnea, bradycardia, and periodic breathing were absent during KMC in a randomized, controlled trial of 33–35-weeks' gestation infants (Ludington-Hoe, Anderson, Swinth, Thompson, & Hadeed, 2004).

Oxygen saturations maintain high levels when babies are in KMC position, and fewer desaturations are seen. Values of less than 90% oxygen saturation were seen in 24% of the standard care recordings compared to only 11% of the KMC recordings ($p < 0.001$) (Bier et al., 1996). Fohe, Kropf, and Avenarius (2000) broke down the study infants into the following three different weight categories: < 1000 grams, 1000–1500 grams, and > 1500 grams. The smallest heart rate increases and highest respiratory rate decreases during STS care were seen in the smallest babies (< 1000 grams). This group also had double the increase in oxygen saturation and transcutaneous pO_2 compared with larger babies during STS care.

However, despite many studies in this area, Charpak et al. (2005) state that the amount of evidence for cardiorespiratory benefits remains low because the studies are "either limited or equivocal" (p. 516). Potential confounders, are, among others, heterogeneity of gestational age and lack of definition of gestational age groups in the study, type and severity of illness both at birth and entry into the study, and the duration and frequency of KMC. A Cochrane systematic review from 2003 found only three randomized trials to include, all from developing countries and of "moderate to poor methodological quality. The most common shortcomings were in the areas of blinding procedures for those who collected the outcomes measures, handling of drop outs, and completeness of follow-up" (Conde-Agudelo,

Diaz-Rossello, & Belizan, 2003). This review highlights the need for further research and randomized, controlled trials in developed countries on all physiological parameters.

Neurodevelopmental Outcomes

Charpak et al. (2005) cite studies from Colombia that demonstrated higher IQs at 1 year of age when continuous KMC occurred compared to control subjects who were given traditional care (KMC 101.1; traditional care 97.4; $p < 0.02$). A higher Griffiths score was found at 1 year corrected age in infants who had been previously diagnosed with "doubtful or overtly abnormal neurological development" (p. 517) at 6 months in the group who had KMC (12.9 points higher). The authors explain that there are several effects of KMC. Mothers experiencing KMC are more sensitive to their infants' needs and respond more rapidly. They also try to provide more stimulating home environment for the infant. Early initiation of the intervention also helps by providing qualitative compensation for lost intrauterine experience and decreases stimulus overload from the extrauterine environment. Higher scores on the Neonatal Behavioral Assessment Scale at 40 weeks' postmenstrual age and on the Bayley Scales of Infant Development and the Carey's Infant Temperament Questionnaire at 6 and 12 months corrected ages were seen in babies held in KMC (Ohgi et al., 2002).

The KMC position itself also provides combinations of sensory experiences for the infant that interact. These include auditory experiences of the mother's voice, olfactory sensations of the mother and her milk, vestibular-kinetic stimulation from being placed on the mother's chest and experiencing her walking about, tactile stimulation from the skin-to-skin contact; and visual stimulation of being able to see the mother's face. Higher breastfeeding rates among mothers giving KMC also may contribute to the higher IQs (Charpak et al., 2005).

Pain Relief

Considerable research has been conducted on pain relief in healthy, term newborns who undergo heel-stick procedures and circumcisions. A review of this literature, conducted by Gray, Watt, and Blass. (2000), summarizes the palliative mechanisms as components of the nursing-suckling process, various tastes and flavors (including sweet solutions, milk, protein, and fat), and body contact. Each appears to be mediated by a different mechanism or pathway, with flavor-associated mediation apparently from an opioid effect.

In their own study of healthy, term infants, Gray et al. found significant reductions in crying (82%) and grimacing (65%) during the heel-stick procedure when infants were held by their mothers STS prior to and during the procedure compared with the control group of infants who were swaddled in a crib. Heart rates of infants in the contact group also remained stable during the procedure, rising only 8–10 heartbeats per minute over the course of the collection, compared to a rise of 36–38 beats per minute to a peak of 160 in the control group. Unlike nonnutritive sucking and flavor-induced analgesia, KMC is context dependent and gradual. It requires that the mother (or person engaging in the STS contact) be relaxed and that the holding begin 10–15 minutes prior to the onset of the painful procedure. The authors conclude that STS is "an effective, easily implemented, and safe intervention against pain in human newborns" (Gray et al., 2000).

Other researchers have documented similar effects of pain control in preterm infants who had blood drawn during KMC versus while they were in the incubator. Crying was less both during the procedure and during the recovery phase when babies were receiving KMC (Castral, Warnock, Leite, Haas, & Scochi, 2008; Kostandy et al., 2008; Ludington-Hoe, Hosseini, & Torowicz, 2005). Heart rate during a heel stick also was decreased during KMC compared to standard care (Castral et al., 2008; Johnston et al., 2008; Ludington-Hoe et al., 2005). Scores for facial changes and behavioral state were significantly lower during KMC (Castral et al., 2008; Ferber & Makhoul 2008; Johnston et al., 2008). Oxygen saturation was better during recovery from the heel stick in KMC babies, and they took significantly less time to recover (a 1-minute difference) than swaddled infants in their incubators. The protective power of the KMC response to pain appears to be moderated by gestational age, however, and the pain response in very preterm infants is not as powerful as the response in somewhat older and more mature infants (Johnston et al., 2008).

Adding rocking, music, and sucking during KMC made no difference in the efficacy of KMC for pain relief (Johnston et al., 2009). In a comparison of KMC and oral glucose for pain management in 28–36-week preterm infants, there was a smaller variation in heart rate and oxygen saturation, a shorter duration of facial responses, and a lower pain profile in the group receiving only KMC (Freire, Garcia, & Lamy, 2008). A coregulatory response of cortisol levels (as an indicator of stress) has been demonstrated between mothers and infants held in KMC, with moderation of this effect by sound levels in the NICU. A quiet environment when mothers and infants are in KMC position is therefore recommended (Neu, Laudenslager, & Robinson, 2008).

State Modulation

Crying

Crying is an indication of stress in an infant—something is not right in the infant's life. In several mammalian species, when babies become separated from their mothers they make a separation distress call that alerts the mother that all is not well and draws her back into close proximity to her infant. Cat owners recognize this in kittens; when the mother leaves the nest to feed herself or take a break, there is much mewing from the kittens who are distressed to be separated from the source of food and warmth. Christensson, Cabrera, Christensson, Uvnas-Moberg, and Winberg (1995) suggest that there is a counterpart in humans when mothers and infants are separated at birth. In a randomized, controlled trial, term infants who were allowed to remain in STS contact for the first 90 minutes after birth cried significantly less than infants who remained in a crib for the first 90 minutes after birth (Christensson et al., 1992). Bergman et al. (2004) refer to the crying elicited during separation as a part of protest-despair behavior. Driven by the sympathetic nervous system, the baby exhibits agitation (disorganized activity) and crying as a protest to being left on its own. The baby is trying to elicit a response from the mother and reunite with the mother. The parasympathetic nervous system, in turn, lowers heart rate and temperature—a despair response—perhaps to increase the possibility of survival in case the mother does not return for an extended period of time.

Anderson (1989) provides a mechanism that explains why crying is harmful in newborns. Crying obstructs return of venous blood flow in the inferior vena cava and reestablishes fetal circulation in the heart. This can happen as soon as the baby cries within the first 4 to 5 days postbirth. When pressure is released, then poorly oxygenated blood flows through the foramen ovale and back into the systemic circulation rather than to the lungs where it would pick up more oxygen. The release of a large bolus of blood also causes large fluctuations in blood flow under high pressure through the foramen ovale, some of which must go to the brain. Venous return in the superior vena cava is also obstructed, and this increases cerebral blood volume and decreasing cerebral oxygenation in a fluctuating pattern. This type of fluctuating pattern is associated with intracranial hemorrhage in preterm infants (Brenner, Perlman, & Volpe, 1988). Anderson (1989) notes that patent foramen ovale has been discovered in 40% of adults under 55 with ischemic strokes who have normal cardiac examination. The hypothesis is that paradoxical emboli can transfer through a patent foramen ovale to the brain and cause the stroke. Anderson suggests that preterm infants are even more vulnerable to crying during this period because it takes longer for the circulatory adaptation to an extrauterine environment to occur. Therefore, more mother–infant contact to prevent crying and distress might be preventive of intracranial hemorrhage, especially in infants whose respiratory systems are compromised by immaturity (Anderson, 1989).

KMC helps to regulate behavioral state by decreasing crying (Anderson, 1991; Ludington-Hoe & Swinth, 1996; Whitelaw, 1986). In a randomized, controlled trial of stable, preterm infants in early KMC (1 day after birth), Chwo et al. (2002) found that KMC infants spent less time crying and had more quiet sleep than the non-KMC control subjects.

Sleep States

A number of observational studies have demonstrated that both the frequency and duration of quiet sleep are increased during KMC in both term and preterm infants. In the case of term infants (Ferber & Makhoul, 2004), all the study infants were initially left skin to skin with their mothers immediately after birth until delivery of the placenta, then taken to the nursery for assessment (a 15–20-minute time frame). The babies in the intervention group were then returned to their mothers in the delivery rooms, where they were placed skin to skin once more and left there for an hour. The control group remained in the nursery. The intervention group spent significantly more time in sleep states (both deep [quiet] and light [active REM] sleep) and significantly less time in the transitional, fussy, crying, and alert states than the control group. The authors suggest that the mother's touch elicits a more competent and adaptive response from the infant and provides a barrier to stimuli that interferes with this adaptation. More quiet sleep also implies better brain stem control and has been shown to be associated with better cognitive abilities and attention in later development (Ferber & Makhoul, 2004).

In the preterm infant, one of the advantages of KMC is that the mother's skin and clothing as well as the blankets placed over both mother and infant provide sound-dampening effects and reduce stimulation in the NICU. Numerous studies have found that preterm infants spend more time in quiet sleep during KMC (Anderson, 1991; Feldman & Eidelman, 2003; Ludington 1990; Ludington-Hoe & Swinth 1996; Messmer et al., 1997). In a review by Charpak et al. (2005), the results of these studies are "uniform . . . for preterm infants, ranging from those who are very small and very immature within the first week of life to those who are nearly at term and medically stable" (p. 516). Preterm infants settle down rapidly when KMC is initiated and usually fall asleep. Active sleep diminishes in KMC, and the infant goes into quiet sleep. Fathers also have this effect on their KMC-held preterm infants, and quiet sleep continues for longer periods with fathers compared to mothers. Long-term differences have also been noted with more mature state organization and sleep-wake cycles in preterm infants at term (Feldman, Weller, Sirota, & Eidelman, 2002).

In another randomized, controlled trial that measured sleep using objective electroencephalographic/polysomnographic measurements, the KMC group had significantly more quiet sleep, less rapid eye movement, fewer arousals, and less indeterminate sleep than the control group in the incubator. The authors suggest that the more mature sleep pattern experienced by the KMC group could be used as an intervention to improve not only sleep organization in preterm infants but also their brain organization (Ludington-Hoe et al., 2006).

Behavioral State

Improved infant state is an outcome of KMC and better brain stem organization. Even when they are awake, preterm infants in STS contact/KMC position are less agitated and remain in a quiet alert state (Charpak et al., 2005). Less energy is therefore expended when infants are STS with their mothers because infants have less random activity that wastes energy. Anderson (1991) reported more alert inactivity in infants during KMC and better growth rates as a result. Feldman and Eidelman (2003) also reported that KMC infants had more alert wakefulness and significantly more mature neurodevelopmental profiles for habituation and orientation. Ludington (1990) refers to KMC as a "simple, cost-effective intervention that reduces activity and state-related energy expenditure" (p. 445).

Thermoregulation

Meta-analyses show that the two physiological outcomes that are clearly altered by KMC are temperature and weight (Charpak et al., 2005). The mother's breasts are very sensitive thermoregulators, warming up when the baby becomes chilled and cooling down when the baby gets too warm. During a 1–2-hour session of KMC, infant body temperature increases approximately 1°C (Charpak et al., 2005).

Bauer et al. (1997) measured rectal and skin temperatures in stable preterm infants < 1500 grams during the first week of life outside the womb, comparing temperatures during incubator care versus 1 hour of KMC. Temperatures at both sites were significantly warmer during the 1 hour of KMC than during the previous hour during incubator care. Once placed back in the incubator, infants cooled down to their original temperatures. It was also noted that there was no significant difference in oxygen consumption during KMC versus incubator care. In a follow-up study, Bauer tried to determine if there is an effect of gestational age on STS care; is there an age at which STS care is not advisable during the first week of life postbirth due to increased stress on the infant from being out of a controlled environment (Bauer, Pyper, Sperling, Uhrig, &Versmold, 1998)? In this second study, infants 25–27 weeks' gestation lost heat when placed STS, but infants 28–30 weeks' gestation did not lose body heat and instead warmed up when STS. By the second week postbirth, the 25–27-week group of infants could maintain a stable body temperature when STS. A prospective study by Fohe et al. (2000) conducted in a pretest (incubator)-test (STS)-posttest (incubator) method on infants weighing less than 1800 grams found no risk of hypothermia, even in the subgroup that weighed less than 1000 grams.

In a randomized, controlled trial, toe temperatures were significantly higher during KMC than when infants were in the incubator, and mothers' breasts met their infants' thermal needs within 5 minutes of initiating KMC (Ludington-Hoe, Nguyen, Swinth, & Satyshur, 2000). In the same study, infants maintained their optimal body temperature even during the 3-hour interfeeding interval.

In shared kangaroo mother care (SKMC), twins receive kangaroo care simultaneously. In two cases of SKMC, each breast responded independently of the other to the thermal needs of the closest infant (Ludington-Hoe et al. 2006). The authors conclude that twins can be held in SKMC without thermal compromise.

WHAT ABOUT FATHERS?

If KMC/STS care is so beneficial for babies, then we should be practicing it. But do fathers practicing KMC/STS care have the same beneficial effects on infant physiology as mothers do? The earliest study to examine paternal STS contact was in Colombia, where KMC originated. Eleven healthy, preterm infants had 2 hours of paternal STS contact within the first 17 hours after birth. Infant physiology and behavioral states, as well as fathers' behaviors, were monitored during this time. Infant heart and respiratory rates increased during paternal STS care as did body temperatures. However, the regulatory process involved in maintaining infant body temperature at optimal levels did not seem to work as well with fathers, and five of the infants became overheated despite cooling measures. Similar to STS care by mothers, infants also slept most of the time when they were held by fathers. Paternal behavior towards the infant was very different, however, and fathers seldom spoke to their infants, touched them, or looked at them for long periods of time (Ludington-Hoe, Hashemi, Argote, Medellin, & Rey, 1992). However, blinded researchers in an unpublished Swedish study found that they could tell from the way the father interacted with the baby months later whether STS care had occurred. The STS fathers were much more interactive and bonded to their infants (M. Vilandia, personal communication, September 7, 1997).

Other differences between mothers and fathers have been noted in a Norwegian study where fathers waited significantly longer times ($p = 0.0004$) postdelivery to hold their infants STS. Fathers held their infants later than mothers, despite having seen the infants much earlier than the mothers did. The mean waiting time for fathers before the first opportunity to hold their infants was 120.9% longer than the mean waiting time for mothers (Gloppestad, 1996).

Fathers also need to learn to be parents and need that bonding time with their infants. If the mother is too ill to provide STS care, then support should be given to the father to provide this essential part of caregiving, including allaying fears of causing harm to the infant.

KMC—THE HOW AND WHEN

When to Practice KMC

There are five different time periods at which KMC can begin for preterm infants—birth, very early, early, intermediate, and late. The definitions of each of these time frames can be seen in **Table 9-3**. Based on information from Ludington-Hoe's book for parents (Ludington-Hoe & Golant, 1993), written during a period of time when there was not a great deal of research available, these time frames of initiation of KMC have specific criteria. For example, hospitals around the world in both developed and developing countries routinely practice KMC at *birth* for older preterm infants (34–36 weeks' gestation) who have APGAR scores of 6 or more at 5 minutes. No adverse effects are seen from this practice when the criteria are observed. *Very early* KMC is practiced on babies who have adapted well to their environment within the first 5–10 minutes postbirth. They are dried off and then handed back to their mothers, usually within 30 minutes of birth while the

Table 9-3 Starting KMC–Time Frame Definitions

Birth
Immediate placement of the infant on the mother's chest prior to the cord being cut. This is used in other countries, especially with infants of 34 to 36 weeks' gestation who have 5-minute APGAR scores of 6 or more.

Very Early
Begins within the first 30 minutes of life after the infant has been assessed for specific medical needs and problems. In several countries, such as France and Sweden, babies of 27 and 28 weeks' gestation are handed back to their mothers within 5 minutes if the assessment has found that the baby has adapted well to its extrauterine environment.

Early
Begins as soon as the baby is stabilized after birth. Early KMC may also begin within the first 24 hours of life.

Intermediate
Begins after the first 7 days in the NICU, when infants have had a chance to stabilize in an incubator. They have been removed from ventilation prior to initiation of KMC.

Late
Begins when a baby is in an open-air crib and is able to breathe room air.

Source: Adapted from Ludington-Hoe & Golant, 1993, pp. 182–189.

delivery is completed. This can happen successfully in some 26–27-weeks' gestation preterm infants, and in older gestational ages it has resulted in competent breastfeeding within 24 hours and shorter hospitalizations because the infants remain in KMC (3.7 days compared to 10 days in the NICU). *Early* KMC can be started even for babies who are on ventilators. According to European experience, even when an infant is not stabilized, there has not been a need to stop KMC because of a clinical problem. *Intermediate* KMC begins when the baby is stabilized and off the ventilator but still in an incubator. *Late* onset of KMC is the type of KMC that had been studied the most as of the writing of Ludington-Hoe's book (Ludington-Hoe & Golant, 1993, pp. 182–189).

Criteria

Criteria for beginning KMC should be based on the individual baby, its stability (which admittedly means different things to different people), and clinical judgment. In Chapter 6, two situations in which KMC is *not* recommended were delineated—babies with skin that is too fragile for handling and babies on pressor medications for blood pressure regulation. The upright position required for KMC may change the blood pressure and therefore alter the medication needs. In the early 1990s, when not a lot was known about how infants responded to KMC, one group of researchers established a series of criteria that are more conservative than current ones (Ludington-Hoe & Galant, 1993; Ludington-Hoe, Thompson, Swinth, Hadeed, & Anderson, 1994). As they conducted more research on younger gestational ages, they relaxed their criteria, recognizing that many of these critically ill babies could tolerate KMC very well (Ludington-Hoe, Ferreira, Swinth, & Ceccardi, 2003). It is now understood that because of the added physiological stability gained when babies are in KMC, many of these criteria were unnecessary.

A comprehensive set of criteria comes from the California Perinatal Quality Care Collaborative (CPQCC) and its revised *Nutritional Care of the VLBW Infant Toolkit* (CPQCC 2008). In Appendix 5–A1, *eligible infants* are defined as those who are on less than 40% oxygen consistently and who tolerate daily weighing well with no adverse events. Ineligible infants may include:

- Infants having severe apnea, requiring more than tactile stimulation to recover
- Infants receiving vasodilators, vasopressors, or analgesics/sedatives via continuous IV
- Infants requiring increasing ventilatory support such as increasing pressures, oxygen requirements, or reintubation

Appendix 5–A2 of the tool kit does not give the criteria for ineligibility, instead focusing on eligibility of stable, preterm infants. *Stable* is defined in this document as "infants who are not requiring frequent changes of respiratory support, with stable vital signs in normal ranges, who will tolerate brief handling with no change, or brief changes, in oxygen saturation. Infants on low dose dopamine may be considered stable, if frequent adjustments of the dosage are not required." (CPQCC, 2008). No weight restrictions appear as part of the following criteria:

- Stable respiratory status. (This includes minimal apnea and bradycardia episodes. O_2 is acceptable and babies who are ventilated or on Nasal Continuous Positive Air Pressure (NCPAP) and stable on those are eligible for KMC.)

- Peripherally Inserted Central Catheter (PICC), Broviac, or umbilical venous catheter lines are permissible.
- Babies with umbilical arterial catheters and peripheral arterial lines may be allowed to receive KMC with an order from a physician or neonatal nurse practitioner.

Transfer Method

Neu, Browne, & Vojir (2000) recommend the parent type of transfer as being the least problematic for NICU infants. Babies served as their own control subjects and were randomly assigned to receive either parent or nurse transfer on two consecutive days. Thermoregulation, oxygenation, and heart rate were monitored, and assessment of behavioral scores for physiologic organization, motor organization, and self-regulation was conducted at each of the transfers. Both methods resulted in some physiologic disorganization, but infants showed more disorganization, less self-regulation, and more need for caregiver facilitation when the nurse transferred the baby to the parent.

With both types of transfer, the nurse assists the mother. The nurse changes all the monitor leads so that they are on the outside of the incubator and ensures that the leads do not become dislodged in any way during the transfer, or that the ventilator becomes dislodged. In the nurse transfer, the mother is already seated in a chair and the nurse places the infant on the mother's chest and the mother covers both herself and the infant so that they both stay warm. In the mother transfer, the mother opens her hospital gown or clothing and leans into the incubator, moving the baby perhaps no more than a foot to her chest. She then covers herself and the baby and the nurse assists the couplet to the chair.

Position

The baby, wearing only a diaper and maybe a hat and booties, is placed on the mother's unclothed chest in a fetal or froglike and flexed position. The baby can lie between the mother's breasts vertically or diagonally across the mother's chest. The fetal position is the most comforting for the infant as it simulates womb position. Once positioned, the baby is covered with a blanket and the mother then wraps her clothing or hospital gown around the blankets and baby. In some countries, special shirts have been designed for KMC that support the weight of the baby if the mother is standing up and walking around doing chores and needs her hands free.

A reclining chair is a must for KMC. If the baby is limp, flaccid, weak, very sick, or very young gestationally, the baby may have difficulty in maintaining its head in an upright position if the mother is sitting in an erect posture. When the baby cannot maintain its head position, the airway may become obstructed and apnea may result. A reclining position for the mother is therefore advantageous. It is also advantageous to have a slightly reclining posture (at about a 60° angle) for about 30–45 minutes if the baby begins KMC right after being fed. This helps prevent regurgitation of the feeding. If the baby has gastroesophageal reflux, then it is important for the mother to remain in a more erect position for at least 45 minutes after the feeding. A semireclined position is also more comfortable for the mother if the infant has a ventilatory tube in place. Once the baby has reached approximately 34 weeks' corrected age, mothers can sit in a more upright position with no ill effects on the infant. Ludington-Hoe and Golant (1993) offer more tips for parents about making themselves comfortable as well.

Duration

Ludington-Hoe, Thompson, Swinth, Hadeed, and Anderson (1994) recommend that the *minimum* time frame for KMC is 1 hour. Transferring infants from incubator to mothers' arms and dressing and undressing infants is physiologically stressful to the infant, so longer durations of KMC allow the infant to acclimate and experience some deep sleep before being stressed again with the transfer back to the incubator. "There is no rationale to support policies limiting or dictating the amount of time spent in KMC. Even though many European sites recommend four to five hours of KMC per session, KMC may be more enjoyable if it is not time-locked . . ." (Ludington-Hoe et al., 1994, p. 25).

Ending KMC Sessions

Appendix 5–A1 from the CPQCC's protocols recommend terminating a KMC session at the parent's request or if the baby shows persistent signs of stress such as apnea, bradycardia, desaturation, or respiratory distress that does not resolve with the usual interventions.

IMPLEMENTING A KMC PROGRAM—ONE HOSPITAL'S EXPERIENCE

Smith (2007) writes of her level 3 NICU's change in practice to using KMC. The implementation was based on published research, current practice within the nursery, and discussions with both staff and parents. Interactive education, support, and ongoing review of unit practices and outcomes were used, with a focus on educating parents and staff about sleep states and cues. Understanding sleep states helped staff to better assess infants and recognize the difference between restful and restless sleep and to accept the parent's role in infant sleep and growth in the NICU to achieve discharge.

SUMMARY

Appendix 9-1 gives a set of model policies for the implementation of step 7. As we have seen in this chapter and in Chapter 6, staff discomfort and lack of understanding about the benefits and how-tos of KMC/STS care looms as a barrier for its implementation. Education about STS care/KMC for both staff and parents should therefore be a top priority. KMC/STS care should also become an integral part of milk production for every breastfeeding mother, but should not be limited only to mothers who have chosen to provide their milk. STS care/KMC should be for *all* new parents, both mothers and fathers.

Staff members and parents should also be informed about how the baby communicates distress or comfort with its environment. As Smith (2007) suggests, information about sleep states should also be included in this education so that parents and staff can recognize when the infant is becoming agitated or restless.

Protocols should include clear procedures describing how to provide STS care/KMC, when to initiate it, and when to terminate it for infants. In Bonnie's case (see Chapter 1), it was the lack of a protocol and clear policies relating to STS care/KMC that frustrated her so much. Every nurse had a different piece of knowledge about STS care/KMC, often incorrect and anecdotal. Physicians also contributed to the confusion with their mixed messages to both nurses and parents. Bonnie and her son were only allowed to be skin to skin for 1 hour maximum. If the STS care was to happen after a feeding, she had to wait for 30 minutes before she could hold him. The premise was that if she held him too soon after feeding that he would get sick, which is not at all research or evidence-based. Bonnie also reported that her son would be placed between her breasts with his legs incorrectly dangling straight down and he would tuck each hand under the closest breast and fall into a deep sleep. Bonnie would read to him and he would stay in the deep sleep until someone came to put him back in the incubator. When she read to him in the incubator, he would open his eyes and look at her, but did not keep them open very long because the amount of light bothered him, but he would listen to the sound of her voice and be awake.

Unfortunately, Bonnie and her son never received the maximum benefits of KMC. Even as he began to gain weight well and his heart and respirations stabilized in the incubator, his sleep patterns were interrupted by the short duration of KMC. He was destabilized by transfers that were too close together and did not allow a lot of recovery time and synchrony with his mother. He was not allowed the analgesic effects of KMC during painful procedures. As his mother struggled to maintain the milk supply that allowed him to grow so well, she was deprived of the benefits of KMC that could have helped increase her supply.

We learned that Bonnie's son cried while he was still in the amniotic sac on the delivery table—a distress cry from separation and getting chilled. Skin-to-skin care would have recreated the experience of the womb for him—hearing his mother's heartbeat, the sound of her voice, and all the while feeling the rocking motion of her body, and the security of containment and being held in a flexed position snuggled up to his mother's body with minimized sensory stimulation from external sources. Technology has taken precedence over the baby and his security. Technology has supplanted our understanding of physiology and the response of mothers' and babies' bodies to each other. As a standard of NICU care, KMC enhances the prematurely born infant's normal biology and the behavioral entrainment of primates that Small describes (Small, 1998).

REFERENCES

Affonso, D., Wahlberg, V., & Persson, B. (1989). Exploration of mothers' reactions to the kangaroo method of prematurity care. *Neonatal Network, 7*(6), 43–51.

Anderson, G. (1989). Risk in mother–infant separation postbirth. *IMAGE: Journal of Nursing Scholarship, 21*(4), 196–199.

Anderson, G. (1991). Current knowledge about skin-to-skin (kangaroo) care for preterm infants. *Journal of Perinatology, 11*(3), 216–226.

Bauer, K., Pyper, A., Sperling, P., Uhrig, C., & Versmold, H. (1998). Effects of gestational and postnatal age on body temperature, oxygen consumption, and activity during early skin-to-skin contact between preterm infants of 25–30 weeks gestation and their mothers. *Pediatric Research, 44*(2), 247–251.

Bauer, K., Uhrig, C., Sperling, P., Pasel, K., Wieland, C. & Versmold, H. (1997). Body temperatures and oxygen consumption during skin-to-skin (kangaroo) care in stable preterm infants weighing less than 1500 grams. *Journal of Pediatrics, 130*(2), 240–244.

Bergman, N., Linley, L., & Fawcus, S. (2004). Randomized controlled trial of skin-to-skin contact from birth versus conventional incubator for physiological stabilization in 1200–2199-gram newborns. *Acta Paediatrica, 93*(6), 779–785.

Bier, J., Ferguson, A., Morales, Y., Liebling, J., Archer, D., Oh, W., et al. (1996). Comparison of skin-to-skin contact with standard contact in low-birth-weight infants who are breastfed. *Archives of Pediatric and Adolescent Medicine, 150*(12), 1265–1269.

Brenner, J., Perlman, J., & Volpe, J. (1988). Muscle paralysis (MP) of infants with blood pressure (BP) fluctuations markedly reduces the incidence of intraventricular hemorrhage (IVH). *Pediatric Research, 23*, 402a [Abstract 1207].

Cadwell, K., & Turner-Maffei, C. (2009). *Continuity of care in breastfeeding: Best practices in the maternity setting.* Sudbury, MA: Jones and Bartlett.

California Perinatal Quality Care Collaborative. (2008). *Nutritional support of the VLBW infant—revised 2008.* Retrieved December 31, 2008, from http://www.cpqcc.org/quality_improvement/qi_toolkits/nutritional_support_of_the_vlbw_infant_rev_december_2008

Castral, T., Warnock, F., Leite, A., Haas, V., & Scochi, C. (2008). The effects of skin-to-skin contact during acute pain in preterm newborns. *European Journal of Pain, 12*(4), 464–471.

Charpak, N., Ruiz, J., Zupan, J., Cattaneo, A., Figueroa, Z., Tessier, R., et al. (2005). Kangaroo mother care: 25 years later. *Acta Paediatrica, 94*(5), 514–522.

Christensson, K., Cabrera, T., Christensson, E., Uvnas-Moberg, K., & Winberg, J. (1995). Separation distress call in the human neonate in the absence of maternal body contact. *Acta Paediatrica, 84*(5), 468–473.

Christensson, K., Siles, C., Moreno, L., Belaustequi, A., De La Fuente, P., Lagercrantz, H., et al. (1992). Separation distress call in the human neonate in the absence of maternal body contact. *Acta Paediatrica, 81*(6–7), 488–493.

Chwo, M., Anderson, G., Good, M., Dowling, D., Shiau, S., & Chu, D. (2002). A randomized controlled trial of early kangaroo care for preterm infants: Effects on temperature, weight, behavior, and acuity. *Journal of Nursing Research, 10*(2), 129–142.

Conde-Agudelo, A., Diaz-Rossello, J., & Belizan, J. (2003). *Kangaroo mother care to reduce morbidity and mortality in low birthweight infants.* Retrieved December 27, 2008, from http://www.cochrane.org/reviews/en/ab002771.html

Engler, A., Ludington-Hoe, S., Cusson, R., Adams, R., Bahnsen, M., Brumbaugh, E., et al. (2002). Kangaroo care: National survey of practice, knowledge, barriers and perceptions. *American Journal of Maternal Child Nursing, 27*(3), 146–153.

Feldman, R., & Eidelman, A. (2003). Skin-to-skin contact (kangaroo care) accelerates autonomic and neurobehavioural maturation in preterm infants. *Developmental Medicine and Child Neurology, 45*(4), 274–281.

Feldman, R., Weller, A., Sirota, L., & Eidelman, A. (2002). Skin-to-skin contact (kangaroo care) promotes self-regulation in premature infants: Sleep-wake cyclicity, arousal modulation, and sustained exploration. *Developmental Psychology, 38*(2), 194–207.

Ferber, S., & Makhoul, I. (2004). The effect of skin-to-skin contact (kangaroo care) shortly after birth on the neurobehavioral responses of the term newborn: A randomized, controlled trial. *Pediatrics, 113*(4), 858–865.

Ferber, S., & Makhoul, I. (2008). Neurobehavioral assessment of skin-to-skin effects on reaction to pain in preterm infants: A randomized, controlled within-subject trial. *Acta Paediatrica, 97*(2), 171–176.

Fohe, K., Kropf, S., & Avenarius, S. (2000). Skin-to-skin contact improves gas exchange in premature infants. *Journal of Perinatology, 20*(5), 311–315.

Freire, N., Garcia, J., & Lamy, Z. (2008). Evaluation of analgesic effect of skin-to-skin contact compared to oral glucose in preterm neonates. *Pain, 139*(1), 28–33.

Furman, L., Minich, N., & Hack, M. (2002). Correlates of lactation in mothers of very low birth weight infants. *Pediatrics, 109*(4), e57.

Gloppestad, K. (1996). Parents' skin-to-skin holding of small premature infants: Differences between fathers and mothers. *Vard i Norden, 16*(1), 22–27.

Gray, L., Watt, L., & Blass, E. (2000). Skin-to-skin contact is analgesic in healthy newborns. *Pediatrics, 105*(1), e14.

Hake-Brooks, S., & Anderson, G. (2008). Kangaroo care and breastfeeding of mother-preterm infant dyads 0–18 months: A randomized, controlled trial. *Neonatal Network, 27*(3), 151–159.

Hurst, N., Valentine, C., Renfro, L., Burns, P., & Ferlic, L. (1997). Skin-to-skin holding in the neonatal intensive care unit influences maternal milk volume. *Journal of Perinatology, 17*(3), 213–217.

Johnston, C., Filion, F., Campbell-Yeo, M., Goulet, C., Bell, L., McNaughton, K., et al. (2008). Kangaroo mother care diminishes pain from heel lance in very preterm neonates: A crossover trial. *BMC Pediatrics, 8,* 13. Available from http://www.biomedcentral.com/1471-2431/8/13

Johnston, C., Filion, F., Campbell-Yeo, M., Goulet, C., Bell, L., McNaughton, K., et al. (2009). Enhanced kangaroo mother care for heel lance in preterm neonates: A crossover trial. *Journal of Perinatology, 29*(1), 51–56.

Kostandy, R., Ludington-Hoe, S., Cong, X., Abouelfettoh, A., Bronson, C., Stankus, A., et al. (2008). Kangaroo care (skin contact) reduces crying responses to pain in preterm infants: Pilot results. *Pain Management Nursing, 9*(2), 55–65.

Ludington, S. (1990). Energy conservation during skin-to-skin contact between premature infants and their mothers. *Heart Lung, 19*(5 Pt. 1), 445–451.

Ludington-Hoe, S., Anderson, G., Simpson, S., Hollingsead, A., Argote, L., & Rey, H. (1999). Birth-related fatigue in 34–36 week preterm neonates: Rapid recovery with very early kangaroo (skin-to-skin) care. *Journal of Obstetric, Gynecologic, and Neonatal Nursing, 28*(1), 94–103.

Ludington-Hoe, S., Anderson, G., Swinth, J., Thompson, C., & Hadeed, A. (2004). Randomized controlled trial of kangaroo care: Cardiorespiratory and thermal effects on healthy preterm infants. *Neonatal Network, 23*(3), 39–48.

Ludington-Hoe, S., Ferreira, C., Swinth, J., & Ceccardi, J. (2003). Safe criteria and procedure for kangaroo care with intubated infants. *Journal of Obstetric, Gynecologic, and Neonatal Nursing, 32*(5), 579–588.

Ludington-Hoe, S., & Golant, S. (1993). *Kangaroo care: The best you can do to help your preterm infant.* New York: Bantam Books.

Ludington-Hoe, S., Hashemi, M., Argote, L., Medellin, G., & Rey, H. (1992). Selected physiological measures and behavior during paternal skin contact with Colombian preterm infants. *Journal of Developmental Physiology, 18*(5), 223–232.

Ludington-Hoe, S., Hosseini, R., & Torowicz, D. (2005). Skin-to-skin contact (kangaroo care) analgesia for preterm infant heel stick. *AACN Clinical Issues, 16*(3), 373–387.

Ludington-Hoe, S., Johnson, M., Morgan, K., Lewis, T., Gutman, J., Wilson, P., et al. (2006). Neurophysiologic assessment of neonatal sleep organization: Preliminary results of a randomized controlled trial of skin contact with preterm infants. *Pediatrics, 117*(5), e909–e923.

Ludington-Hoe, S., Nguyen, N., Swinth, J., & Satyshur, R. (2000). Kangaroo care compared to incubators in maintaining body warmth in preterm infants. *Biological Research for Nursing, 2*(1), 60–73.

Ludington-Hoe, S., & Swinth, J. (1996). Developmental aspects of kangaroo care. *Journal of Obstetric, Gynecologic and Neonatal Nursing, 25*(8), 691–703.

Ludington-Hoe, S., Thompson, C., Swinth, J., Hadeed, A., & Anderson, G. (1994). Kangaroo care: Research results, and practice implications and guidelines. *Neonatal Network, 13*(1), 19–27.

McCain, G., Ludington-Hoe, S., Swinth, J., & Hadeed, A. (2005). Heart rate variability responses of a preterm infant to kangaroo care. *Journal of Obstetric, Gynecologic, and Neonatal Nursing, 34*(6), 689–694.

Messmer, P., Rodriguez, S., Adams, J., Wells-Gentry, J., Washburn, K., Zabaleta, I., et al. (1997). Effect of kangaroo care on sleep time for neonates. *Pediatric Nursing, 123*(4), 408–414.

Neu, M., Browne, J., & Vojir, C. (2000). The impact of two transfer techniques used during skin-to-skin care on the physiologic and behavioral responses of preterm infants. *Nursing Research, 49*(4), 215–223.

Neu, M., Laudenslager, M., & Robinson, J. (2008). Coregulation in salivary cortisol during maternal holding of premature infants. *Biological Research for Nursing, 10*(3), 226–240.

Ohgi, S., Fukuda, M., Moriuchi, H., Kusumoto, T., Akiyama, T., Nugent, K., et al. (2002). Comparison of kangaroo care and standard care: Behavioral organization, development, and temperament in healthy, low-birth-weight infants through 1 year. *Journal of Perinatology, 22*(5), 374–379.

Ramanathan, K., Paul, V., Deorari, S., Taneja, U., & George, G. (2001). Kangaroo mother care in very low birth weight infants. *Indian Journal of Pediatrics, 68*(11), 1019–1023.

Small, M. (1998). *Our babies, ourselves: How biology and culture shape the way we parent.* New York: Anchor Books, Doubleday.

Smith, K. (2007). Sleep and kangaroo care: Clinical practice in the newborn intensive care unit: Where the baby sleeps . . . *Journal of Perinatology and Neonatal Nursing, 21*(2), 151–157.

Suman, R., Udani, R., & Nanavati, R. (2008). Kangaroo mother care for low birth weight infants: A randomized controlled trial. *Indian Pediatrics, 45*(1), 17–23.

Swinth, J., Anderson, G., & Hadeed, A. (2003). Kangaroo (skin-to-skin) care with a preterm infant before, during, and after mechanical ventilation. *Neonatal Network, 22*(6), 33–38.

Whitelaw, A. (1986). Skin-to-skin contact in the care of very low birth weight babies. *Maternal Child Health, 7*, 242–246.

APPENDIX 9-1

STEP 7

Promote early and continued skin-to-skin contact for mothers and their premature and/or compromised infants with full mechanical breastmilk expression.

Policies 7.1–7.7

Title

Optimizing benefits of skin-to-skin contact for both NICU/SCN babies and their parents.

Purpose

To provide parents with education and support to facilitate close contact with their infants for up to 24 hours per day.

Supportive Data

Premature and/or compromised infants held skin to skin have improved physiologic stability and feeding tolerance (Bergman, Linley, & Fawcus, 2004). Skin-to-skin contact increases milk production and the establishment and maintenance of breastfeeding for longer periods in NICU/SCN mothers and babies (Hurst, 1997). Skin-to-skin contact may facilitate bonding and attachment (Kirsten, Bergman, & Hahn, 2001).

Rationale

The presence of parents is the most fundamental basic security that an infant can have, especially when separated from parents due to prematurity and/or medical fragility. Skin-to-skin care is associated with increased amounts of milk, longer duration of breastfeeding, and breastfeeding success (Anderson, 1991; Furman, Minich, & Hack, 2002; Hurst, Valentine, Renfro, Burns, & Ferlic, 1997; Kirsten et al., 2001).

Scope

These policies apply to all NICU/SCN personnel including the medical director, nursing director, nursing supervisors, licensed staff, ancillary staff, and volunteers.

Policy 7.1

Staff should be educated regarding benefits of kangaroo mother care (KMC) and skin-to-skin (STS) care for the physiological and psychological well-being of both mother and baby.

Policy 7.2

Parents should be informed about the benefits of skin-to-skin contact and encouraged to practice skin-to-skin contact during visits, as soon as the infant's physical condition allows.

Procedure 7.2.1
Staff should educate parents about the benefits of skin-to-skin care including:

Neonatal

- Thermal synchrony—mother's body temperature rises and falls to maintain the infant in a neutral state.
- Cardiopulmonary—adequate or improved oxygenation; fewer episodes of periodic breathing, apnea, and bradycardia.
- Breastfeeding—increased incidence and length; increased milk supply.
- Behavioral—increased alert activity, *en face* positioning, and deep sleep; decreased or no crying; reduction in perception of pain during painful procedures.
- Earlier discharge—increased weight gain; no increased infection; decreased severity of infection and mortality; out of incubator earlier.
- Long term—increased length and head circumference at 9 month/1 year of age; more consistent and appropriate maternal responses at 15 month of age; less crying at 6 months of age.

Parental

- Increase in maternal self-confidence, competence, and self-esteem.
- Enhancement of parent–infant attachment.
- Initiation and maintenance of maternal interactive behavior.
- Acquisition of positive and personally beneficial experience.
- Promotion of positive parental identity and knowledge of infant.
- Increase in confidence in meeting infant's needs.
- Promotion of parental eagerness for infant's discharge.

Procedure 7.2.2
Staff should demonstrate skin-to-skin care with the parents and return demonstration should be documented in the medical record.

Process

- Nurse transfers all leads and monitors and prepares all parties and physical setting.
- Instruct parent to wear front-opening shirt or patient gown open in front (mothers should remove bra for infant comfort). Infant wears only a diaper and hat as needed to minimize temperature loss.
- Provide a chair with arms and pillows as needed for comfort, as well as a footstool if available. Reclining chairs are preferable.
- Have parent take care of personal needs (hunger, thirst, use of bathroom facilities) before initiating skin-to-skin contact.
- Initiate skin-to-skin care using the standing transfer technique preferentially. For standing transfer, parent stands directly in front of infant in bed with nurse assisting (two NICU/SCN staff members if the infant is intubated). Parent leans into incubator and lifts baby and places the infant gently against his or her chest. Parent is assisted to chair by nurses and seated.
- Position the infant so that the parent supports buttocks with hands, tucking lower extremities into flexion so that the infant feels secure. Infant is covered with parent's shirt, gown, and/or blanket. Head and neck are positioned to protect the airway.
- Terminate skin-to-skin contact immediately at parent's request or if the infant exhibits any of the following:

  sustained desaturations
  color changes
  respiratory distress
  heart rate instability
  unrelenting irritability
  other signs of intolerance noted by parents and/or staff

Policy 7.3

To improve maternal milk supply, ensure that mothers practice STS care frequently throughout the infant's NICU stay. Maternal practice of STS care should be *preferentially encouraged* over father until adequate milk volumes are attained.

Policy 7.4

Parents should be taught infant approach and avoidance behaviors.

Policy 7.5

The medical and nursing staff should conduct minor procedures whenever possible while the baby is on either parent's chest (e.g., heel stick, vital signs, assessment, etc.).

Policy 7.6

The hospital should provide space and opportunity in the NICU/SCN for the parents to be in close contact with their baby both at the bedside and, when the baby is more stable, in private parents' sleep or day rooms. Privacy should be provided as necessary with the judicious use of screens. Interruptions should be minimized.

Policy 7.7

NICU/SCN units should maintain an open and welcoming parental visitation policy. It is expected that as part of the team working toward optimal infant outcome, parents should be with their infants frequently and practicing skin-to-skin care as much as possible. Periods in which the unit is closed to parents should be rare and brief.

REFERENCES

Anderson, G. (1991). Current knowledge about skin-to-skin (kangaroo) care for preterm infants. *Journal of Perinatology, 11*(3), 216–226.

Bergman, N., Linley, L., & Fawcus, S. (2004). Randomized controlled trial of skin-to-skin contact from birth versus conventional incubator for physiological stabilization in 1200- to 2199-gram newborns. *Acta Paediatrica, 93*(6), 779–785.

Furman, L., Minich, N., & Hack, M. (2002). Correlates of lactation in mothers of very low birth weight infants. *Pediatrics, 109*(4), e57.

Hurst, N., Valentine, C., Renfro, L., Burns, P., & Ferlic, L. (1997). Skin-to-skin holding in the neonatal intensive care unit influences maternal milk volume. *Journal of Perinatology, 17*(3), 213–217.

Kirsten G., Bergman, N., & Hann, F. (2001). Kangaroo mother care in the nursery. *Pediatric Clinics of North America, 48*(2), 443–452.

chapter ten

Step 8: Transitioning the Baby to Full Breastfeeding

The WHO/UNICEF Ten Steps for Successful Breastfeeding, step 8, specifies that the infant should be breastfed on demand (on cue), while step 9 specifies that breastfed infants should not be given any artificial teats, meaning bottle nipples and pacifiers. For the purposes of this book, these two steps have been combined and placed opposite the ABI Step 8 for the preterm infant. Step 8 states that initiation of breastfeeding should be developmentally appropriate and early and that transition to full breastfeeding occur as soon as possible (see **Table 10-1**).

STEPS 8 AND 9 FOR THE HEALTHY, TERM INFANT

For the healthy, term infant step 8 means that babies should be exclusively breastfed on their own schedules at their best times. According to Cadwell and Turner-Maffei (2009), scheduled feedings have distinct disadvantages for the healthy, term infant, including:

- Lower weight gain when compared to infants fed on cue
- Shorter duration of breastfeeding
- Increased likelihood of supplementation
- Increased risk of jaundice

All of these negative outcomes can be minimized when mothers demonstrate knowledge of feeding and satiety cues and understand that irregular time intervals between feedings are expected. Allowing the infant

Table 10-1 Side-by-Side Comparison of Three Models

Principle	*WHO/UNICEF Ten Steps to Successful Breastfeeding for the Healthy Term Newborn*	*ABI's Ten Steps for the NICU/SCN*	*Nyqvist and Kylberg (2008) Swedish Mothers' 13 Steps*	*Danish Ten Steps to Successful Breastfeeding of Preterm Infants*
Baby-led feeding	Step 8. Encourage breastfeeding on demand.*	Step 8. Foster early developmentally appropriate initiation and transition to full breastfeeding.	Step 7. Encourage and support mothers in early initiation of breastfeeding, with infant stability as the only criterion. Give mothers individual support. Step 9. Encourage breastfeeding on demand as early as possible, with semidemand breastfeeding as a transitional strategy for preterm infants (the mother nurses when an infant shows signs of interest, and in addition offers her infant the breast in order to reach a breastfeeding frequency per 24 hours that is sufficient for adequate infant milk intake).	Step 3. Parents are prepared to breastfeed a preterm infant. Step 5. The mother gets the support and information she needs to facilitate breastfeeding. Step 7. The mother is guided in positioning and attachment of the infant at the breast.
Pacifier use	Step 9. Give no artificial teats or pacifiers (also called dummies or soothers) to breastfeeding infants.		Step 10. Offer the infant a pacifier for relief of pain, stress and anxiety, and for stimulating the uptake of nutrients during tube feeding. Introduce bottle-feeding when there is a reason.	Step 9. Parents are prepared to continue breastfeeding/milk expression after discharge.

* Should be read as "on cue."

to practice unrestricted feeding, determining when it wants to breastfeed and when it wants to end the feeding should extend breastfeeding duration and exclusivity.

When healthcare providers integrate these basic tenets of successful breastfeeding into their practices, they are better able to translate this information for the mother. Many misconceptions about unrestricted breastfeeding exist. The following are accurate statements that refute the misconceptions:

- Sore nipples are *not* the result of unrestricted feeding (they are most commonly the result of suboptimal breastfeeding practices and poor attachment that lead to increased incidence of engorgement, sore nipples, and other breast and nipple problems).
- The breast is not a bladder and does *not* need to fill, store, and rest between feedings in order for the infant to have adequate nutrition (in fact, the opposite is true—milk is produced faster when it is efficiently removed from the breast frequently).
- Crying is *not* a feeding cue (it is an indication that all of the baby's other feeding cues have been missed! See **Table 10-2** for a list of feeding cues).

Healthy, term infants are fabulous little communicators if we only take the time to listen and observe. They are programmed to feed in an unrestricted way—it is an innate method of survival.

In step 9 of the Ten Steps for the healthy, term infant, the expectation is that pacifier use and the use of bottles and nipples be avoided for breastfed infants in the hospital. Pacifiers and nipples have been observed to create difficulties for some infants when they are first learning to breastfeed. The mechanisms of feeding on the human breast versus a bottle with a nipple on it are very different, as explained next.

- In breastfeeding, the infant must open his mouth very wide and get as much of the breast as possible into his mouth to create the space and negative pressure required to remove milk; the reverse is true for bottle-feeding, where the baby makes his mouth as small as possible when he sucks on the teat like a straw.
- The shape and feel of the mother's nipple in the baby's mouth are very different from the shape and feel of an artificial nipple, which is firmer and less pliable.

Table 10-2 Early Feeding Cues (in the Healthy, Term Infant)

- Rooting, turning the head, especially with searching movements of the mouth
- Increasing alertness, especially rapid eye movement under closed eyelids
- Flexing of the legs and arms
- Bringing or attempting to bring a hand to the mouth (the baby does not have to be successful)
- Sucking on a fist or finger
- Mouthing motions of the lips and tongue
- Head bobbing

Source: Cadwell & Turner-Maffei, 2009, p. 96. Used with permission.

According to the World Health Organization and UNICEF, cup feeding is the preferred method of providing supplemental feedings to breastfed infants. This is largely for reasons of sanitation and cost—cups are standard feeding utensils found in virtually every household in the world and they are more easily cleaned than bottle teats and bottles. The mechanism of bottle-feeding, as mentioned previously, is different, and research on term infants cited in Cadwell and Turner-Maffei (2009) indicates that bottle-feeding is more stressful physiologically on the infant than breastfeeding. Infants have lower oxygen saturations and higher heart and respiratory rates when supplements are given via the bottle.

Evidence shows that routine pacifier use in healthy, term infants may have a negative association, in a dose-dependent way, on breastfeeding. The more frequently a pacifier is used, the shorter the duration of breastfeeding. Exclusive breastfeeding is also negatively impacted with more frequent supplementation given to babies who use pacifiers routinely. Cause and effect have not been established, however, and the issue remains whether a mother uses a pacifier more frequently *because* she is already have breastfeeding problems, or whether the use of the pacifier *causes* the breastfeeding problems. Cadwell and Turner-Maffei (2009) give a comprehensive evidence-based review of the effects of pacifiers on breastfeeding.

MODIFICATIONS FOR THE PRETERM INFANT

Step 8 for the hospitalized, preterm infant has been modified to state that NICUs/SCNs should foster early developmentally appropriate initiation and transition to full breastfeeding. The goal is to work toward the preterm infant feeding at the breast efficiently and effectively at every feeding. When the infant cannot be breastfed from the moment of birth because of premature birth and lack of mature, stable, and optimally functioning organ systems, the process of achieving breastfeeding at every feeding is a long and sometimes arduous journey. The ability to successfully achieve breastfeeding is directly related to the type of practices that occur (or do not occur) in the NICU from the beginning of the baby's journey to wellness. In Bonnie's case (see Chapter 1) she was never able to feed her son at breast even though she succeeded in providing him with her milk at every feeding for more than 7 months. NICU practices that were directly related to her son's difficulty in achieving full breastfeeding were limiting skin-to-skin contact, not allowing skin-to-skin contact during a feeding and for an hour after each feeding, insistence on the baby being able to bottle-feed before he could go to breast, etc. The model policy presented in **Appendix 10-1** demonstrates how a NICU implementing the policy might avoid some of the problems Bonnie and her son experienced.

Early Feeding Practices: Use of Colostrum, Trophic Feedings

According to the World Health Organization, low birth weight (< 2500 g) and very low birth weight (< 1500 g) may contribute, either directly or indirectly, to 60–80% of all neonatal deaths globally. Among other practices such as early detection and treatment of infections and maintaining thermal stability, appropriate infant feeding practices can "substantially reduce excess mortality" in these infants (WHO, 2009, p. 51). As stated previously in Chapter 8, the best choice for feeding a preterm infant who cannot go directly to the breast is the mother's expressed milk, beginning with colostrum used either as oral care or fed through a tube, depending on the volume available. If the mother's own expressed colostrum or mature milk is unavailable or the quantity is inadequate, then donor milk should be used, either as the entire feeding or as a supplement. WHO (2009) reinforces this recommendation and also recommends that infants less than 32 weeks' gestation be fed every 1–2 hours beginning within the first 12–24 hours of life (see also Chapter 8). For very-low-birth-weight infants (< 1250 g) "who do not show feeding readiness," (WHO, 2009, p. 53) beginning with trophic feedings of 1–2 ml every 1–2 hours is recommended by WHO. WHO recommends that low-birth-weight babies less than 32 weeks' gestation receive 60 ml/kg on day 1 of life outside the womb, increasing by 10–20 ml per day over the first 7 days of life with a minimum of eight feedings in a 24-hour period. If the infant received an increase of 15 ml/day, by day 7 postbirth, the baby would be receiving 160 ml/kg/d. After the first 7 days postbirth, WHO recommends that the quantity be increased further on a daily basis until the infant reaches 180 ml/kg/d. However, if the baby is not achieving what WHO deems a satisfactory weight gain of more than 15 g/kg each day, then the volume should be increased further until 200 mg/kg/d is reached (WHO, 2009). (See **Tablc 10-3** and **Table 10-4**.) However, when practicing more aggressive nutrition for the preterm infant, these recommendations of exclusive human milk may appear to be on the conservative side in some NICUs.

Nonnutritive Sucking: Gavage Feeding While at the Breast and Use of a Pacifier

In a video entitled *Breast is Best*, produced by the Norwegian National Breastfeeding Committee, there is a section on breastfeeding the preterm infant. A 30-weeks'-gestation infant is being held by his mother for the very first time. They are skin to skin and he looks at his mother and demonstrates mouthing movements. When placed at the breast his lower jaw drops and he attaches to the nipple. Although he doesn't really know how to suck, when his mother hand expresses some colostrum he laps it up off her nipple, hugging the breast while doing so. A care provider then provides his feeding through a tube while he is at the breast, so the he will "associate the feeling of a full stomach with being at the breast" (*Breast is best*, 1994). The care

Table 10-3 Feeding the Preterm Infant: What, When, How, and How Much?

	< 32 Weeks' Gestation	*32–36 Weeks' Gestation*	*Late Preterm**
What	Expressed human milk—either mom's own or donor	Human milk—expressed or suckled depending on skills of the infant	Suckled human milk supplemented with expressed human milk or donor milk as needed
How	Nasogastric tube while at breast or skin to skin	Cup, spoon, *paladai* if not breastfeeding	Breastfeeding
When	Begun 12–24 hours after birth	Start within 1 hour of birth or as soon as the infant is clinically stable	Start with first hour of life
How much	Depends on birth weight	Depends on birth weight	Feed on cue

* Late preterm infants are those born between 37 and 40 weeks' gestation.

Source: Modified from WHO, 2009.

Table 10-4 Advancing Feedings in the First 7 Days Postbirth[a]

Day of Life Postbirth	*1000–1500 g (Fed q°2)*[b]	*1500–2000 g (Fed q°3)*[b]	*2000–2500 g (Fed q°3)*[b]
Day 1	60 ml/kg/d (6 ml/feed)	60 ml/kg/d (12 ml/feed)	60 ml/kg/d (17 ml/feed)
Day 2	70 ml/kg/d (7 ml/feed)	75 ml/kg/d (16 ml/feed)	80 ml/kg/d (22 ml/feed)
Day 3	80 ml/kg/d (8 ml/feed)	90 ml/kg/d (20 ml/feed)	100 ml/kg/d (27 ml/feed)
Day 4	90 ml/kg/d (9 ml/feed)	115 ml/kg/d (24 ml/feed)	120 ml/kg/d (32 ml/feed)
Day 5	110 ml/kg/d (11 ml/feed)	130 ml/kg/d (28 ml/feed)	140 ml/kg/d (37 ml/feed)
Day 6	130 ml/kg/d (13 ml/feed)	145 ml/kg/d (32 ml/feed)	150 ml/kg/d (40 ml/feed)
Day 7	150 ml/kg/d (16 ml/feed)	160 ml/kg/d (35 ml/feed)	160 ml/kg/d (42 ml/feed)

[a]Amounts are given as the total fluid intake per day (recommended volumes for each feeding). If infants are being cup fed, an additional 5 ml per feeding should be added to allow for spilling and feeding differences in infant appetite.

[b]The shorthand used here, as in q°2, refers to a feeding every two hours; q°3 would refer to feeding every 3 hours. This assumes scheduled feeding rather than baby-led or cue-based feeding, which larger babies should be capable of depending on gestational age.

Source: Modified from WHO, 2009.

provider uses a syringe attached to the feeding tube and hand pushes the feeding into the baby's stomach, paying careful attention all the time for any indication that the baby might be under stress and that the feeding is occurring too rapidly. Many care providers in Scandinavia feel that using a syringe system without using an automatic pump to deliver the feeding is an advantage, as the nurse can immediately tell when the baby is being compromised or decompensating. With the use of an infusion pump system, close attention may not be paid to the infant while he is being fed. Signs of distress may be missed when an infusion pump set-up is used.

Besides the additional monitoring that the infant receives from this close attention, there are clear advantages to this type of individualized feeding. First, the baby and mother are skin to skin, which helps foster that mother–infant interaction that is so crucial to the well-being of both of them.

The peripheral nerve stimulation that occurs during STS contact elevates beneficial gastrointestinal hormones such as gastrin and cholecystokinin and improves the absorption of nutrients from a feeding (see Chapter 8). STS care also helps calm the baby and helps the mother to increase her milk supply (see Chapter 9).

Second, if the infant is being fed while at the mother's breast, he does learn that the smell of her milk and the taste of it are associated with being fed, especially if he can lick colostrum or hand-expressed milk off the nipple. Even if his mouth is surrounding the nipple and he sucks on the breast occasionally, this is practice and learning by association. One group of researchers has found that the smell of breastmilk increases the total number of sucks as well as the number of sucking bursts (Bingham, Abassi, & Sivieri, 2003; Bingham, Churchill, & Ashikaga, 2007). In the first study, breastmilk (with fortifier added) odor was directed to the nose using a specially modified pacifier. As the suck occurred, a pressure pulse was recorded to indicate the suck. Simultaneously, the suck led to the release of odor via nasal ports created in the pacifier. The experiments were conducted during a tube feeding. The odor of the breast milk was compared to the odor of formula or water (as a sham observation). Combining the results of the human milk group and water group gave a highly statistically significant difference when compared to exposure to formula alone. In a 10-minute observation period, the human milk group combined with the water group had 260.4 sucks and 41 bursts of sucking compared to the formula group, which had 144.8 sucks and 27.4 suck bursts (Bingham et al., 2003). The second study used an olfactometer with tube-fed, premature infants and found that six out of seven preterm infants responded to the smell of human milk with an increased number of sucks (Bingham et al., 2007).

Narayanan and colleagues describe nonnutritive sucking (NNS) at the breast as follows:

> The mother was asked to express the milk as completely as possible from both breasts (in the unit manual expression was practiced as is common in developing countries); the infant was then put to breast in a warm room and allowed to suckle. Finally the full calculated volume of milk was given by intermittent bolus by the orogastric route. (Narayanan, Mehta, Choudhury, & Jain, 1991, p. 241)

The intervention began when preterm infants were 10 days old. Tiny, preterm infants are described as merely mouthing the nipple when initially put to breast, but soon established well-sustained sucking with bursts of sucking activity. Exclusive and total breastfeeding durations postdischarge were longer in the group that received the NNS on the emptied breast. The intervention helped the mother improve her milk supply and supplied infants with sucking experience and practice while avoiding nutritional compromise. For Narayanan (1990), use of the emptied breast for NNS is preferable to use of a pacifier, primarily because of concerns related to infection with pacifier use in developing countries.

Nonnutritive Sucking with a Pacifier

In developed countries, nonnutritive sucking (NNS) on a pacifier is thought to be beneficial to preterm infants, decreasing significantly the time for tube feeding as well as gastric retention when used during tube feeding. Somatostatin levels are significantly reduced in connection with NNS, and the gastric hormones released during NNS stimulate gastric motor functions and facilitate digestion and absorption of nutrients, resulting in better growth (Widstrom et al., 1988). Field et al. (1982) found that preterm infants offered pacifiers during the feedings averaged 27 fewer tube feedings, started bottle-feeding 3 days earlier, had a greater average daily weight gain, and were discharged from the hospital eight days earlier. Baghat and Elsayed (1999) found that their NNS (pacifier) cohort of preterm infants had an accelerated development of the sucking reflex, and this cohort also shifted to oral feedings earlier and were discharged from the hospital earlier. Gill, Behnke, Conlon, and Anderson (1992) reported that the infants' behavioral state was significantly affected by pacifier use for 5 minutes both before bottle-feeding and after routine caregiving. Infants given pacifiers had more sleep and fewer restless states. The authors state: "When self-regulatory feeding policies based on early hunger cues are not allowed, nonnutritive sucking for 5 minutes pre-feeding is simple, brief, and appropriate for busy intensive care units" (p. 3). Another benefit of NNS on a pacifier may be sudden infant death syndrome prevention via protection of the upper airway. Tonkin et al. (2007) report that in preterm infants who suck on a pacifier, there is significant forward movement of the lower mandible and tongue, which does not change very much when the pacifier is removed. This forward movement helps open up the upper airway. Stress from bottle-feeding, as measured by heart rate and oxygen saturation rate in infants between 26 and 34 weeks, was reduced when NNS occurred for 5 minutes before and 5 minutes after feeding. Higher feeding performance scores were also seen after NNS (Pickler, Higgins, & Crummette, 1992). A Cochrane Database Systematic review of NNS on pacifiers in preterm infants by Pinelli and Symington (2005) found little consistent benefit of pacifier use in terms of weight gain, energy intake, heart rate, oxygen saturation, intestinal transit time, age at full oral feeds, or behavioral state. However, significantly shorter hospital stays as well as better transition from tube to bottle feeding were found when NNS on pacifiers was in place. Better bottle-feeding performance was also found. They also point out the need for further research, particularly on long-term outcomes related to pacifier use. If NNS occurred at the emptied breast, would similar benefit in the transition from tube to breastfeeding rather than bottle-feeding be seen?

Physiological Differences Between Breastfeeding and Bottle-Feeding

Many NICUs have policies that mandate that preterm infants, when transitioning from tube feedings to oral feedings, must "pass" bottle-feeding before they can advance to feeding at the breast. Because discharge from the NICU is predicated upon feeding competency, the rationale for passing bottle-feeding is that the infant can then be discharged as soon as he is feeding well on the bottle (all other factors being in place) (Nye, 2008). However, there is no scientific evidence to support these policies (Marinelli & Hamelin, 2005), and there is ample evidence to indicate that bottle-feeding is much more stressful for the preterm infant than breastfeeding. Meier (1988) monitored feeding sessions in five preterm infants who served as their own control subjects, bottle-feeding at one feeding and breastfeeding at another feeding. Transcutaneous oxygen pressure and temperature differed significantly in the infants between the two feeding types, with breastfeeding preserving better oxygen saturation levels—higher immediately postbreastfeed and 10 minutes after breastfeeding than during bottle-feeding. Infants also became significantly warmer during breastfeeding than during bottle-feeding. Similar findings were obtained in a larger study population of preterm infants by Chen, Wang, Chang, and Chi (2000). Observations of body temperature, oxygen saturation, heart rate, and respiratory rate were recorded every minute during a 20-minute feeding period. Body temperatures were significantly higher during the entire feeding period when the preterm infants were breastfed compared to being bottle-fed. Oxygen saturation levels decreased initially during bottle-feeding, but then recovered during the last half of the 20-minute feeding period. There were two episodes of apnea during bottle-feeding (none during breastfeeding) and 20 episodes of oxygen desaturations during bottle-feeding (none during breastfeeding). Pulse rate was more stable during breastfeeding (Chen et al., 2000). Given the more positive physiological outcomes of breastfeeding compared to bottle-feeding, it is surprising that so many NICUs still insist on bottle-feeding and putting preterm infants at risk for apnea, bradycardia, and oxygen desaturations. Meier (1996) also found that infants continued to breathe fairly regularly during breastfeeding within long sucking bursts, but did not breathe during long sucking bursts at the bottle. Meier suggests that either the flow of milk was slower at the breast or that the infant could *control* the rate of flow of milk better at the breast than when feeding from a bottle.

One short paper by Stine (1990) provides a protocol for the NICU to transition preterm babies directly to the breast. The babies were introduced to the breast as early as possible and supplementation was provided by gavage feedings. Among the mothers who had intended to breastfeed at discharge, most of them had achieved exclusive breastfeeding at discharge with this bottle-free protocol. In the Kliethermes, Cross, Lanese, Johnson, and Simon study (1999), the group who were transitioned to full breastfeeding without the use of bottles (feedings were given by gavage) were significantly more likely to be breastfeeding both at discharge and 3 months and 6 months postdischarge. A Cochrane review finds fault with the methodology of these studies, however, and therefore fails to endorse tube-feeding strategies as a method of avoiding bottles until more research can be done (Collins, Makrides, Gillis, & McPhee, 2008).

Transition to Breastfeeding—Earlier Rather Than Later

Nyqvist, Sjoden, and Ewald (1999) found early development of breastfeeding behaviors in preterm infants when they were allowed to go to the breast and practice. Breastfeeding was initiated in 71 infants at postmenstrual age of 27.9–35.9 weeks. At first contact with the breast, all infants demonstrated rooting and sucking behavior, regardless of gestational age. Efficient rooting, areolar grasp, and latch were observed at 28 weeks with repeated sucking bursts of $\geq$ 10 sucks and maximum bursts of $\geq$ 30 sucks at 32 weeks' postmenstrual age (PMA). Nutritive sucking appeared at about 30.6 weeks. At hospital discharge, 67 of the 71 infants were breastfeeding, with 57 of them establishing full breastfeeding at a mean of 36 weeks PMA. Nyqvist and colleagues interpret the early establishment of sucking behavior as the result of learning. In a later study by Nyqvist (2008), 15 mothers used the Preterm Infant Breastfeeding Behaviour Scale to assess their infants' oromotor behavior, and breastfeeding was initiated from a PMA of 29 weeks at which time obvious rooting, efficient areolar grasp, and repeated short sucking bursts were observed. Longer sucking bursts and repeated swallowing was observed from 31 weeks' PMA. Full breastfeeding was achieved at a median of 35 weeks (range 32–38 weeks), indicating that very preterm infants can develop oral motor competence and full breastfeeding at an early PMA.

Cue-Based Feeding—Hunger Cues

In bottle-feeding studies of premature infants fed on cue (demand) rather than on a schedule, cue-fed infants were discharged earlier than schedule-fed infants (Collinge, Bradley, Perks, Rezny, & Topping, 1982) and reached full oral feedings 6 days earlier than control subjects (Kirk, Alder, & King, 2007). Using a semidemand method of feeding (bottle-fed infants), McCain (2003) achieved hospital discharge 5 days earlier. The semidemand method was described as combining nonnutritive sucking to promote waking behavior for feeding, identifying feeding behaviors and readiness state, and observation of infant responses to feeding so that feedings could be terminated when the infant showed signs of distress or had had enough.

Signs that indicate interest in feeding are rhythmic sucking on a pacifier or a fist, mouthing movements, and a quiet alert state with an attentive and focused gaze, and they may include reaching movements when placed at or near the breast (Isaacson, 2008). If the infant begins to show signs of stress during a feeding, then a pause should occur to allow the baby to reorganize. If reorganization does not occur and the baby remains stressed or overstimulated, the feeding should be stopped and the baby should be fed the balance of intake by gavage.

The Developmental Phases of Transition to Full Breastfeeding

Dougherty and Luther (2008) have delineated the following five phases of breastfeeding development: (1) kangaroo care (see Chapter 9); (2) lick and sniff; (3) nibble and swallow; (4) milk transfer; and (5) full breastfeeding. These steps progress as the infant gains maturation, each infant having her own time frame. In the KMC phase, the mother provides physiological stabilization for the infant. This phase should accompany each of the following phases and should not be considered completed and checked off the checklist once the baby goes on to the second phase of lick and sniff. In the lick and sniff phase, the infant laps up milk on the end of the nipple that the mother has manually expressed and then may fall asleep at the breast. During this phase the mother may be asked to pump her breasts immediately before the session so that if she has a letdown during the licking and mouthing, the flow of milk will not overwhelm the infant and cause choking. Phase three is the nibble and swallow phase, during which the infant has brief periods of quiet alert time when learning is optimal. The beginning of a coordinated suck-swallow-breathe pattern may be seen during the later parts of this phase. It is advisable, according to Dougherty and Luther, to continue to have the mother express her milk prior to putting the infant to the breast. During the milk transfer phase, the baby can sustain a short sucking burst, with a pause to breathe, and some milk transfer is seen, although the volume may be quite small in the early stages of this phase. As the infant matures and his stamina improves, more and more milk will be transferred until the baby can occasionally transfer an entire feeding. This usually occurs by 36–37 weeks but may occur earlier. In the final phase, the infant has enough coordination, stamina, and strength to take all of its feedings at the breast, usually by discharge (Dougherty and Luther, 2008).

Positioning the Infant at the Breast

The two most effective positions for breastfeeding the preterm infant are the football hold and the cross-cradle hold. Both positions compensate for the infant's lack of muscle tone and help support the infant and maintain proper alignment so that the airway is not compromised. Lack of good support can result in the baby sliding off the breast and tiring easily from trying to stay latched (Marinelli & Hamelin, 2005; Isaacson, 2006). In both positions, the mother can control the head with one hand and support her breast and massage it with the other hand. Marinelli and Hamelin (2005) cite the need for keeping the infant on the nipple/areola by supporting the baby's head at the nape of the neck. In both positions, the baby is held close to the mother's body in a slightly flexed position. In each case, the mother should position the baby at the breast by bringing the baby to her breast, not leaning into the infant so that the breast touches the baby's mouth. Only after she has positioned the baby correctly should pillows be placed to support her arms and back and assist her in supporting the infant. According to Marinelli and Hamelin (2005), the cradle-hold or "Madonna" position that seems natural for mothers to use while breastfeeding is not appropriate for preterm infants or other infants with low muscle tone.

Marinelli and Hamelin (2005) also offer tips for helping an infant achieve a good latch. Lightly brushing the nipple across the infant's mouth will cause the infant to spontaneously open her mouth. When the mouth is open, the mother gently guides the infant onto the nipple/areola so that the nipple is in the upper half of the baby's mouth and the infant looks off center. If the mother's nipple is flat or otherwise not very elongated, it may be helpful for her to manipulate the nipple to shape a teat for the baby. The mother can do this by rolling her nipple between her thumb and forefinger or briefly using an electric pump just prior to the feeding session. Another suggestion to help make feedings more effective is to learn the infant's sleep/wake pattern. If the mother tries to feed the baby every afternoon at the same time when the baby is sound asleep, transition to breastfeeding may not progress. But if she changes her visiting schedule to be with the baby when he is more alert and awake and in an optimal state for learning, perhaps in the evenings or at night, then on-cue feedings can advance in number, and progress in the transition to full breastfeeding may be much more rapid.

When infants slow down at the breast during a feeding and do not swallow as often, the mother can frequently encourage more transfer of milk by either switching breasts or by doing breast massage and compression. The compression should occur during a sucking to stimulate the baby's interest and keep her actively sucking for a longer period of time (Marinelli & Hamelin, 2005).

Use of Nipple Shields to Assist in Transitioning the Infant to Breast

In a few examples in the literature, ultrathin silicone nipple shields have been used to assist in transitioning the preterm infant to breastfeeding. In a retrospective chart review, Clum and Primomo (1996) measured actual intake of milk at breast the first time the nipple shield was used and compared it to the prescribed amount the infant was supposed to be getting at each feeding. Sixty percent of infants consumed 50% or more of the prescribed amount. Infants who succeeded in removing greater than 50% of their feedings were found to have attempted feedings at an earlier age and to be heavier at birth, suggesting that these infants might have been slightly more mature and stronger than their counterparts whose intake was less than half the prescribed amount. Clum and Primomo note that time constraints in the NICU may have been a factor, since 67% of the infants were discharged after only 18 days or fewer between the first oral feed and discharge, indicating limited opportunities for learning and practicing on the part of the infants since mothers could not always be there to participate in oral feedings. Mothers in this study reported that their confidence in breastfeeding increased with use of the shield; others reported reduction in frustration levels surrounding getting the baby latched on and feeding.

In the Meier et al. (2000) report, milk transfer in two consecutive breastfeedings was compared, one with nipple shield use, one without. All 34 infants in the comparison consumed more milk when the nipple shield was in place. The influence of nipple shield use on breastfeeding duration was also examined. The mean duration of breastfeeding was 169.4 days with mean duration of nipple shields use 32.5 days—approximately 24% of the total breastfeeding experience. The author suggests that this indicates that there was no significant association of nipple shield use with shortened duration of breastfeeding.

Isaacson (2008) presents a number of reasons for using a nipple shield in a preterm population. If the infant has trouble staying awake at the breast and maintaining attachment, the nipple shield can assist the infant in maintaining attachment. The shield helps maintain the shape of the nipple in the baby's mouth during pauses in sucking, lessening the chance that the infant will slide off. Isaacson also notes that if the mother's nipple is large and/or flat, the use of a nipple shield also helps the infant to attach. Premature infants who may benefit from the use of a silicone nipple shield when learning how to breastfeed are "those with short inefficient bursts of sucking, limited energy and low suction at the breast, who fall asleep quickly at the breast, or whose mothers have flat or ill-defined nipples . . ." (Marinelli & Hamelin, 2005, p. 435). However, the size of nipple shield used should fit the size of the infant's mouth. If the mother's nipple is quite large and the infant's mouth very small, will the nipple shield fit the mother's nipple well? Dougherty and Luther (2008) indicate that the need for a nipple shield is demonstrated when infants show active feeding behaviors but frequent, repeated attempts to latch on are unsuccessful.

Isaacson (2008) states that the nipple shield is commonly used until the infant's approximate due date. By that time, the infant should have learned how to maintain attachment with enough suction pressure to maintain the shape of the nipple. Marinelli and Hamelin (2005) state that it is preferable to wean the baby from the nipple shield prior to discharge. If the infant must be discharged still using a nipple shield, then experienced lactation support must be available to ensure that the baby weans from the shield and that neither the mother's milk supply nor the infant's weight gain is compromised by continued use of the shield.

Supplementing the Breastfeeding, Preterm Infant

There are a number of ways to supplement a breastfeeding, preterm infant, several of which have been used by nurses in the absence of the mother. These include bottle-feeding (see discussion on the physiological differences between breastfeeding and bottle-feeding earlier in this chapter), continuing to tube feed (see previous discussion on nonnutrive sucking), finger feeding, and use of a cup. There is no data to evaluate or support the use of finger feeding as an alternative feeding method (Marinelli & Hamelin, 2005). These authors state that there is concern about finger feeding in that it introduces a hard surface into the baby's mouth, which is unlike the malleable and stretchable nipple of the mother's breast. Isaacson (2008) discusses the types of noxious oral stimuli that are frequent in the preterm infant's environment that can lead to oral aversion where the infant identifies anything in the mouth as being painful. Does invasion of the oral cavity by a large adult finger for the purposes of feeding present one more noxious stimulus to an infant trying to transition to full breastfeeding?

Many protocols that avoid bottles utilize cup feeding as one means of providing the balance of the prescribed volume when infants do not take the entire feeding at breast. According to Nye (2008), the National Association of Neonatal Nurses does not endorse the use of cup feeding in preterm infants. However, there are several studies that have looked at cup feeding in the preterm population and found it to be beneficial. Marinelli, Burke, and Dodd (2001) found that there was a tenfold increase in desaturation episodes during bottle-feeding compared to cup feeding. Preterm infants were physiologically more stable when cup feeding; however, they took smaller volumes over a greater period of time. Despite this drawback, the authors concluded that cup feeding was a safe alternative to bottle-feeding when infants were learning to breastfeed. Dowling, Meier, DiFiore, Blatz, and Martin (2002) found that cup-fed infants maintained physiologic stability when being fed, but bottle-fed infants did not maintain physiologic stability. However, spilling/drooling was high (range of loss to the bib = 6.7–63.2%; average loss 38.5%), and actual intake much less than anticipated. These authors concluded that cup feeding had questionable efficacy and efficiency.

Cup-fed infants are reported to be significantly more likely to be breastfeeding at discharge from the hospital when they were cup fed compared to those being bottle fed. Rocha, Martinez, and Jorge (2002) found a higher incidence of breastfeeding at 3 months in a cup-fed group of preterm infants compared to a bottle-fed group (cup feeding = 68.4% vs. bottle-feeding

33.3%; p = 0.04). Collins et al. (2004) found that cup-fed infants (compared to bottle-fed infants) were significantly more likely to be fully breastfeeding upon discharge, but had an overall longer hospital stay. Another study (Abouelfettoh, Dowling, Dabash, Elguindy, & Seoud, 2008) found that infants cup fed in the NICU developed significantly more mature breastfeeding behaviors than their bottle-fed peers at 6 weeks postdischarge, and as a result were significantly more likely to be exclusively breastfed 1 week postdischarge. In a Cochrane review, however, Flint, New, and Davies (2007) do not recommend cup feeding for supplemental feedings in infants unable to fully breastfeed because they found no differences in the number of infants who were fully or partially breastfeeding whether the supplementation was done by cup, bottle, or feeding tube.

When the mother is available, use of at-breast supplementers that have feeding tubes attached have been found to be effective in supplementing infants. For infants with a good latch who are able to transfer some milk but not an adequate volume, the supplementer is a way of delivering extra milk. Use of a supplementer also has the added advantage of helping to increase the mother's milk supply. According to Marinelli the device reinforces the position and latch of breastfeeding while reducing energy output in the infant. The tip of the tube should be placed close to the end of the nipple. The feeding-tube portion of an at-breast supplementer can also be placed inside a nipple shield to assist a baby with milk transfer (Marinelli & Hamelin, 2005).

Monitoring Intake

Clinical indices such as audible infant swallowing and measuring the number of swallows during a breastfeeding are not adequate measures of intake in the premature population (Meier, 1996). Highly skilled assessors of maternal and infant breastfeeding activity have been fooled by these indicators; for example, when transfer has been assessed by listening to the swallowing and then assessed immediately after, under identical conditions, using a digital scale, documentation of zero transfer has been seen. Babies have been swallowing their own saliva! What is needed to assess milk transfer is a digital scale that is accurate to 2 grams, as the weight in grams of milk consumed is the equivalent of the number of ccs of milk transferred. Weighing the infant before and after the feeding without changing clothing, blankets, diapers, bibs, leads, or tubes is the only way that one can assess the effectiveness of a feeding (Marinelli & Hamelin, 2005). The difference between the infant's actual intake and the prescribed volume can then be calculated, and the balance of the feeding given by gavage or cup, depending on the skills of the infant.

SUMMARY

There are many challenges for both the mother and the preterm baby in transitioning from the use of expressed breastmilk to full breastfeeding. Strict routines in the hospital, scheduled feedings, and limits on the amount of time spent at the breast work against feeding on cue/demand and establishing a successful at-breast feeding routine. Use of bottles and emphasis on measuring the baby's intake increases the mother's anxiety about her ability to establish breastfeeding successfully. Mothers also may get discouraged when attempts to transition the infant to the breast are not successful or take a much longer period of time than the mother expected. Weaning from the bottle of expressed milk may frequently go directly to bottle-feeding formula, especially after mothers get their infants home and find that the transition is even more difficult when they lack the support of the NICU staff (Buckley & Charles, 2006).

This chapter has been about the NICU practices and professional skills that can foster success at transitioning the infant to full breastfeeding. We must do a better job at getting babies to the "breastaurant" so that they associate the smell of the breast and the milk with something pleasurable, like a full tummy. More effort should be made to tube feed infants while they are at the breast as a standard of practice. We must also provide more opportunities for preterm infants to have early learning experiences at the breast, to learn and practice coordinating latching, sucking, swallowing, and breathing skills. Although not particularly addressed in this chapter, opportunities for mothers to really live with their infants and care for them for longer periods of time (along the lines of Levin's model—see Chapter 1) must be provided. The occasionally provided 24-hour rooming in that occurs in some NICUs immediately prior to discharge is not sufficient time and practice to instill confidence in a mother. Support for the mother while she learns to care for and feed her baby totally on her own should be provided. While this may be difficult for most hospitals to accomplish given space and staff limitations, a priority should be time for mothers and babies to really learn how to breastfeed and for the mothers to learn how to care for their infants and feed them exclusively at the breast prior to discharge.

REFERENCES

Abouelfettoh, A., Dowling, D., Dabash, S., Elguindy, S., & Seoud, I. (2008). Cup versus bottle feeding for hospitalized late preterm infants in Egypt: A quasi-experimental study. *International Breastfeeding Journal, 3*(1), 27.

Bahgat, R., & Elsayed, E. (1999). Effect of non nutritive sucking on the behavioral state and physiological change in premature infants before feeding. *Journal of the Egyptian Public Health Association, 74*(1–2), 81–96.

Bingham, P., Abassi, S., & Sivieri, E. (2003). A pilot study of milk odor effect on nonnutritive sucking by premature newborns. *Archives of Pediatric and Adolescent Medicine, 157*(1), 72–75.

Bingham, P., Churchill, D., & Ashikaga, T. (2007). Breast milk odor via olfactometer for tube-fed, premature infants. *Behavioral Research Methods, 39*(3), 630–634.

Breast is best. Norwegian National Breastfeeding Committee. VHS. Video-Vital, 1994.

Buckley, K., & Charles, G. (2006). Benefits and challenges of transitioning preterm infants to at-breast feedings. *International Breastfeeding Journal, 1*, 13.

Cadwell, K., & Turner-Maffei, C. (2009). *Continuity of care in breastfeeding: Best practices in the maternity care setting.* Sudbury, MA: Jones and Bartlett.

Chen, C., Wang, T., Chang, H., & Chi, C. (2000). The effect of breast- and bottle-feeding on oxygen saturation and body temperature in preterm infants. *Journal of Human Lactation, 16*(1), 21–27.

Clum, D., & Primomo, J. (1996). Use of a silicone nipple shield with premature infants. *Journal of Human Lactation, 12*(4), 287–290.

Collinge, J., Bradley, K., Perks, C., Rezny, A., & Topping, P. (1982). Demand vs. scheduled feedings for premature infants. *Journal of Obstetric, Gynecologic, and Neonatal Nursing, 11*(6), 362–367.

Collins, C., Makrides, M., Gillis, J., & McPhee, A. (2008). Avoidance of bottles during the establishment of breast feeds in preterm infants. *Cochrane Database of Systematic Reviews, 4*, CD005252.

Collins, C., Ryan, P., Crowther, C., McPhee, A., Paterson, S., & Hiller, J. (2004). Effect of bottles, cups, and dummies on breast feeding in preterm infants: Randomized controlled trial. *British Medical Journal, 329*(7459), 193–196.

Dougherty, D., & Luther, M. (2008). Birth to breast—a feeding care map for the NICU: Helping the extremely low birth weight infant navigate the course. *Neonatal Network, 27*(6), 371–377.

Dowling, D., Meier, P., DiFiore, J., Blatz, M., & Martin, R. (2002). Cup-feeding for preterm infants; mechanics and safety. *Journal of Human Lactation, 18*(1), 13–20.

Field, T., Ignatoff, E., Stringer, S., Brennan, J., Greenberg, R., Widmayer, S., et al. (1982). Nonnutritive sucking during tube feedings: Effects on preterm neonates in an intensive care unit. *Pediatrics, 70*(3), 381–384.

Flint, A., New, K., & Davies, M. (2007). Cup feeding versus other forms of supplemental enteral feeding for newborn infants unable to fully breastfeed. *Cochrane Database of Systematic Reviews, 2*, CD005092.

Gill, N., Behnke, M., Conlon, M., & Anderson, G. (1992). Nonnutritive sucking modulates behavioral state for preterm infants before feeding. *Scandinavian Journal of Caring Science, 6*(1), 3–7.

Isaacson, L. (2008). Steps to successfully breastfeed the premature infant. *Neonatal Network, 25*(2), 77–86.

Kirk, A., Alder, S., & King, J. (2007). Cue-based oral feeding clinical pathway results in earlier attainment of full oral feeding in premature infants. *Journal of Perinatology, 27*(9), 572–578.

Kliethermes, P., Cross, M., Lanese, M., Johnson, K., & Simon, S. (1999). Transitioning preterm infants with nasogastric tube supplementation: Increased likelihood of breastfeeding. *Journal of Obstetric, Gynecologic, and Neonatal Nursing, 28*(3), 264–273.

Marinelli, K., Burke, G., & Dodd, V. (2001). A comparison of the safety of cupfeedings and bottlefeedings in premature infants whose mothers intend to breastfeed. *Journal of Perinatology, 21*(6), 350–355.

Marinelli, K., & Hamelin, K. (2005). Breastfeeding and the use of human milk in the neonatal intensive care unit. In M. MacDonald, M. Mullet, & M. Seshia (Eds.), *Avery's neonatology: Pathophysiology and management of the newborn* (6th ed., pp. 413–444). Philadelphia: Lippincott Williams & Wilkins.

McCain, G. (2003). An evidence-based guideline for introducing oral feedings to healthy preterm infants. *Neonatal Network, 22*(5), 45–50.

Meier, P. (1988). Bottle- and breast-feeding: Effects on transcutaneous oxygen pressure and temperature in preterm infants. *Nursing Research, 37*(1), 36–41.

Meier, P. (1996). Suck-breathe patterning during bottle and breastfeeding for preterm infants. In T. David (Ed.), *Major controversies in infant nutrition.* (International Congress and Symposium Series No. 215). London: Royal Society of Medicine Press Limited.

Meier, P., Brown, L., Hurst, N., Spatz, D., Engstrom, J., Borucki, L., et al. (2000). Nipple shields for preterm infants: Effect on milk transfer and duration of breastfeeding. *Journal of Human Lactation, 16*(2), 106–114.

Narayanan, I. (1990). Sucking on the 'emptied' breast—a better method of non-nutritive sucking than the use of a pacifier. *Indian Pediatrics, 27*(10), 1122–1124.

Narayanan, I., Mehta, R., Choudhury, D., & Jain, B. (1991). Sucking on the 'emptied' breast: Non-nutritive sucking with a difference. *Archives of Disease in Childhood, 66*(2), 241–244.

Nye, C. (2008). Transitioning premature infants from gavage to breast. *Neonatal Network, 27*(1), 7–13.

Nyqvist, K. (2008). Early attainment of breastfeeding competence in very preterm infants. *Acta Paediatrica, 97*(6), 776–781.

Nyqvist, K., Sjoden, P., & Ewald, U. (1999). The development of preterm infants' breastfeeding behavior. *Early Human Development, 55*(3), 247–264.

Pickler, R., Higgins, K., & Crummette, B. (1992). The effect of nonnutritive sucking on bottle-feeding stress in preterm infants. *Journal of Obstetric, Gynecologic, and Neonatal Nursing, 22*(3), 230–234.

Pinelli, J., & Symington, A. (2005). Non-nutritive sucking for promoting physiologic stability and nutrition in preterm infants. *Cochrane Database of Systematic Reviews, 4*, CD001071.

Rocha, N., Martinez, F., & Jorge, S. (2002). Cup or bottle for preterm infants: Effects on oxygen saturation, weight gain, and breastfeeding. *Journal of Human Lactation, 18*(2), 132–138.

Stine, M. (1990). Breastfeeding the premature newborn: a protocol without bottles. *Journal of Human Lactation, 6*(4), 167–170.

Tonkin, S., Lui, D., McIntosh, C., Rowley, S., Knight, D., & Gunn, A. (2007). Effect of pacifier use on mandibular position in preterm infants. *Acta Paediatrica, 96*(10), 1422–1436.

World Health Organization (WHO). (2009). Appropriate feeding in exceptionally difficult circumstances. In *Infant and young child feeding: Model chapter for textbooks for medical students and allied health professionals* (pp. 51–64). Geneva, Switzerland: Author. Retrieved April 12, 2009, from http://www.who.int/nutrition/publications/infantfeeding/9789241597494.pdf

Widstrom, A., Marchini, G., Matthiesen, A., Werner, S., Winberg, J., & Uvnas-Moberg, K. (1988). Nonnutritive sucking in tube-fed preterm infants: Effects on gastric motility and gastric contents of somatostatin. *Journal of Pediatric Gastroenterology and Nutrition, 7*(4), 517–523.

APPENDIX 10-1

STEP 8

Foster early developmentally appropriate initiation and transition to full human milk feeding/breastfeeding.

Policies 8.1–8.15

Title

Early feeding practices and transitioning to full human milk feedings/exclusive breastfeeding.

Purpose

There are two purposes for these policies. The first is to employ early, antibody-rich colostrum for oral care in the infant who is not yet being fed orally, to stimulate metabolic and gastrointestinal adaptations to extrauterine nutrition, and to stimulate hormone production and secretion, enhance gastrointestinal motor activity, and promote intestinal growth and development. The second is to encourage mothers to put their premature and/or compromised infants to the breast as soon as the infant's medical condition warrants, so that the mother/infant dyad will become competent at feeding at the breast and be able to breastfeed exclusively without the need for bottle supplements by hospital discharge.

Supportive Data

During medically indicated periods when oral feeding is impossible in these vulnerable babies, oral care is traditionally done with sterile water. Alternatively, colostrum should be used not only to provide oral care, but also to begin to protect the oral mucosa with the high concentration of antibodies found in colostrum. The early use of colostrum is also associated with positive effects on the mother who feels she is providing an important part of her baby's care.

Suboptimal nutrition, starting early in the neonatal period, contributes to the accumulation of growth deficits early in postnatal life (Ziegler, Thureen, & Carlson, 2002). Infants provided only glucose solutions as nutrition in the first few days rapidly develop large protein and essential fatty acid deficits, with the smallest, most immature infants suffering the worst postnatal malnutrition (Thureen, 1999). Also, postnatal gut luminal starvation, after active GI activity in utero, results in nutritional deficits, morphological and developmental changes in the gut, and reduced host resistance to infections. Early introduction of feedings shortens the time to full feeds as well as the length of hospitalization and does not lead to an increase in NEC incidence (Ziegler et al., 2002). Feedings of human milk lead to an actual decrease in NEC (Lucas & Cole, 1990).

Early at-breast experiences, irrespective of current gestational age or weight, are valuable learning experiences even if calories are not transferred by the infant. Mothers are able to practice holding and positioning their infants without the pressure of needing to meet caloric requirements. If nasogastric (NG) feeds are given concurrently, infants are imprinted with how it feels, looks, smells, and tastes as their stomachs fill. Although it is quite variable, babies have been documented to transfer measurable amounts of milk as early as 28 weeks' gestational age (Nyqvist, 2008; Nyqvist, Sjoden, & Ewald, 1999).

Rationale

Premature infants on early enteral feedings have improved metabolic function and feeding tolerance without increased morbidity. Other advantages include the following:

- Shortened time to regain birth weight
- Reduced duration of parenteral nutrition
- Reduced need for IV access
- Reduced incidence of secondary line sepsis, subcutaneous IV infiltration, and need for central line placement
- Enhanced enzyme maturation
- Reduction of intestinal permeability
- Improved GI motility
- Matured hormone responses
- Improved mineral absorption and bone mineralization
- Lowered incidence of parenteral nutrition-associated cholestasis
- Reduced duration of phototherapy

Sucking and swallowing at the breast is less stressful than the utilization of the oral motor skills required for bottle-feeding (Meier, 1988, 1996).

Scope

These policies apply to all NICU/SCN personnel, including the medical director, nursing director, nursing supervisors, licensed staff, ancillary staff, and volunteers.

Policy 8.1

In the absence of oral feedings, maternal colostrum used as oral care should be initiated within hours of birth as listed next, irrespective of the infant's gestational age or medical stability. Colostrum or early milk is collected into small-volume containers to avoid waste.

- NICU/SCN staff or parents place a sterile swab into the colostrum container.
- Swab colostrum over tongue and oral mucosa.
- Use a fresh swab each time mouth care is done. Do not place a used swab into the colostrum container.
- Mouth care may be done as often as every 4 hours during cluster care.
- Record *colostrum mouth care* on NICU daily flow sheet.

Policy 8.2

Minimal enteral feedings of colostrum or donor human milk should begin within the first 2 hours after birth or as soon as medically possible. If infants are healthy enough or gestationally developed enough to begin breastfeeding, this should also begin within the first 2 hours after birth or as soon as medically possible.

Procedure 8.2.1

Enteral feedings should be administered via orogastric (OG) or NG tube until the infant is able to coordinate and tolerate suck and swallow.

Procedure 8.2.2

As soon as the infant begins minimal enteral feeds, colostrum should be used for that purpose if available. Use of frozen colostrum is preferable to fresh, more mature milk because it is developmentally appropriate for the immature gut.

Policy 8.3

Full-strength human milk, either colostrum, milk from the mother, or pasteurized donor milk, should be used for enteral feeds unless medically contraindicated. It should not be diluted. If full-strength human milk cannot be used, the reason should be documented in the medical record.

Policy 8.4

For infants who are NPO or on minimal enteral feedings, nonnutritive sucking should be offered so that gastric motility can begin as soon as possible.

Procedure 8.4.1
Infants who are NPO should be offered a pacifier during touch times with staff or parents or any time feeding cues are observed.

Procedure 8.4.2
Infants who are receiving minimal enteral feedings via tube should be offered a pacifier at the onset of each feeding. Pacifiers may be dipped in mother's colostrum, mature milk, or donor milk.

Policy 8.5

Volume of feedings (Kcal/kg/day) should be individualized to meet the infant's nutritional needs. No upper limit should be placed on oral feeds unless there are obvious medical complications with high volumes.

Policy 8.6

Infants who are not yet on oral feeds should be placed at the breast while being tube fed.

Policy 8.7

The NICU/SCN staff should provide the infant with time at the breast as soon as his/her condition permits.

Policy 8.8

Infants should be fed on cue, recognizing signs that indicate feeding readiness or hunger.

Procedure 8.8.1
Mothers should be taught to recognize hunger cues and signs of satiety.

Policy 8.9

No restrictions should be placed on the frequency or length of time at the breast unless the infant becomes unstable at the breast.

Procedure 8.9.1
Infants who demonstrate avoidance behaviors as documented per visual assessment and vital signs should be removed from the breast.

Policy 8.10

Evidence-based protocols and procedures for the use of supplemental feeding devices should be developed and indications for their use outlined.

Policy 8.11

The NICU/SCN staff and/or lactation staff should educate mothers about the process of breastfeeding.

Procedure 8.11.1
Mothers should be taught correct latch, correct body position and holding, and signs of milk transfer and satiety.

Policy 8.12

The NICU/SCN and/or lactation staff should assess each breastfeeding session and document each feeding in the medical record.

Procedure 8.12.1
The PIBBS assessment tool should be used by NICU/SCN staff and/or mother at least once daily.

Policy 8.13

Prebreastfeeding and postbreastfeeding weights should be used to assess baseline milk transfer and possible need for supplementation.

Procedure 8.13.1
A hospital-grade electronic gram scale (accurate to 1–2 g) should be used for weights.

Procedure 8.13.2
Prebreastfeeding and postbreastfeeding weights should be done intermittently at the onset of breastfeeding sessions to document progress. Once infants are transferring milk at the majority of feeds, weights should be done with each feed at breast and volumes transferred counted toward daily intake.

Procedure 8.13.3
The prebreastfeeding and postbreastfeeding weight information should be given to the mother as a baseline volume approximation of milk transfer by her infant.

Procedure 8.13.4
Mothers should be educated that even small volumes transferred are very positive signs that the infant is beginning to mature to a coordinated suck-swallow-breathe cycle.

Procedure 8.13.5
Initially, as infants are practicing at breast, daily fluid intake should be calculated based on energy and fluid requirements and given by NG feeds. As infants begin to transfer measurable quantities of milk, these volumes should be included with daily intake while the remainder is given by NG/OG. As infants begin to transfer appreciable amounts of milk, they should be placed on an ad lib or demand feeding plan and not supplemented unless growth begins to falter.

Policy 8.14

Mothers should be encouraged to assume total care for their infants during a rooming-in period prior to discharge.

Procedure 8.14.1
NICU/SCN nursing staff should be readily available if needed by the mother during these rooming-in periods.

Procedure 8.14.2
During this time, feeding should be ad lib or on demand unless the infant medically requires supplementation.

Procedure 8.14.3
The NICU/SCN and/or lactation staff should assist the mother in overcoming breastfeeding problems and maximizing learning.

Procedure 8.14.4
The following should be noted, documented by the mother, and provided to NICU/SCN staff for documentation in the infant's medical record.

- Hunger cues
- Avoidance behaviors
- Signs of milk transfer
- Signs of satiety
- Stools and voids

Policy 8.15

A designated healthcare professional should ensure that prior to the infant's discharge from the NICU/SCN, a qualified staff member explores with each mother, family members, or support persons the mother's plans for feeding after discharge.

Procedure 8.15.1
Feeding plans, along with growth and intake data, should be central to the development of a postdischarge feeding plan made by the mother and necessary medical team members.

REFERENCES

Lucas, A., & Cole, T. (1990). Breast milk and neonatal necrotising enterocolitis. *The Lancet, 336*(8730), 1519–1523.

Meier, P. (1988). Bottle- and breast-feeding: Effects on transcutaneous oxygen pressure and temperature in preterm infants. *Nursing Research, 37*(1), 36–41.

Meier, P. (1996). Suck-breathe patterning during bottle and breastfeeding for preterm infants. In T. David (Ed.), *Major controversies in infant nutrition* (International Congress and Symposium Series No. 215). London: Royal Society of Medicine Press Limited.

Nyqvist, K. (2008). Early attainment of breastfeeding competence in very preterm infants. *Acta Paediatrica, 97*(6), 776–781.

Nyqvist, K., Sjoden, P., & Ewald, U. (1999). The development of preterm infants' breastfeeding behavior. *Early Human Development, 55*(3), 247–264.

Thureen, P. J. (1999). Early aggressive nutrition in the neonate. *Pediatric Reviews, 20*(9), e45–e55.

Ziegler, E. E., Thureen, P. J., & Carlson, S. J. (2002). Aggressive nutrition of the very low birthweight infant. *Clinics in Perinatology, 29*(2), 225–224.

chapter eleven

Step 9: Addressing Issues of Conflict of Interest

IMAGINE THIS (PART 1) . . .

You have just spent the last 10 days in the hospital recuperating from a heart attack. Hospital staff, from nurses to dietitians to physicians, have talked to you about your need for a health behavior change that will improve your prognosis and decrease the risk of future heart attacks. You are told that you must stop smoking. You will need to lose the salt shaker and avoid high-sodium foods. You will need to cut back on fats in your diet and replace butter with olive oil. You must begin exercising and lose weight. Finally, you are ready to go home and a nurse from the cardiac unit gives you one more thing to take home—a gift bag from the hospital—a thank you for being a patient in their facility. When you get home you open the gift bag and find the following: a T-shirt with a tobacco company logo on it, a sample packet of salt substitute, a schedule of classes for recovering cardiac patients at a local health club, a list of names of nutrition counselors in your area who do independent consultations and help with diet plans, a pamphlet containing information from the Heart Association on having sex after a heart attack, and a coupon for a discount on butter from the local dairy.

IMAGINE THIS (PART 2) . . .

You have just delivered a 32-weeks'-gestation baby girl via emergency cesarean section. The nurses on the postpartum unit have been very helpful in setting you up with an electric breast pump, and you have been supplying your milk for your daughter, Amanda. The neonatologist has made a point of telling you that Amanda's health can be optimized and major problems decreased if you will supply your milk to feed Amanda. Breastfeeding is best feeding. You are really pleased to be included in the care of Amanda in this way and have spent a lot of time in the NICU talking and singing to Amanda and holding her in a KMC position. On day 4 postpartum, you are discharged from the hospital. You are sad to be leaving Amanda behind, but you know that she will be getting your milk when you are not there. At discharge, you are given a gift—a discharge bag. It has little animals on it and would make a nice lunch box since it is insulated. You might even use it to bring your milk into the NICU. Inside the bag are coupons for disposable diapers and baby wipes, advertisements for vitamin D solutions, sample bra pads, a small tube of a lanolin product for sore nipples, a book that a formula company has produced about all the problems that can occur with breastfeeding, and a bottle of ready-to-feed formula plus coupons for formula purchase in the grocery store.

CONFLICTS OF INTEREST WITH COMMERCIAL ENTITIES: HOW HEALTH CARE IS INFLUENCED

Across the country there is a growing awareness that large multinational pharmaceutical companies hold a tremendous amount of influence over the way health care is provided and on the access that patients have to equipment, devices, and drugs (see Angell, 2005). This discussion has turned into a heated ethical debate. Because of aggressive marketing practices including education and gifts, "big pharma" has increased the cost of drugs, both prescription and over the counter, to consumers. In addressing the excessive spending of drug companies on educational offerings, the chief executive officer of the Accreditation Council for Continuing Medical Education, Dr. Murray Kopelow, is quoted as saying that "The quality of the educational opportunity is dependent on how well designed the education is and how well matched it is to the needs of the learners. The quality of the amenities and the meal are not critical to that" (Moynihan, 2003, p. 1163). He cites an example of a seminar that cost over $100,000, but for which only about $20,000 was actually spent on speakers, renting space for the seminar, and advertising it. The rest of the more than $100,000 was spent on amenities and gifts, visual aids like displays and packaged samples, drug promotion, meals, and entertainment (Moynahan, 2003). In 2003, approximately $1.4 billion was spent on accredited continuing medical education, over half of which was funded by drug companies and device manufacturers (see also Lexchin and Cassels, 2005).

Recent regulations approved by the Massachusetts Department of Public Health ban pharmaceutical and medical device companies "from providing gifts to physicians, limiting when companies can pay for doctors' meals, and requiring companies to publicly disclose payments over $50 to doctors for certain types of consulting and speaking engagements" (Kowalczyk, 2009). At the time of this writing, Massachusetts is the only state to require disclosure from device makers as well as drug companies, making it the state with the most comprehensive rules in the nation. Even so, these regulations have been watered down in their final form and continue to allow companies to provide financial assistance to medical residents and others so that they may attend conferences and educational courses (Kowalczyk, 2009).

Margolis (1991) discusses the ethics of accepting gifts from pharmaceutical companies and, by extension, their formula company subsidiaries. First, the duty of fidelity (role fidelity) is violated when gifts are accepted. The gift represents a conflict of interest between serving the patient and serving the commercial entity, and the acceptance of the gift makes the donee an agent of the commercial donor. Veracity is also violated in this gift relationship because patients usually do not know about the gift and therefore do not understand all the ramifications of the relationship and how it might affect them as patients. Acceptance of gifts also violates the principle of justice in that the donee is clearly benefiting from the gift. Margolis sees this as a particular problem for pediatricians, for example, who may have a patient population that could not afford the same type of meal that the pediatrician is being treated to by the commercial sponsor. Margolis continues, saying that the physician and other healthcare providers have an obligation to continue their training and enhancement of practice skills. The acceptance of the gift as an incentive to take part in continuing education "suggests that physician regard for the importance of self-improvement has eroded ... Education that is acquired through commercial relationships may not be as effective as that acquired through noncommercial scientific presentations more dependent on a physician's self-motivation" (p. 1236). He continues to point out that the resources utilized to promote a product actually come directly from the patient who uses the product. The ethical principle of autonomy is violated when healthcare providers become agents of drug companies, and this loss of autonomy may have untoward consequences. Finally he states, "The gift relationship undermines several of the fundamental duties, nonmaleficence, fidelity, justice, and self-improvement of physicians" (p. 1236). (For a more in-depth discussion of the ethics of care in the NICU, see Chapter 17.)

In the past, formula companies have provided similar types of gifts to hospitals and individuals to ensure that their brand would continue to be the formula the hospital uses—doughnuts, pizzas, and other types of food brought to the nurses' station or doctors' lounge along with the advertising materials; free seminars on infant feeding that invariably provide information about their product to the exclusion of other products; all-expense-paid junkets that have some sort of quasi-educational component to them; parent gift bags and free formula for the hospital; money for physicians to use for educational purposes, often held as a departmental discretionary fund; designs and building funds for new NICUs and nurseries that are separated from the postpartum unit, sometimes by several hospital floors (see Palmer 1988, p. 8; see also Baumslag and Michels 1995, pp. 171–174). Furthermore, the formula company pays the hospital large sums of money for the privilege of providing discharge bags to hospitals; in doing so the companies are guaranteeing the right to use the hospital's name and reputation as a stamp of authority and endorsement of the company's product. This method of advertising directly to parents via the gifting of discharge bags sends very clear messages to parents that the hospital and its nurses and doctors endorse this brand of formula as the best.

The International Code of Marketing of Breast-milk Substitutes (the Code) attempts to address these violations of ethical principles by restricting the manner in which formula companies, manufacturers of feeding bottle sets and teats, and producers of complementary foods and supplements can market their products. While all of these items have their place, it is the inappropriate marketing of these items as substitutes for breastfeeding that are "just as good as breastfeeding" that is the issue. The Code is an implicit part of step 6 of the Ten Steps to Successful Breastfeeding for healthy, term infants, and hospitals that are trying to earn Baby-Friendly status must follow the principles of the Code. The criteria for step 6 specify that the maternity care facility must purchase all formula and feeding bottle sets at fair market value, must cease distribution of formula discharge bags, and must purge the hospital of all advertising and proprietary logos that mothers might see. The hospital or birth center must also have vendor policies in place that prevent marketing representatives from having physical access to staff or mothers on the postpartum unit and prevent staff from accepting gifts from the company representatives. Regarding the distribution of formula gift packs, Cadwell and Turner-Maffei (2009) state:

Table 11-1 Side-by-Side Comparison of Three Models

Principle	*WHO/UNICEF Ten Steps to Successful Breastfeeding for the Healthy Term Newborn*	*ABI's Ten Steps for the NICU/SCN*	*Nyqvist and Kylberg (2008) Swedish Mothers' 13 Steps*	*Danish Ten Steps to Successful Breastfeeding of Preterm Infants*
Conflicts of interest	A subobjective of step 6 states that a business relationship should be established with manufacturers that aligns with the International Code of Marketing of Breast-milk Substitutes.	Step 9. Use ethical, evidence-based breastfeeding practices free of conflicts of interest.	Step 2. Treat every mother with sensitivity, empathy, and respect for her maternal role. Support her in taking informed decisions about milk production and breastfeeding according to her own wishes.	

> Nowhere else in the healthcare system are commercial gift packs distributed to patients at discharge. In return for giving the discharge bag to new mothers, the health system receives kickbacks from the company for the right to advertise to patients. This kind of arrangement is at odds with modern healthcare ethics. (p. 77–78)

The discussion in hospitals about formula marketing and the role the hospital plays should be part of the larger discussion that is currently going on in many medical schools, nursing schools, teaching hospitals, and professional journals about the role of large, multinational pharmaceutical companies and the way they market drugs and influence medical practice. The principles of the Code have been incorporated into the American Breastfeeding Institute (ABI)'s step 9 for the NICU (see **Table 11-1**), because this is an issue of such crucial importance that it needs a policy and step of its own. A model policy is given in **Appendix 11-1**.

THE CODE AND ITS APPLICATIONS FOR THE NICU

How the Code Came to Be

In 1939, Dr. Cecily Williams presented a talk to the Singapore Rotary Club entitled "Milk and Murder" that focused attention on the link between inappropriate marketing of baby formulas and death from malnutrition and diarrhea. Termed *commerciogenic malnutrition* by Dr. Derrick Jelliffe in 1968, publicity about the problem became more widespread, and various grassroots organizations and nongovernmental organizations began to take up the cause of stopping the spread of marketing of infant formula, particularly in traditionally breastfeeding underdeveloped areas of the world with extreme poverty and lack of infrastructure that would support the safe preparation practices required for infant formula. This culminated in 1977 with the U.S. launch of a boycott of Nestlé products to protest that company's unfair marketing practices. Particularly egregious was the practice of using sales representatives who misrepresented themselves to mothers as mothercraft nurses and promoted formula feeding as the most modern and best way to feed one's baby. The boycott spread to other countries and grew rapidly at the grassroots level until 1984 when it was suspended as Nestlé agreed to implement the Code in developing countries (Baby Milk Action, n.d.). Other producers of formula were also targeted, but Nestlé, being the best known of the multinational corporations, was selectively targeted.

In 1979, WHO and UNICEF convened a joint meeting on infant and young child feeding that was attended by approximately 150 representatives from individual governments, international organizations from within the United Nations, nongovernmental organizations, the infant food industry, and experts in related disciplines. Of the five areas discussed, the fifth one, appropriate marketing and distribution of breastmilk substitutes, resulted in a statement and recommendations that were taken to the 1980 World Health Assembly, where the recommendations were endorsed in their entirety, leading to the drafting of an international code of marketing for infant formula and other products related to feeding infants manufactured milks. The 34th World Health Assembly adopted the fourth iteration of this code in May 1981 by a vote of 118 votes in favor, 1 against (the United States), and 3 abstentions.

The resolution of the World Health Assembly (WHA34.22) that adopts the Code urges all member states to "give full and unanimous support" (WHO, 1981, p. 18) to the implementation of the Code in all those states by translating the Code "into national legislation, regulations or other suitable measures" (p. 18) and to involve all social and economic segments of the society in this implementation. Member states are also urged to monitor the compliance of companies to the Code in their own individual countries.

The Intent and Scope of the Code

The Code is intended to be applied globally and establishes a universal set of marketing conditions that formula companies should meet *at a minimum* (Armstrong & Sokol, 2001). This means that countries may enact regulations that are stricter than those in the Code itself. Some countries chose to implement the Code through legal measures; others chose to make compliance with the Code voluntary, leaving the success of the measures dependent on the will of the companies involved. The strength of the Code in any given country is dependent on the community or government agencies that "monitor compliance, publicize deviations, and impose sanctions" (Armstrong & Sokol, 2001, p. 6).

The focus of the Code is on *marketing practices* that give companies an unfair advantage over breastfeeding. It does not attempt to eliminate the availability of formula or the right of a mother to choose to formula feed, but instead tries to assure that mothers are not subjected to undue influence and interference in their decision making but are supported in breastfeeding as optimal infant and young child nutrition (with appropriate complementary foods added after 6 months of age) for as long as the mother and baby mutually desire.

The Code also covers much more than just infant formula because the term *breastmilk substitutes* has a very broad definition and includes any food that replaces breastfeeding, such as teas, follow-up milks, sugar or fruit drinks, processed baby foods, and cereals, especially if the product is packaged so that it could be fed easily in a bottle. The Code also covers the implements used to feed the breastmilk substitute. Armstrong and Sokol point out that breast pump companies may also violate the Code in this regard by promoting the nipples and feeding bottle sets in the breast pump supplies with false advertising, such as nipples being close to mothers' own.

The first two articles of the Code are reproduced in **Box 11-1** and define the aim of the document and the scope of it (WHO, 1981). Equally important are the definitions given in Article 3, which clearly define the meaning of various terms used within the Code.

How the Code Applies to the NICU

Articles 4, 5, 6, and 7 of the Code apply directly to activities that occur in NICUs/SCNs. The last four articles (8-11) apply more directly to individual responsibilities of commercial representatives, the companies themselves,

Box 11-1 Articles 1 and 2 of the International Code of Marketing of Breast-milk Substitutes

Article 1. Aim of the Code
The aim of this Code is to contribute to the provision of safe and adequate nutrition for infants, by the protection and promotion of breast-feeding, and by ensuring the proper use of breast-milk substitutes, when these are necessary, on the basis of adequate information and through appropriate marketing and distribution.

Article 2. Scope of the Code
The Code applies to the marketing, and practices related thereto, of the following products: breast-milk substitutes, including infant formula; other milk products, food and beverages, including bottle-fed complementary foods, when marketed or otherwise represented to be suitable, with or without modification, for use as a partial or total replacement of breast milk; feeding bottles and teats. It also applies to their quality and availability, and to information concerning their use.

Source: WHO, 1981.

and government entities in the implementing, monitoring, and reporting processes. The following discussion relies heavily on the Code itself as a source (WHO, 1981) and the interpretive materials written by Armstrong and Sokol (2001).

Article 4

Since the United States has not enacted any portion of the Code, its government does not play a role in any of these articles, leaving it up to individual institutions to implement the intent as they see fit. Article 4 concerns information and education given to pregnant women and mothers of young children, and that this information should contain clear and concise messages about:

a) the benefits and superiority of breastfeeding;
b) maternal nutrition, and the preparation for and maintenance of breastfeeding;
c) the negative effect on breastfeeding of introducing partial bottle-feeding;
d) the difficulty of reversing the decision not to breastfeed; and
e) where needed, the proper use of infant formula, whether manufactured industrially or home prepared. (WHO, 1981, p. 10)

If and when information about infant formula needs to be given, topics such as the social and financial implications of its use should be included as well as the health hazards associated with inappropriate foods and feeding methods. No text or pictures that idealize the use of breastmilk substitutes are to be present in the information. To comply with this part of the Code, NICUs would have to carefully prepare materials for mothers that would support breastfeeding and the use of human milk as the norm and standard and carefully explain the hazards of infant formulas as they relate to the infant's preterm status, explaining to the parents that sometimes formula is necessary in this population, but that every attempt will be made to lessen the use of formulas and bovine-based fortifiers and that introduction will be delayed until full enteral feedings of human milk are established to gain maximum benefit of human milk. Staff will also be able to clearly and accurately explain the meaning of labels on these commercial products and be able to explain the difference between a bovine-based human milk fortifier and a human milk-based fortifier. Any pictures included in these materials would not show happy babies being bottle-fed—they would show premies being breastfed. Company logos on educational materials would also be absent. In many cases, this translates into the NICU developing and creating its own handouts with the hospital logo on it to avoid marketing for a pump company or a formula company, in particular pamphlets and brochures about storage and handling of expressed milk. Clinical protocol No. 14 from the Academy of Breastfeeding Medicine (2006) on how a physician's office practice could become breastfeeding friendly delineates the type of information that should be available that is helpful to mothers and recommends that these educational offerings, whether written or visual aids, should not be commercial and should not have logos or other advertisements for companies that produce bottles, teats, or breastmilk substitutes. Model policies and protocols discussed in previous chapters will help support this article of the Code.

In a study by Hayden, Nowacek, Koch, and Kattwinkel (1987) that examined discharge pack distribution in the hospital, 95% of the hospitals surveyed gave out the discharge packs even though only 66% of the pediatricians surveyed actually approved of the practice. Furthermore, in most cases the hospital medical staff had not voted on whether to distribute the packs or not—the decision had been made totally without medical input. Parents were also not being informed of the source and intent of the packs. Perhaps this might lead parents to think that the hospital just wanted to give a thank-you gift for using their facility. Education then requires that parents be told about the intent and sources of the packs and why the formula companies work so hard at distributing them. When mothers who intended to breastfeed exclusively were interviewed in a nationally representative sample, 74% of first-time mothers and 61% of multiparas were given discharge formula sample packs (Declercq, Labbok, Sakala, & O'Hara, 2009). When the state of Massachusetts was attempting to abolish promotional discharge packs in all hospitals as a public health measure, one hospital reported that they had temporarily ceased giving them out but had returned to the practice when mothers complained on their patient satisfaction surveys that they did not get their free gift and thought it was their right to get the bag (Smith, 2006).

Article 5

Article 5 is about marketing commercial products directly to the public. According to the Code, advertisements of this nature are not allowed and samples of products cannot be given to mothers to entice them to use a particular brand, including discount coupons for products within the scope of the Code. In the NICU setting, this means that all items with a proprietary label or logo on them need to be purged, including the less obvious things such as crib cards; badge holders and lanyards for staff IDs; canvas tote bags that nurses received at seminars; posters of babies being fed formula; measuring tapes; conversion charts; prescription pads; pens and pencils; ways to sign up for formula company-sponsored new moms' clubs; use of formula company tapes and DVDs on breastfeeding in the hospital TV system; etc. One hospital, as part of becoming baby friendly, conducted a scavenger hunt to see which staff member could come up with the most items that had formula company logos on them. Staff were surprised at the multiple ways in which formula companies had injected themselves into the healthcare setting.

In a study by Chezem, Friesen, Montgomery, Fortman, and Clark (1998), receipt of formula samples and supplementation in the hospital were examined to see if they influenced breastfeeding duration in women who were planning on returning to work. Of note were that 59% received free formula from the hospital in the form of discharge packs, 30% received free formula from a physician's office, and 51% received free formula in the mail. Receipt of formula samples by mail was associated with reduced incidence of breastfeeding at 6 weeks postpartum and shortened duration of breastfeeding. Women receive formula by mail as a result of signing up for new mothers' clubs. They see an ad for these clubs in a parenting magazine and think they will be receiving coupons for diapers, baby wipes, or clothing, not realizing that it is a formula company that sponsors the magazine, writes all its content, and supplies the magazines for free to the physician's office. The mail-in cards to join these clubs routinely ask the pregnant women to designate whether they intend to feed formula, practice mixed feeding, or exclusively breastfeed. Women who check that they are choosing only formula feeding do not receive the free formula by mail as they are already a captive market. The formula company markets largely to those women who are intending to or have initiated breastfeeding.

Article 5 also prohibits the distribution of free samples of products within the scope of the Code. It is inappropriate and a violation of the Code to give mothers free samples of formula at discharge. Studies show that when mothers receive free formula samples in the form of commercial hospital discharge bags, they have shorter durations of exclusive breastfeeding (Rosenberg, Eastham, Kasehagen, & Sandoval, 2008) and may start offering inappropriate solids earlier than 6 months when compared to mothers who did not receive discharge packs (Cadwell & Turner-Maffei, 2009; Donnelly, Snowden, Renfrew, & Woolridge, 2000). It is also inappropriate for mothers to come in contact with sales representatives from companies within the scope of the Code, so sales representatives should be restricted in their access to the hospital and physicians and nurses on the floor of the unit. Of course, Health Insurance Portability and Accountability Act (HIPAA) violations may easily occur if company representatives are in places other than the purchasing department. For the physician's office that has formula available in case an infant has an immediate need for feeding, the formula should be stored out of sight (ABM, 2006). The NICU and attending neonatologists should also store formula out of sight. Howard et al. (2000) found that office advertising of formula and products covered in the Code were associated with increased breastfeeding cessation in the first 2 weeks postpartum. These types of advertisements need to be eliminated from NICU-associated practices to encourage continued milk expression and transition to full breastfeeding.

Article 6

Article 6 covers healthcare systems and their responsibilities under the Code. According to this article, the healthcare system should:

- Give appropriate information and education to healthcare workers
- Avoid promoting infant formula or other products within the scope of the Code

- Avoid displaying or providing visual aids or literature from the companies about products that fall within the scope of the Code
- Disallow personnel in the healthcare system to be used for marketing purposes
- Demonstrate safe feeding techniques for formula use only to the family members who need to use it, and use only trained and skilled staff to teach the method
- Use donations or low-priced sales from manufacturers only for infants who must be fed on breastmilk substitutes
- Ensure that low-cost supplies can be continued as long as the infant in question needs them
- Not allow materials that are donated to refer to any proprietary product within the Code

Many of these restrictions have already been mentioned. Of particular interest to the NICU, however, is the fact that techniques for mixing formula and how to conduct formula feeding safely must be taught by a trained caregiver. Since many preterm infants are discharged receiving formula supplements or other components that must be either fed by themselves or mixed with expressed milk, it is incumbent on NICU staff to ensure that mothers know how to mix and prepare the feeding correctly. In this way, causing harm to the baby by providing an inappropriately reconstituted formula or a contaminated feeding is avoided. It is also incumbent on the healthcare facility to ensure that NICU care providers are well trained in ways to support breastfeeding and that everyone is giving appropriate and nonconflicting information. This element was clearly missing in Bonnie's case in Chapter 1, where staff perpetrated incorrect information, conflicting information, and non–evidence-based information.

Article 7

Article 7 delineates the responsibilities of healthcare workers as individuals. They must know what their responsibilities are under the Code. When commercial entities provide information to staff, this information should be free of messages that imply that bottle-feeding is equivalent or superior to breastfeeding. Under the Code, healthcare workers and their families are not allowed to receive any gifts or financial inducements to promote the products that are within the scope of the Code, nor are they allowed to receive samples of any of the products within the scope of the Code. They should not give out free samples to families either. Any contributions made for the purposes of fellowships, study tours, research grants, attendance at professional conferences, etc. should be reported to the institution by the recipient and the company providing the benefit.

SUMMARY

The NICU environment has an ethical obligation to protect mothers from undue influence of the formula companies and has an obligation to implement the International Code of Marketing of Breast-milk Substitutes while still recognizing that some preterm infants will need formula and fortifiers whose sole source is the pharmaceutical industry and their subsidiary formula companies. NICUs should not accept gifts of any kind from manufacturers of products that are within the scope of the Code and avoid having products and advertisements in sight of the mothers. The message must be consistent that breast is absolutely the best. Behavior of staff in this regard should be exemplary in their own lives, and they should not accept products that parents might use in their NICU as gifts from sales representatives.

A particularly egregious violation of ethical marketing practices is the NICU nurse who accepts a free breast pump from the sales representative who wants to ensure that the hospital will remain with that brand of breast pump for the foreseeable future. While breast pumps may be acceptable and needed in the NICU by mothers, the mothers do not know that a staff member is benefiting personally from their inability to have access to more than one brand of equipment.

REFERENCES

Academy of Breastfeeding Medicine (ABM). (2006). ABM clinical protocol # 14: Breastfeeding-friendly physician's office, part 1: Optimizing care for infants and children. *Breastfeeding Medicine, 1*(2), 115–119.

Angell, M. (2005). *The truth about the drug companies: How they deceive us and what to do about it.* New York: Random House.

Armstrong, H., & Sokol, E. (2001). *The international code of marketing of breast-milk substitutes: What it means for mothers and babies worldwide.* Raleigh, NC: International Lactation Consultant Association.

Baby Milk Action. (n.d.). *Briefing paper: History of the campaign.* Retrieved April 21, 2009, from http://www.babymilkaction.org/pages/history.html

Baumslag, N., & Michels, D. (1995). *Milk, money, and madness: The culture and politics of breastfeeding.* Westport, CT: Bergin & Garvey.

Cadwell, K., & Turner-Maffei, C. (2009). *Continuity of care in breastfeeding: Best practices in the maternity care setting.* Sudbury, MA: Jones and Bartlett.

Chezem, J., Friesen, C., Montgomery, P., Fortman, T., & Clark, H. (1998). Lactation duration: Influences of human milk replacements and formula samples on women planning postpartum employment. *Journal of Obstetric, Gynecologic, and Neonatal Nursing, 27*(6), 646–651.

Declercq, E., Labbok, M., Sakala, C., & O'Hara, M. (2009). Hospital practices and women's likelihood of fulfilling their intention to exclusively breastfeed. *American Journal of Public Health, 99*(5), 929–935.

Donnelly, A., Snowden, H., Renfrew, M., & Woolridge, M. (2000). Commercial hospital discharge packs for breastfeeding women. *Cochrane Database Systematic Review, 2*, CD002075.

Hayden, G., Nowacek, G., Koch, W., & Kattwinkel, J. (1987). Providing free samples of baby items to newly delivered parents. An unintentional endorsement? *Clinical Pediatrics, 26*(3), 111–115.

Howard, C., Howard, F., Lawrence, R., Andresen, E., DeBlieck, E., & Weitzman, M. (2000). Office prenatal formula advertising and its effect on breastfeeding patterns. *Obstetrics and Gynecology, 95*(2), 296–303.

Kowalczyk, L. (2009, March 12). State bans drug firm gifts to doctors. *The Boston Globe*. Retrieved April 21, 2009, from http://www.boston.com/news/local/massachusetts/articles/2009/03/12/state_bans_drug_firm_gifts_to_doctors

Lexchin, J., & Cassels, A. (2005). Does the C in CME stand for "continuing" or "commercial"? *Canadian Medical Association Journal, 172*(2), 160–162.

Margolis, L. (1991). The ethics of accepting gifts from pharmaceutical companies. *Pediatrics, 88*(6), 1233–1237.

Moynihan, R. (2003). Drug company sponsorship of education could be replaced at a fraction of its cost. *British Medical Journal, 326*(7400), 1163.

Palmer, G. (1988). *The politics of breastfeeding*. London: Pandora.

Rosenberg, K., Eastham, C., Kasehagen, L., & Sandoval, A. (2008). Marketing infant formula through hospitals: The impact of commercial hospital discharge packs on breastfeeding. *American Journal of Public Health, 98*(2), 290–295.

Smith, S. (2006, May 8). Some hospitals forgo baby-formula handout: State considers ban on gift bags. *The Boston Globe*. Retrieved April 23, 2009, from http://www.boston.com/business/healthcare/articles/2006/05/08/some_hospitals_forgo_baby_formula_handout

World Health Organization (WHO). (1981). *International code of marketing of breast-milk substitutes*. Geneva, Switzerland: Author. Retrieved April 22, 2009, from http://whqlibdoc.who.int/publications/9241541601.pdf

APPENDIX 11-1

STEP 9

Employ ethical, evidence-based breastfeeding practices free of conflicts of interest.

Policies 9.1–9.3

Title

The institutional philosophy regarding ethical practice free of conflicts of interest.

Purpose

To ensure that all materials distributed or displayed in the facility, particularly those given to or used with breastfeeding mothers, shall be free of messages that promote or advertise infant nutrition other than human milk or discourage the provision of human milk to infants in the NICU/SCN.

Supportive Data

Obstetricians, pediatricians, family practitioners, and hospital staff may unintentionally undermine breastfeeding by providing formula company access to patients via commercial literature and formula marketing strategies (Howard et al., 2000; Donnelly, 2003). Public display of policies supporting breastfeeding reinforces their importance to staff, patients, and the public.

Rationale

Patient education materials and gifts are attractive and perceived as free. In reality, formula prices include the costs of those materials and gifts in their pricing. Marketing practices clearly influence physician choice (Wazana, 2000). The American Medical Association, American College of Obstetricians and Gynecologists, American Academy of Pediatrics (AAP), and other professional societies have developed ethical guidelines that recognize and advise how to mitigate the influence of pharmaceutical company marketing messages and gifts. The AAP's policy statement, "Breastfeeding and the Use of Human Milk," asks physicians "to work actively toward eliminating hospital practices that discourage breastfeeding (e.g., infant formula discharge packs and separation of mother and infant)" (AAP, 2005, p. 501).

Scope

These policies apply to All NICU/SCN personnel including the medical director, nursing director, nursing supervisors, licensed staff, ancillary staff, and volunteers.

Policy 9.1

The institutional philosophy regarding the purchase and promotion of human milk substitutes should be displayed in all areas that serve mothers and their premature and/or compromised infants in the NICU/SCN.

Procedure 9.1.1

The hospital should implement the following strategies:

- Do not allow donation or sale of patient lists/contact information to formula or marketing companies, as this is a potential violation of HIPAA.
- Do not use formula company materials as patient education materials.
- Do not allow/accept formula company gifts to staff on the unit, e.g., pens, mugs, notepads, food, etc.
- Provide visual cues (artwork, posters, calendars not sponsored or provided by a commercial company) that actively support breastfeeding.
- Support breastfeeding patients and staff by providing space and supplies for pumping and breastfeeding.

Policy 9.2

The hospital should review and revise current practices regarding vendors and their educational materials and/or supplies.

Procedure 9.2.1

Marketing representatives of formula companies or other commercial entities shall not be allowed on the unit because of the potential for violations of HIPAA and the undue influence such representatives have on staff.

Procedure 9.2.2

All feeding supplies should be purchased by the facility at a fair market value in the same competitive manner as other food and medical supplies purchased. The hospital should not accept or distribute free or subsidized supplies of human milk substitutes or feeding implements or supplemental devices. (See also Policy 6.6 in Appendix 8-1 for step 6.)

Policy 9.3

Educational materials used should be free of messages that promote or advertise manufactured infant nutrition as substitutes for human milk. These materials should not refer to any proprietary products or bear any product logos.

Procedure 9.3.1
All healthcare staff should review all promotional or educational materials displayed or distributed to parents of babies in the NICU/SCN, including but not limited to measuring tapes, conversion charts, crib cards, pens, prescription pads, pamphlets, artwork, etc.

Procedure 9.3.2
No promotional or educational materials given to mothers should promote the use of formula or specific brand of equipment over another brand, such as breast pumps.

REFERENCES

American Academy of Pediatrics (AAP). (2005). Breastfeeding and the use of human milk. *AAP Policy, 115*(2), 496–506.

Donnelly, A., Snowden, H., Renfrew, M., & Woolridge, M. (2000). Commercial hospital discharge packs for breastfeeding women. *Cochrane Database Systematic Review, 2*, CD002075.

Howard, C., Howard, F., Lawrence, R., Andresen, E., DeBlieck, E., & Weitzman, M. (2000). Office prenatal formula advertising and its effect on breastfeeding patterns. *Obstetrics and Gynecology, 95*(2), 296–303.

Wazana, A. (2000). Physicians and the pharmaceutical industry: Is a gift ever just a gift? *Journal of the American Medical Association, 283*(3), 373–380.

chapter twelve

Step 10: The Role of the NICU in Providing Breastfeeding Support

According to the World Health Organization (WHO, 2003), there are three strategies that help individual mothers achieve breastfeeding success. These three strategies—promotion, protection, and support—also help local communities, states, and countries achieve increases in breastfeeding initiation and duration. Each of the Ten Steps to Successful Breastfeeding encompasses one or more of these three strategies.

Breastfeeding promotion involves educating women as well as the general public about the advantages of breastfeeding. Examples of promotion include media campaigns such as the National Breastfeeding Awareness Campaign that the U.S. Department of Health and Human Services ran in 2005 or a one-on-one discussion about breastfeeding between a pregnant client and her prenatal healthcare provider. Breastfeeding promotion may involve talking about breastfeeding as an economical and natural way of feeding babies in a high school health class, or it may involve a public campaign such as the one in Marin County, California, where life-size cardboard cutouts of women breastfeeding in public were placed around the county. The discreetly breastfeeding mother in each cutout held a small sign that said, "When breastfeeding is accepted, it won't be noticed" (Farooq, 2009). In the Ten Steps to Successful Breastfeeding for the healthy, term infant, breastfeeding promotion is seen in steps 2 and 3 where staff and pregnant women are all educated about the benefits of breastfeeding.

Breastfeeding protection involves leveling the playing field between breastfeeding and commercial interests that interfere with breastfeeding. Legislation that restricts marketing practices of formula companies in compliance with the International Code of Marketing of Breast-milk Substitutes is an example of protection. In the United States, which has not enacted any specific legislation to address the International Code of Marketing of Breast-milk Substitutes, other laws protect nursing mothers and their right to breastfeed. As of this writing, 43 states, the District of Columbia, and the Virgin Islands have laws that protect a woman's right to breastfeed in any public or private location, and 28 states, the District of Columbia, and the Virgin Islands exempt breastfeeding from prosecution under public indecency laws. Only West Virginia and the territories of American Samoa and Guam have no law about breastfeeding in public (National Conference of State Legislatures [NCSL], 2009). Additionally, 23 states, the District of Columbia, and Puerto Rico have laws that protect a mother's right to breastfeed or collect her milk while working. These laws specify, among other things, that employers must provide unpaid breaks for women to either nurse their infants or express their milk in a clean place that is not a bathroom. Twelve states and Puerto Rico exempt a woman from serving on a jury if she is breastfeeding. In Puerto Rico, any mother who is breastfeeding a child under 24 months of age is exempt. Two states, Louisiana and Mississippi, have laws that prohibit childcare facilities from discriminating against breastfed babies, and Maryland exempts the sale of personal equipment used in "initiating, supporting or sustaining breastfeeding" from sales tax (NCSL, 2009, p. 2). In September 1999, President Bill Clinton signed the Treasury Postal Appropriations bill that included New York Representative Carolyn Maloney's Right to Breastfeed Act (HR 1848), which assures a woman's right to breastfeed on federal property.

Protection of breastfeeding involves more than legislation, however, and is seen in the development of hospital policies that improve birth practices that foster the establishment and maintenance of breastfeeding and decrease the opportunities for supplementation and exposure to formula marketing. Steps 1, 2, 4, 5, 6, 7, 8, and 9 all contain elements of protection. By helping breastfeeding get off to a good start, mothers are less likely to experience problems that may lead to early supplementation and weaning. Initiation and duration rates are therefore positively impacted when protection is in place. As Cadwell and Turner-Maffei (2009) point out, "What happens during the maternity stay has a profound long-term effect on feeding outcomes

Table 12-1 Side-by-Side Comparison of Three Models

Principle	*WHO/UNICEF Ten Steps to Successful Breastfeeding for the Healthy Term Newborn*	*ABI's Ten Steps for the NICU/SCN*	*Nyqvist and Kylberg (2008) Swedish Mothers' 13 Steps*	*Danish Ten Steps to Successful Breastfeeding of Preterm Infants*
Breast-feeding protection and support	Step 10. Foster the establishment of breastfeeding support groups and refer mothers to them on discharge from the hospital or clinic.	Step 10. Foster the establishment of NICU/SCN breastfeeding support groups and postdischarge community programs, and refer mothers to them.	Step 11. Provide a family-centered and supportive physical environment. Step 12. Support the father's presence without restrictions as the mother's main supporter and the infant's caregiver. Step 13. Plan the infant's discharge by early transfer of the infant's care in the neonatal unit to the parents. Inform the mother about where she can obtain breastfeeding support after discharge by staff or members of breastfeeding support groups with adequate knowledge.	Step 8. Parents are encouraged to use their social network. Step 10. Parents are supported if they choose not to breastfeed or if they are unable to make breastfeeding work.

whether or not the staff provide linkage between the mother and breastfeeding resources outside the facility" (p. 120).

The last strategy, support, is what step 10 is all about (see **Table 12-1**). The concept of support is a broader concept than many people believe. Support is not just education as some would define it. It is also the kind of emotional cheerleading support for a mother who may be having a crisis in confidence. This type of encouragement also involves good counseling skills that emphasize listening and empathy for the mother. For the healthy, term mother–infant dyad, most support will be required outside the hospital setting. The hospital should be identifying and addressing any problems that arise and then ensuring that women have access to breastfeeding support systems immediately after they are discharged. Community-based resources may be in the form of visits from home healthcare agencies like the Visiting Nurse Association, peer counselors in Women, Infants, and Children programs, lactation consultants working privately, or volunteer mother-to-mother support groups such as La Leche League, to name but a few. In resource-poor areas, the hospital may find that it has to create a support system for breastfeeding mothers. Support may come in the form of assistance with problem solving and/or in the form of appropriate encouragement and praise.

For the term infant and mother, the most critical period of time for support is in the first 2 weeks postdischarge. Studies are consistent in showing that the fastest drop-off in breastfeeding is in the first 2 weeks after discharge from the hospital (Ertem, Votto, & Leventhal, 2001; Hawkins, Nichols, & Tanner, 1987; Taveras et al., 2003). Taveras et al. (2003) also found that lack of confidence in breastfeeding during the hospital stay and early breastfeeding problems were key reasons for discontinuation of breastfeeding by 2 weeks. The primary reason why women discontinue breastfeeding in these first 2 weeks is that they believe they do not have enough milk (Ahluwalia, Morrow, & Hsia, 2005; Li, Fein, Chen, & Grummer-Strawn, 2008). As their milk supply settles down to what the baby needs and the breast softens compared to the normal fullness in the early stages of breastfeeding, it is not unusual for mothers to think that they are losing their milk even though they are feeding 10–12 times in a 24-hour period and the baby is gaining sufficient weight. A community-based support person will encourage the mother to observe her baby and believe what the baby is telling her, reassuring the mother that she has plenty of milk.

Many breastfeeding problems can be prevented when hospital practices facilitate rooming in, skin-to-skin contact, breastfeeding on cue, no nonmedical separation of mother and baby in the first hours of life, supplementation with the mother's own milk as a first choice and with formula only if there is a medical indication, and lack of routine pacifier use. Hospital staff require education and skills in order to implement these practices. What appears to be protection of breastfeeding also becomes support when these practices are routine—staff educate as well as problem solve breastfeeding issues preventively. Practice becomes prophylaxis. When these practices and skill sets are lacking, community support becomes even more essential, in terms of both management of breastfeeding problems and inspiring confidence in the mother in her ability to succeed.

Barriers to a continuum of support prenatally, in hospital and in the community, are fragmentation of the healthcare system; lack of awareness of what is available in the community, as well as limitations on community resources; and difficulty in providing proactive services, i.e., breastfeeding help before and while it is needed, not after the mother has already begun to wean. Cadwell and Turner-Maffei (2009) provide a case of a community that developed a breastfeeding referral system that tracked mothers from prenatal care through hospital care and into the community. Wide dissemination of the tool, continuous refinement, and annual in-service sessions occur to solve the fragmentation of care issue and provide continuity of care so that mothers get the help that they need.

HOW DOES THIS APPLY TO THE NICU?

As with the mother of a term infant, the mother of a preterm infant needs to be supported in the process of becoming a parent. Hospital policies that foster more contact with the infant and provide mothers with accurate and timely information as well as opportunities for mothers to demonstrate new learning are essential. Cleveland (2008) conducted a systematic review of the literature to examine the needs of NICU parents and the nursing behaviors that are most supportive of parents. She found sixty studies that met her inclusion criteria. Mothers in the NICU needed to be:

- Included in the care of their infants;
- Provided with accurate information and education;
- Able to protect and watch over the infant;
- Given frequent opportunities to touch or hold the infant;
- Perceived in a positive light by nursing staff;
- Provided with individualized care; and
- Able to sustain a therapeutic relationship with nurses.

The nursing behaviors that best assisted parents in meeting these needs were:

- Emotional support;
- Empowerment of parents through teaching and doing;
- A NICU environment that welcomed parents and had policies supportive of parenting; and
- Education with an opportunity to practice new skills under supervision.

For the mother of a preterm, hospitalized infant, the need for support is unique and more intense than that required for the mother of a term infant. She needs knowledgeable support that addresses her emotional needs as well as physical needs. The mother also needs support in three distinct time frames—the peripartum period when she is hospitalized, the postpartum period when she has been discharged but the baby remains hospitalized, and the postdischarge period when both she and her infant are at home. Each of these time frames will be discussed separately.

The Peripartum Period

In the peripartum period, support comes in the form of both education as well as physical and emotional support. If the mother has been assigned to antepartum bed rest, it works best if she has been approached by the neonatologist, who initiates a discussion of how important her milk is for her infant and the specific benefits that could accrue to her infant. If she has not been hospitalized prior to the birth of the infant, the neonatologist needs to raise this subject early and the mother should be taught about milk expression and how to establish and maintain an adequate milk supply for her infant. However, this may not always happen, as in Bonnie's case in Chapter 1, when a mother delivers in a hospital that does not have special care facilities and the baby gets transported to a different city or even state. While she recovers postpartum prior to discharge, she may be, like Bonnie, the victim of fragmentation of care, where the postpartum hospital was ill equipped to provide her with information or assistance in milk expression. In Bonnie's case, there was no communication between the delivering hospital and the special care hospital about how to assist mothers with the initiation of milk expression, although presumably this is not the first time a special care baby had been transferred from one hospital to the other. Every community hospital should have policies in place on how to get a mother started expressing her milk if the baby has to be transported to a different facility. Furthermore, it is incumbent on the receiving hospital to make sure that all community hospitals in its catchment area be informed of what to do and how the NICU wants mothers to be cared for in terms of breastfeeding support.

In-hospital breastfeeding support for new mothers of preterm infants may be seen as the domain of the NICU nurses, not the postpartum nurses, and little effort may be made to help a mother initiate milk expression in a timely fashion. In one hospital, women who delivered prematurely were put on the floor with all the gynecological surgeries. The idea was that they should be protected from all those healthy babies on the postpartum floor so that they did not have to be reminded of their own loss of a normal birth and healthy, term infant. However, nurses on the surgical/medical floor had not received training in how to help preterm mothers express and collect their milk. They did not know how to procure a pump from the hospital, they did not know how to set one up, and they did not know the protocols and procedures for mothers to follow. Fortunately for the mothers in this hospital there was a lactation consultant whose job it was to visit mothers with babies in the NICU. She was notified of all births each morning when she came in and would start her rounds, beginning with the women on the surgical floor. Coverage, however, was limited to weekdays. Because we know that the best time to establish an adequate milk supply using mechanical means is within the first 6 hours of life (Furman, Minich, & Hack, 2002), then other staff need to be able to provide mothers with this type of education and assistance in the middle of the night and on weekends.

Nyqvist, Sjoden, and Ewald (1994) also found that physical support of mothers in-hospital was very important. New mothers experience pain and physical exhaustion, especially if they have been on extended bed rest and have lost muscle tone and strength. Mothers reported that having to walk between the postpartum unit and the NICU added to their physical exhaustion and pain, especially after a cesarean section, prolonged delivery, or vacuum extraction. In many cases, they were dependent on others for assistance with transportation to the NICU and felt helpless when they were told by nurses that they would have to wait until a family member could take them because the nurse was too busy. Hospital routines in the postpartum unit frequently coincided with similar routines in the NICU and mothers had to choose, for example, between eating or going to feed the infant in the NICU. NICUs and postpartum units need to do a better job of coordinating not only the teaching they do with postpartum mothers, but the logistics of care so that the mother and baby can be together as much as possible without interrupting the care of either party.

Support in the NICU After the Mother Is Discharged

Once the mother is discharged, optimally she will be with the infant continuously or as near to that as possible. What happens, however, if she lives in a community that is a great distance from the baby's care facility? Good counseling skills are required of staff. They must listen to the mother and her concerns, try to read between the lines, and ask appropriate open-ended questions to explore the mother's full range of emotions and feelings. According to Nyqvist et al. (1994) "mothers emphasized the need for the nurse to be an observer and empathetic supporter, on whom mothers can rely" (p. 241).

The goal in every NICU should be to support the mother in becoming a mother—to try to include her in the caregiving as much as possible so that she will feel competent in the care of her baby once the baby is discharged. This means that attitudes, policies, and procedures must be accommodating of the mother's role as a parent. Relating to breastfeeding, McGrath (2007) states:

> Supporting breastfeeding in the NICU can be time-intensive for the bedside nurse. More to the point, there are many patterns of caregiving in the NICU that decrease the likelihood that mothers will be encouraged or supported to provide breast milk or to breastfeed their high risk preterm infant. . . . Nurses are at the crux of the institutional culture in the NICU, which is regulated through policies and procedures both written and unwritten. Furthermore, the NICU culture often rewards technical proficiency and adherence to policies and procedures that may encourage a less-than-optimal family engagement than is often necessary to promote and support successful initiation of a milk supply and maintenance of breastfeeding. (p. 184)

One of the strategies McGrath cites as being effective in helping mothers to breastfeed their preterm infants is the provision of support through the use of peer mentors, family members, and nurses.

Use of Nurses and Lactation Consultants for Support

If we acknowledge that NICU nurses caring for preterm infants have a heavy workload and cannot be all things to all patients and their parents, then we must also acknowledge that in the case of breastfeeding and breastfeeding support it is essential to have a team of individuals who specialize in lactation who can do much of the education of the mother, some of the assisting with STS care/KMC and help with the transition from expressed milk to at-breast feeding. While nurses caring for the baby need to know basic information so that they are not giving incorrect or conflicting information to the mother, it would be more efficient to have a specialty team that does most things related to lactation counseling and support. Castrucci, Hoover, Lim, and Maus (2007) compared breastfeeding rates among mothers with preterm infants and whether the delivering hospital had an International Board Certified Lactation Consultant (IBCLC) or not. The adjusted odds ratio of breastfeeding initiation prior to hospital discharge was 1.34 times greater in hospitals with an IBCLC. Among mothers of preterm infants in the NICU, breastfeeding rates were nearly 50% (IBCLCs present) compared to 36.9% (no IBCLCs present).

Gonzalez et al. (2003) conducted a preintervention versus postintervention analysis of the effectiveness of a lactation support service in increasing the rates of breastfeeding/milk expression in a NICU. The objective of the service was to provide "educational and clinical support to mothers during their infants' hospitalization and prepare them to continue breastfeeding following discharge" (p. 287). Two IBCLCs and one in training, all of whom were registered nurses, provided the service. The following elements were part of the service:

- Contact all mothers of preterm infants within 24 hours of birth to discuss feeding options.
- Develop individualized feeding plans for mothers who choose to express their milk.
- Establish a pumping regimen.
- Meet daily with mothers to answer any questions.
- Be present for two infant feeding sessions during their 11-hour presence.
- Establish a telephone help line for NICU mothers.

Rates of providing mother's own milk (MOM) increased from 31% preintervention to 47% postintervention. Similar increases were seen in the number of infants who continued to receive MOM after discharge (23% versus 37%). Prior to the intervention, nurses were responsible for providing education and support to mothers who were expressing their milk. However, many of the nurses had little training in lactation and less time available to support mothers. Implementation of the lactation support service provided the support that mothers needed and also began training of their fellow nurses to bring them up to date. Although the effects of such a program using other professionals (without the IBCLC certification) with evidence-based training in lactation management and counseling skills have not been studied, similar outcomes would most likely result.

Sisk, Lovelady, Dillard, and Gruber (2006) also found that milk expression increased among NICU mothers of very-low-birth-weight babies (≥ 700 g and ≤ 1500 g) who had initially chosen to formula feed but who changed their minds when provided lactation counseling services. Breastmilk intake was greater in infants whose mothers had intended to breastfeed, but infant milk intake increased in the first 3 weeks in both groups. Despite the lower total number of days of receiving breastmilk in the formula intent group, those babies still received about 50% of their total intake from their own mothers in the first 3 weeks of life outside the womb. In the 4th week, this dropped to 48.8% and to 32.8% of total enteral intake for the entire hospitalization. Of note is that all mothers said they were glad that staff had helped them with milk expression. Providing lactation counseling did not increase the mothers' anxiety. In Sisk and colleagues' study, the counseling was provided by a registered dietitian who was also a lactation consultant.

These two studies (Gonzalez, et al., 2003 and Sisk, et al., 2006) discuss only the provision of expressed milk and do not discuss the transition to breastfeeding and support during this phase. However, one qualitative study from Sweden looks at the way breastfeeding support is provided during this transition and examines the mothers' feelings and experiences. Weimers, Svensson, Dumas, Maver, and Wahlberg (2006) examined how maternal confidence and knowledge can be enhanced or hindered by the type of breastfeeding experience and the type of support they are given at the first attempt to breastfeed. The authors had observed that many nurses were using a hands-on approach to helping mothers, in which they would unexpectedly touch the mother's breast and the baby's head, neck, or back with their hands to get the baby on the breast. Other nurses demonstrated hand expression by milking the mother's breast for her. In long interviews, mothers expressed their feelings that the hands-on assistance was "slightly brutal, unpleasant, and that it violated their integrity" (Weimers et al., 2006, p. 6). They did not want the experience of having the breast squeezed into the baby's mouth repeated. They particularly did not like this type of help in the NICU in plain sight of other parents and nurses, and they did not understand what the purpose of it was. They felt their breasts became objects. Mothers wanted a hands-off approach, with the nurse sitting next to them and explaining how to do it, especially if it could be modeled with the nurse using a doll and cloth breast model. Weimers et al. (2006) state:

> . . . the hands-on approach may be quicker to perform, but may hinder mother's confidence in her capacities in the long run. In fact, if more time was spent on support and information in the first place, mothers would feel respected and guided into becoming more competent to care for their special baby; they could quickly become

> more knowledgeable and more autonomous. In this study it was the opposite for eight mothers out of ten; they felt their integrity was not respected by the hands-on approach which had not been explained before being performed. (p. 9)

Therefore, the hands-on approach, even when permission is given, seems to be counterproductive, causing a decrease in maternal confidence, and perhaps causing an increase in infant reluctance to go to the breast if he is forced onto it.

In Nyqvist and Kylberg's (2008) application of baby-friendly principles to NICU care, it is noteworthy that mothers themselves wanted a lot more empathetic care from nurses and NICU staff. This engendered Nyqvist and Kylberg's step 2, which states: "Treat every mother with sensitivity, empathy, and respect for her maternal role. Support her in making informed decisions about milk production and breastfeeding according to her own wishes" (p. 256). While many of us expect that sensitivity, empathy, and respect are an inherent part of all interactions within the heathcare system, this is not the case when the healthcare system is financially constrained and understaffed and trying to meet the needs of an ever-larger population. This is certainly the case for neonatal intensive care. While sensitivity, empathy, and respect should be part of the culture of every unit in the hospital, it appears that many care providers, including those in the NICU, need to be reminded often of this culture (see Chapter 3).

One of the nursing care models examined in the Weimers et al. (2006) study cited earlier is Gustafsson's SAUC model where SAUC stands for sympathy expressing, acceptance establishing, understanding, and competence manifesting. This model fits well with Nyqvist and Kylberg's step 2 (2008). Expressions of sympathy/empathy, respect, and sensitivity to the mother's concerns will enable her to be a more competent parent and caregiver for her own infant. Having witnessed many examples such as Bonnie's, I believe that many mothers or preterm infants in the United States take their infants home feeling a great sense of inadequacy and fear about how they will care for the baby after discharge. Little sympathy or understanding has been extended to the mother, and there is an underlying expectation among staff that the mother will not be a good parent. Small wonder—she hasn't been helped to become one and feel competent in her ability to care for the baby while it was still in the NICU. Attitudes and beliefs of individual nurses and differences in quality of care depending on the parents' socioeconomic status exacerbate the problem.

Use of Peer Counselors for Support

In several cases, peer counselors have been utilized as support systems for mothers in the NICU. Ideally, peer counselors should be peers in every sense of the word—be about the same age, have had babies in the NICU for about the same amount of time, be in similar economic circumstances, be experienced at milk expression and transitioning to breastfeeding, etc. In one study in an inner city hospital (Merewood et al., 2006), peer counselors did not necessarily have NICU experience but did have breastfeeding experience and came from the neighborhood in which the hospital and its patients were located. Two of the five peer counselors used in the randomized, controlled trial were U.S.-born African American women, one was U.S.-born White, one was U.S.-born White/Native American, and one was non–U.S.-born Mexican. Two of these women were former teenage mothers. The peer counselors had a specialized course of training in breastfeeding management and were also trained in the hospital about NICU procedures. Study subjects were enrolled in the study within 72 hours of birth and randomly assigned to either the intervention (peer counselor assignment) or control group (no peer counselor). Peer counselors also visited the intervention mothers in the hospital within the first 72 hours of birth, prior to the mother's hospital discharge. All mothers received access to standard of care treatment, which included access to breast pumps, referrals to a lactation consultant when needed, access to three breastfeeding classes a week, and staff who were well trained in lactation management. The group assigned to the peer counselors also got weekly visits from the peer counselor for 6 weeks. These contacts were face-to-face meetings that lasted at least 30 minutes and were conducted in the NICU when the mother was there. If the infant had been discharged, then telephone contact was substituted. Peer counselors discussed and/or provided the following: pumping techniques, companionship while visiting the NICU, help with actual breastfeeding, and help with KMC/STS care.

Infant feeding status was then assessed by a researcher who was blinded to the mother's assignment group at 2, 4, 8, and 12 weeks postpartum. At 12 weeks, women who had peer counselor contact were 181% more likely to be providing any breast milk to their infants compared to the standard of care group. In the analysis of the subgroup of African American infants at 12 weeks, the odds of receiving any breast milk were 249% greater in the peer counselor group. A carefully orchestrated and supervised peer counselor program in the NICU can be very effective in increasing the amount of mother's own milk that NICU infants receive over the long term.

The Rush Mothers' Milk Club also makes use of peer counselors who are former NICU mothers and who became certified as peer counselors through La Leche League's peer counselor training program (Meier, 2003). At weekly luncheons of the Milk Club, peer counselors share their experiences with new mothers of preterm infants, answer questions about breastfeeding problems, and help mothers make decisions about when and how long to express milk and whether to transition to breastfeeding. Peer counselors make phone calls to all new mothers and can make home visits if needed. Transportation for these home visits is provided to peer counselors via the Mothers' Milk Club Taxi, which also picks mothers up at their homes and brings them to the weekly luncheons free of charge and then takes them home afterward. The Rush Mothers' Milk Club model, however, is more of an educative model, with the weekly luncheons devoted to

> . . . sharing the science of lactation and human milk feedings . . . Mothers learn the scientific principles, coming away using terminology such as Interleukin 10, density of the prolactin receptors and statistics about how their milk protects their babies from feeding-related morbidity. This is combined with using each mother's clinical questions as examples for which the scientific principles are articulated. Mothers of all educational, income, and ethnic backgrounds appreciate and understand these principles. (Meier, quoted in Brown, n.d.)

The Rush Mothers' Milk Club appears to be extremely successful. In a retrospective analysis of 24 months of NICU admissions (1997–1998) covering 207 NICU admissions whose mothers were eligible to provide their milk, African Americans (44.9%), Whites (35.7%), and Latinas (17.9%) accounted for 98.5% of the study population (Meier, Engstrom, Mingolelli, Miracle, & Kiesling, 2004). The lactation initiation rate was 72.9%, with the initiation rates for African American mothers among the highest reported in the literature. The initiation rate is very close to the goal of 75% initiation recommended in the Healthy People 2010 goals (CDC, 2008). The mean dose of MOM received over the first 15, 30, and 60 days postbirth was 81.7%, 80.1%, and 66.1% respectively. The success of this milk club, however, may be due more to the peer counselors, the free lunch, the free taxi service, and the free or subsidized electric breast pumps that are provided than to the educational material offered, although the manner in which the education is offered—relating it to the mother's own questions—may be helpful. Education by itself is not the warm and empathetic experience of counseling.

Community Support Postdischarge

Once both mother and baby have been discharged from NICU care, follow-up care and support in the community are equally important to ensure that breastfeeding continues/improves and the baby is not compromised. Preterm infants consume smaller volumes than their term counterparts, and intake needs to be monitored closely to prevent loss of weight and failure to thrive (Baker & Rasmussen, 1997). Meier (2003) points out that in many countries, preterm infants are discharged from the hospital only after they have demonstrated that they can gain weight while consuming all feedings at breast. They are older and heavier as well at discharge. This is not the case in the United States, where preterm infants are discharged in many cases smaller, less mature, and prior to reaching term. They are also usually discharged before they are able to breastfeed efficiently. All too often, we see the mother being helped to breastfeed for the first time 2 or 3 days before the baby goes home. Of course the baby cannot breastfeed successfully at the breast at every feeding with this short of a learning curve. Furman et al. (2002) found that one of the biggest factors contributing to early cessation of breastfeeding is the failure to adequately transition the baby from breastmilk feedings to at-breast feedings and putting the baby to the breast for the first time after 35 weeks' corrected age. Preterm infants are therefore more vulnerable to being fed inadequate amounts of milk postdischarge and need more careful monitoring and follow-up. Mothers, therefore, need increased support as well as access to accurate scales that will measure milk intake at each feeding in test weights.

Mothers of newly discharged preterm infants have concerns about their milk supplies and whether they will be able to provide their infants with enough milk (Baker & Rasmussen, 1997). In a qualitative study of breastfeeding duration at NICU discharge (to a lower level of hospital care), at discharge home, and at 1, 3, 6, and 12 months corrected age (or until weaning), Callen, Pinelli, Atkinson, and Saigal (2005) examined the barriers to breastfeeding in very-low-birth-weight infants (≤ 1500 g). At NICU discharge, low milk volume was the greatest barrier. The infant's compromised physical status was the biggest barrier from discharge home and at 1 and 3 months' corrected age. Nipple and breast problems were barriers at NICU discharge and discharge home, and poor technique was a barrier at 1 month. Many of these issues could have been addressed with access to quality lactation counseling that was sensitive to the special considerations and needs of preterm mothers and infants.

One hospital has developed a documentation form for lactation support that is used by multiple lactation care providers (Baker & Rasmussen, 1997). The form is kept in the infant's bedside chart so that all providers can refer to it. It contains information about the mother and the infant, has a teaching checklist, a breastfeeding assessment grid, and discharge planning information. When the infant is discharged from the NICU or transferred to another step-down unit, a copy of the record is sent to the pediatric care provider or the receiving hospital so it is available for the first visit by mother and baby. The original is kept by the NICU lactation service so that early postdischarge follow-up can be accomplished and proactive solutions to problems can be provided. This is a method of providing continuity of care across the system as all providers can see what the lactation history of this dyad is and what preventive actions that will ensure breastfeeding success have occurred. However, the form alone does not substitute for the personalized care and encouragement that each mother needs postdischarge.

The type of support is also important, and the individual(s) providing the support for the preterm mother in the community need to have some specialized knowledge of the needs and problems of the preterm infants. For this reason, NICU follow-up clinics would be the ideal place for monitoring breastfeeding skills and weight gain in the baby, provided the follow-up care began immediately after the discharge and continued frequently. If follow-up clinic nurses are also trained in breastfeeding management techniques specifically geared to the preterm infant, they should be able to help the mother resolve any problems that arise, as well as ensure that the infant is not nutritionally compromised.

Most of all, the mother needs mothering herself when she is in this vulnerable stage of her infant's development and progress. In this regard, a combination of peers or lay counselors and professional support systems working in tandem would provide the mother with praise, encouragement, and support.

SUMMARY

The third strategy for increasing breastfeeding initiation and duration rates is support. **Appendix 12-1** provides a model policy for the provision of support to mothers of preterm infants. Two main types of support are needed—educative and emotional/physical. The two types are different and can be supplied by different types of helpers. Offering only one type of support is not adequate; for the biggest impact on breastfeeding rates, both types need to be offered. Inherent in both the educative model and the encouragement model is the ability of the support person to counsel the mother effectively. The support person does not tell the mother what to do; instead she listens to what the mother is saying and feeling and then suggests evidence-based options that might work for this mother, allowing the mother to make the choice based on what will work best for her situation.

Individualized support for the mother of a preterm infant needs to be offered more intensively over a longer period of time than support for the mother of a healthy, term infant. It should also occur in three distinct time frames—while the mother is hospitalized in the peripartum period; while the baby remains hospitalized after the mother is discharged; and postdischarge when both mother and baby are home. Much of this support will be needed in the hospital setting. For true continuity of care, hospitals need to form support groups and systems for mothers in the hospital setting that can be utilized not only while the baby is still in house, but also after the baby is discharged, since many communities lack support systems and services for mothers of discharged preterm infants. The healthcare team can thus ensure that the health of the baby is not compromised while breastfeeding becomes better established and maintained postdischarge and that mothers of preterm infants improve their parenting skills.

REFERENCES

Ahluwalia, I., Morrow, B., & Hsia, J. (2005). Why do women stop breastfeeding? Findings from the pregnancy risk assessment and monitoring system. *Pediatrics, 116*(6), 1408–1412.

Baker, B., & Rasmussen, T. (1997). Organizing and documenting lactation support of NICU families. *Journal of Obstetric, Gynecologic, and Neonatal Nursing, 26*(5), 515–521.

Brown, T. (n.d.). *The Rush Mothers' Milk Club: Providing parents of preemies with the support to breastfeed*. Retrieved May 8, 2009, from http://www.breastfeed.com/articles/breastfeeding-advocacy/the-rush-mothers-milk-club-2783/#

Cadwell, K., & Turner-Maffei, C. (2009). *Continuity of care in breastfeeding: Best practices in the maternity setting*. Sudbury, MA: Jones and Bartlett.

Callen, J., Pinelli, J, Atkinson, S., & Saigal, S. (2005). Qualitative analysis of barriers to breastfeeding in very-low-birthweight infants in the hospital and postdischarge. *Advances in Neonatal Care, 5*(2), 93–103.

Castrucci, B., Hoover, K., Lim, S., & Maus, K. (2007). Availability of lactation counseling services influences breastfeeding among infants admitted to neonatal intensive care units. *American Journal of Health Promotion, 21*(5), 410–415.

Centers for Disease Control and Prevention (CDC). (2008). *Breastfeeding among U.S. children born 1999—2005, CDC National Immunization Survey*. Retrieved, June 5, 2009, from http://www.cdc.gov/breastfeeding/data/NIS_data/index.htm

Cleveland, L. (2008). Parenting in the neonatal intensive care unit. *Journal of Obstetric, Gynecologic, and Neonatal Nursing, 37*(6), 666–691.

Ertem, I., Votto, N., & Leventhal, J. (2001). The timing and predictors of the early termination of breastfeeding. *Pediatrics, 107*(3), 543–548.

Farooq, S. (2009). *New breastfeeding campaign turns heads: Group introduces unique ad campaign*. Retrieved May 6, 2009, from http://www.nbcbayarea.com/around_town/the_scene/Lactating-Women-Getting-Second-Looks-in-Marin.html

Furman, L., Minich, N., & Hack, M. (2002). Correlates of lactation in mothers of very low birth weight infants. *Pediatrics, 109*(4), e57.

Gonzalez, K., Meinzen-Derr, J., Burke, B., Hibler, A., Kavinsky, B., Hess, S., et al. (2003). Evaluation of a lactation support service in a children's hospital neonatal intensive care unit. *Journal of Human Lactation, 19*(3), 286–292.

Hawkins, L., Nichols, F., & Tanner, J. (1987). Predictors of the duration of breastfeeding in low-income women. *Birth, 14*(4), 204–209.

Li, R., Fein, S., Chen, J., & Grummer-Strawn, L. (2008). Why mothers stop breastfeeding: Mothers' self-reported reasons for stopping breastfeeding during the first year. *Pediatrics, 122*(Suppl. 2), S69–S76.

McGrath, J. (2007). Breastfeeding success for the high-risk infant and family: Nursing attitudes and beliefs. *Journal of Perinatal and Neonatal Nursing, 21*(3), 183–185.

Meier, P. (2003). Supporting lactation in mothers with very low birth weight infants. *Pediatric Annals, 32*(5), 317–325.

Meier, P., Engstrom, J., Mingolelli, S., Miracle, D., & Kiesling, S. (2004). The Rush Mothers' Milk Club: Breastfeeding interventions for mothers with very-low-birth weight infants. *Journal of Obstetric, Gynecologic, and Neonatal Nursing, 33*(2), 164–174.

Merewood, A., Chamberlain, L., Cook, J., Philipp, B., Malone, K., & Bauchner, H. (2006). The effect of peer counselors on breastfeeding rates in the neonatal intensive care unit: Results of a randomized controlled trial. *Archives of Pediatric and Adolescent Medicine, 160*(7), 681–685.

National Conference of State Legislatures. (2009). *50 state summary of breastfeeding laws*. Retrieved May 6, 2009, from http://www.ncsl.org/programs/health/breast50.htm

Nyqvist, K., & Kylberg, E. (2008). Application of the Baby Friendly Hospital Initiative to neonatal care: Suggestions by Swedish mothers of very preterm infants. *Journal of Human Lactation, 24*(3), 252–262.

Nyqvist, K., Sjoden, P., & Ewald, U. (1994). Mothers' advice about facilitating breastfeeding in neonatal intensive care unit. *Journal of Human Lactation, 10*(4), 237–243.

Sisk, P., Lovelady, C., Dillard, R., & Gruber, K. (2006). Lactation counseling for mothers of very low birth weight infants: Effect on maternal anxiety and infant intake of milk. *Pediatrics, 117*(1), e67–e75.

Taveras, E., Capra, A., Braveman, P., Jensvold, N., Escobar, G., & Lieu, T. (2003). Clinician support and psychosocial risk factors associated with breastfeeding discontinuation. *Pediatrics, 112*(1 Pt. 1), 108–115.

Weimers, L., Svensson, K., Dumas, L., Maver, L., & Wahlberg, V. (2006). Hands-on approach during breastfeeding support in a neonatal intensive care unit: A qualitative study of Swedish mothers' experiences. *International Breastfeeding Journal, 1*, 20.

World Health Organization (WHO). (2003). *Global strategy for infant and young child feeding.* Geneva, Switzerland: Author.

APPENDIX 12-1

STEP 10

Foster the establishment of NICU/SCN breastfeeding support groups and postdischarge community programs and refer mothers to them.

Policies 10.1–10.3

Title

Establishment of predischarge and postdischarge NICU/SCN breastfeeding support groups.

Purpose

To provide support to breastfeeding mothers whose infants are in the NICU/SCN or have been discharged and to help the NICU/SCN team to develop a discharge plan.

Rationale

Proactive support helps to ensure that breastfeeding NICU mothers will have better breastfeeding outcomes and longer durations of breastfeeding. Support groups need to be established so that mothers can have questions answered during the infants' hospitalization and after discharge from the NICU/SCN. Interventions that provide breastfeeding mothers with support at critical times increase the duration of breastfeeding as well as its exclusivity.

Scope

These policies cover all NICU/SCN personnel including the medical director, nursing director, nursing supervisors, licensed staff, ancillary staff, and volunteers.

Policy 10.1

The facility should establish and facilitate an in-house NICU/SCN breastfeeding peer support group, and staff should refer parents to the support group.

Procedure 10.1.1
The peer support group should meet at least weekly and on site.

Procedure 10.1.2
The peer support group should be available to the mother and/or father during the infant's entire hospitalization.

Procedure 10.1.3
The peer support group should be facilitated by a staff member(s) who is knowledgeable about breastfeeding in the NICU and who can answer questions the group may have.

Procedure 10.1.4
NICU/SCN "graduate" mothers should be invited back to attend the support group, discuss solutions to breastfeeding problems, and provide a postdischarge perspective to mothers/fathers still in the NICU/SCN.

Policy 10.2

The NICU/SCN staff should be able to identify postdischarge support groups both within the facility and in the community that provide culturally specific breastfeeding support services, without ties to commercial interests, and refer mothers to them during discharge planning.

Procedure 10.2.1
Should community support services be lacking, it is incumbent upon the hospital to establish and maintain support services where parents can return for assistance and counseling.

Policy 10.3

Mothers should be educated regarding the importance of pediatric visits including weight checks according to current AAP guidelines.

Procedure 10.3.1
Prior to discharge home, an appointment should be made with the pediatric care provider within 48 hours of discharge.

Procedure 10.3.2
Mothers should be referred to facility and community support groups through written materials or counseling. These support groups may include, but not be limited to:

- Women, Infants, and Children breastfeeding support services
- La Leche League

- Lactation clinics
- Home health services, e.g., Visiting Nurse Association
- Telephone hotlines or warm lines
- Pediatricians
- Neonatologists
- Other healthcare providers
- NICU follow-up clinics

Part IV

The Case for Banked Donor Human Milk in the NICU

chapter thirteen

Use of Banked Donor Human Milk as an Alternative to Formula

In the previous sections I have discussed the significant differences in outcome human milk contributes to the preterm infant and how a mother can be supported in supplying her own milk for her hospitalized infant. Yet even in the ideal, supportive NICU setting, a mother may be challenged in her ability to maintain a milk supply. In addition to her exhaustion, muscle atrophy from prolonged bed rest, worry about her infant, family obligations, and perhaps a return to work in order to save her maternity leave for after the baby comes home, the mother who is expressing milk for her baby may have performance anxiety. With each milk collection she wonders, "Is it enough?" "Will I be able to keep up as the baby's needs increase?" "What if my milk isn't enough, and I don't want my baby to get formula?" "Is there another option?"

Sometimes a mother has decided not to breastfeed only to learn that her baby has an illness or condition that would improve with human milk. Sometimes the mother has weaned from the breast only to find out that her baby is allergic to or intolerant of formula. What are the options for feeding these infants? Safe use of milk from other mothers is the answer. Safe use means full knowledge and support of the physician caring for the baby. Safe use means donor human milk from a milk bank (see **Box 13-1**).

Donor human milk banking is the collection, storage, processing, and distribution of human milk according to established guidelines. Donor milk has been voluntarily expressed by mothers who are not biologically related to the recipient. It is dispensed and distributed by prescription from a physician,

Box 13-1 The Hazards of Informal Sharing of Milk

Periodically, stories circulate about women buying human milk over the Internet or borrowing it from a friend or person they might or might not know who is a friend of a friend. Found on the Internet and in local newspapers, these stories seem to be growing in numbers and visibility. When a mother's milk supply starts to falter or she has a condition that precludes breastfeeding (e.g., double mastectomies for breast cancer prevention or treatment), a woman may turn to the Internet or other sources for human milk for her baby.

This risky behavior is not recommended by the U.S. Breastfeeding Committee and other health organizations. Unlike the numerous checks and balances that ensure that donated human milk from a Human Milk Banking Association of North America member milk bank, informal sharing arrangements or purchase of human milk from the Internet has no oversight. Donor screening procedures are not in place, for example. Even if a mother thinks she knows the donor well, the donor herself may be unaware of a potential health hazard. Family members may be among the most secretive about sharing potential risky behaviors with each other. HIV may be transmitted through informal sharing that lacks screening, as can other, less lethal viruses such as herpes—lethal if transmitted to a premature baby, a sick infant, or other compromised individual.

There are no tested and proven methods that provide uniform and minimal effects on the milk without proper equipment and oversight such as a milk bank provides. Using a stovetop and a regular pot, the milk is subjected to uncontrolled temperatures and the damaging effects of high temperatures. Even if the donor is screened, the added protection of pasteurization is missing.

An unanswered question with informal sharing is the legal liability of the donor if the recipient contracts an infection that can be traced to the milk. Liability could increase for the donor if milk from several donors is being given to the baby. Donor milk banks provide anonymity to the donor, and recipients and donors usually do not meet or get to know each other.

When women purchase milk over the Internet the anonymity is certainly there, but the chance of fraud increases. Is it really human milk that is being shipped or is it some other animal milk? Has the milk been diluted to make more money for the seller? How clean is the milk? What drugs might the infant be exposed to? (See http://www.usbreastfeeding.org/LinkClick.aspx?link=Position-Statements%2fDonor-Milk-Statement-2008-06-18-USBC.pdf&tabid=70&mid=393)

nurse practitioner, or other licensed healthcare provider with prescriptive powers. A nominal processing fee is charged by the milk bank to partially defray the costs of donor screening, labor, and overhead costs.

THE ALGORITHM

As represented in the flow chart in **Figure 13-1**, donor human milk banking is a complex process with safety checks and balances. It is also labor intensive, time consuming, and relatively expensive.

It begins with a volunteer mother who wants to donate her milk with the hope that it will help other babies be healthy (Azema & Callahan, 2003;

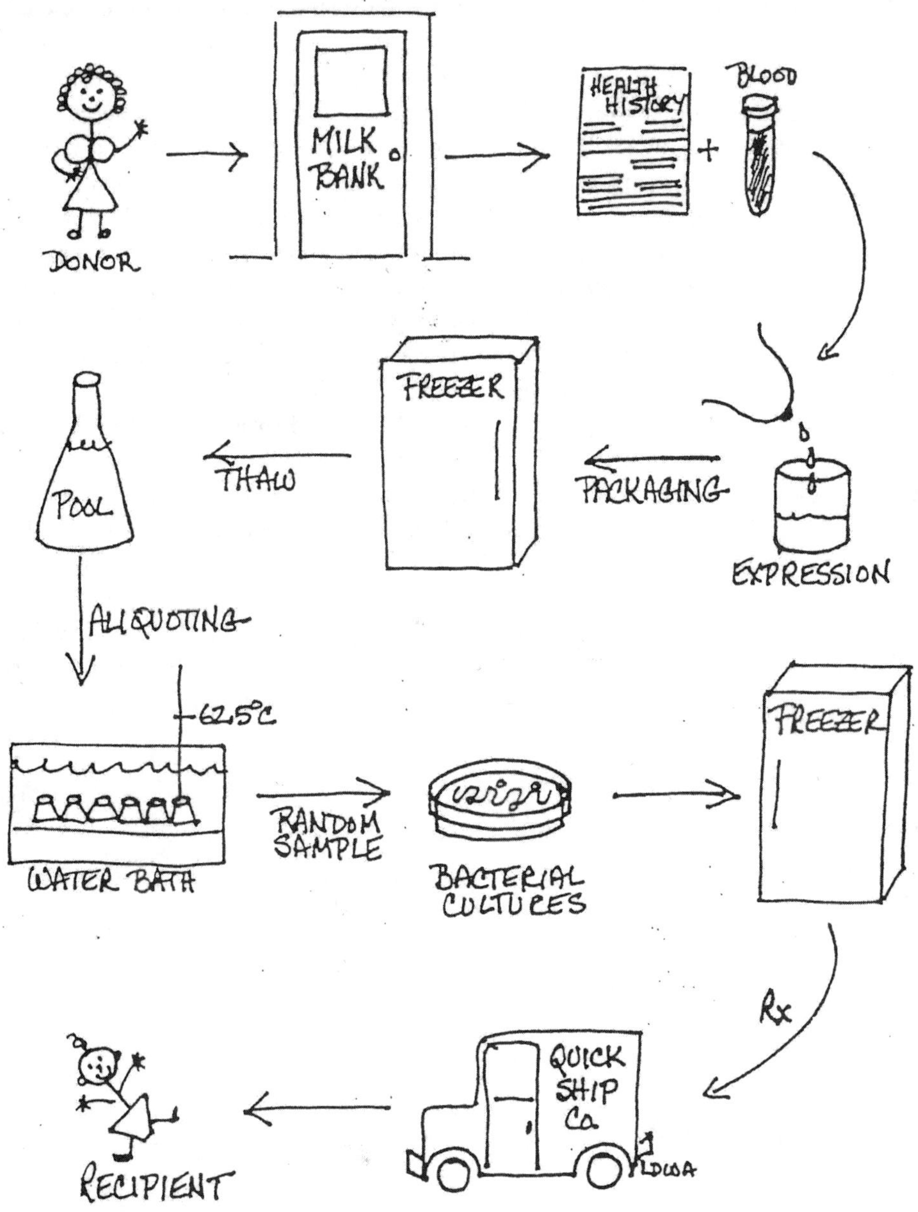

Figure 13-1 Flow chart showing how donated milk is screened and processed for distribution to premature and sick infants. Used with permission of the author and Health Education Associates.

Osbaldiston & Mingle, 2007; Pimenteira Thomaz, Maia Loureiro, da Silva Oliveira, Furtado Montenegro, Dantas Almeida, Fernando Rodrigues Soriano, et al., 2008). In Brazil, the encouragement of a health professional had the most significant impact on the decision to donate, with 61.3% of donors surveyed citing that as a reason for donating. However, repeat donors and those with educational attainment of secondary school or higher ranked the needs of the infants they were helping as the primary motivator for donating, followed by the recommendation of the health professional. A sense of social responsibility was also a motivating factor (Pimenteira Thomaz et al., 2008) Occasionally milk is donated by women who have preterm infants and an excess of milk or by women who have had a fetal demise or a perinatal loss, perhaps from a baby born with a birth anomaly incompatible with life. For these women, donation is a therapeutic part of grieving (Tully, 1997). (See **Boxes 13-2** and **13-3.**)

Once the donor contacts the milk bank, she is thoroughly and systematically screened. A health history based on the screening tool used by the American Association of Blood Banks and serological screening for HIV-1 and -2, human T-cell leukemia virus (HTLV-1 and -2), hepatitis B, hepatitis C, and syphilis are the first steps followed by the mother's primary care provider certifying that she is in good health. The pediatric care provider certifies that the baby (if living) is also in good health and that there is nothing that contraindicates this mother from becoming a donor.

Box 13-2 My Story

I had actually never heard of a donor milk bank when my daughter was born in 1978 in Honolulu. Fortunately, my sister, a pediatric nurse practitioner trained in Boston and Baltimore, had heard of them. She took one look at my dripping breasts and my Michelin-tire-baby daughter and said, "Lois, you could feed the Russian Army with all this milk!" She went directly to the phone book and found the Hawaii Mothers' Milk Bank (HMMB) and I was soon a donor.

One thing led to another, and with my baby on one hip and a cooler on the other, I collected frozen milk all over Honolulu. Then I added office volunteer work to my duties. I did bulk mailings, answered the phone, and wrote the newsletter. I learned how to do donor intakes, gave breastfeeding advice to mothers, rented electric breast pumps, learned to pasteurize milk, and drove milk samples to the Department of Health for bacteriological testing. Then the HMMB hired me as its assistant administrator!

I added bookkeeping and grant writing to my job description and represented HMMB at the founding meeting of HMBANA in 1985. I left my position with HMMB in 1987 to return to school for a maternal and child health-focused master's in public health from the University of Hawaii, a great difference from my undergraduate degree in zoology and my jobs as a marine biologist and research assistant. Having children and breastfeeding them changes lives!

Box 13-3 Hallie's Story

Hallie had waited a long time to become pregnant with her second child, and at 5 months' gestation, she suffered a fetal demise. Heartbroken over the loss of her little girl, Hallie was compelled to find something positive in this tragic event. She called the milk bank in Honolulu several days later as her milk was coming in. The donor screening paperwork was completed over the phone and arrangements were made to have the blood work done. I drove sterile containers in a shipping container to the airport where one of the inter-island airlines transported the bottles free of charge to a neighbor island where they were picked up by Hallie's husband. Instructions for expressing and freezing her milk were included.

Several days later, Hallie called the milk bank again saying that she had filled the bottles and was ready to ship them back to Honolulu. Could the milk bank please send more bottles and larger ones this time? She was filling them rather rapidly. I again drove to the airport with new sterile bottles (bigger and more of them) in several containers. I collected the incoming frozen milk and shipped the new coolers and bottles on the return flight. The airline agreed to continue shipping the milk and empty bottles free of charge as part of its community service. Over a period of 4 months, Hallie donated an average of 36 ounces a day, necessitating twice weekly trips to the airport.

Islanders learned what Hallie was doing and she became the focus of several articles about the milk bank and what local people were doing to help their communities. She became a celebrity in her own community. She was using a cylinder hand pump to express her milk. Her 10-year-old son took it to school one day for show and tell and told all his classmates (who in turn told their parents) about what his mom was doing for the tiny babies in Honolulu. Hallie's husband was given time off with pay by his boss at the local garage to take the milk to the airport and pick up the empty bottles. His boss also supplied all the ice for shipping free of charge. Hallie got letters from people she had never met, and the milk bank received monetary donations to help with its work as a result of the publicity. An added bonus were the amazing drawings by Hallie's son of airplanes flying milk from one island to another that soon decorated the milk bank office. Out of a tragic event came great love and aloha. While Hallie will always grieve for the loss of her daughter, she told me that she could move on with her life—something very good had come out of her tragedy.

Source: Arnold, 2005. Used with permission of the author.

If milk collection is being initiated by the donor specifically for the milk bank, the milk bank provides the containers and instructions for expression. Some mothers, however, have been collecting milk for their own infant and find that they have an overstock well beyond what their baby will need. This previously collected and frozen milk may be donated on a one-time bulk basis. Each container must carry the date of expression and the name of the donor (or unique identifying code number).

After a substantial amount of milk has been collected and frozen, the milk is transported to the milk bank. Some milk banks require that milk be transported every 2 weeks, while others leave it up to the mother to determine when she should send it. Milk banks use different transportation methods. Some have a system of depots in the state or geographic region and milk is brought to the depot freezer by the donor and then transported from the depot to the milk bank by volunteers or a courier service. Other milk banks have volunteer collectors who drive milk routes and pick up milk directly from donors for transport to the milk bank. Some donors are located too far away for easy local transport, in which case milk is shipped frozen overnight in special containers. The milk bank pays the cost of the shipping.

Once in the milk bank, records are verified and the milk is thawed. The milk from several different donors is mixed together in a pool. The rationale for this pooling process is to distribute fat more evenly. Simple observation of stored milk provides evidence that there is a wide variation in milk fat content from one donor to another. Milk banks pool containers of milk that have a thick visible layer of fat with those from another donor whose fat layer is much thinner. Milk from mothers of preterm infants is also segregated and pooled with milk from other mothers of preterm infants. This milk will then be more appropriate compositionally for a preterm infant.

Once pooled and separated as aliquots into small bottles with water-tight lids, milk has been traditionally pasteurized (heat treated) for 30 minutes at 62.5°C. This process destroys all bacteria and most viruses, including HIV, herpes, and cytomegalovirus (CMV) (Dworsky, Stagno, Pass, Cassady, & Alford, 1982; Eglin & Wilkinson, 1987; Friis & Andersen, 1982; Orloff, Wallingford, & McDougal, 1993; Wallingford, 1987). Some milk banks use automated human milk pasteurizers that maintain the temperature of the water bath in which the bottles of milk are submerged for pasteurization and then flush the hot water out and replace it with chilled water in order to stop the heat reaction with milk components. Other milk banks rely on constant temperature water baths, which require the manual removal of bottles for chilling.

Other methods of pasteurization (different times at different temperatures) have been explored. Currently the one commercial entity that processes milk is using a high temperature short time (HTST) method of pasteurization. Although available for use in the dairy industry, equipment for processing the comparatively smaller volumes of human milk in this way is not the standard and is reportedly expensive to develop. In the past, this HTST methodology has only been utilized for small research studies looking into the effectiveness and safety of feeding infants milk that was pasteurized in this way, and HTST pasteurizers are not yet available for milk banks to purchase.

Pasteurization does have negative effects on milk quality. The rule of thumb is that the higher the heat and the longer the processing time, the more the composition changes. From the studies listed in **Table 13-1**, one can see

Table 13-1 Effects of Time and Temperature on Milk Components During Pasteurization

	% Retention (Range)	*Temperature*	*Duration*	*Reference*
Immune components				
C3 complement	0%	73°C	30 min.	Evans, Ryley, Neale, Dodge, & Lewarne, 1978
IgA (total or secretory)	0%	73°C	30 min.	Evans et al., 1978
	0–27%	70–73°C	15–30 min.	Bjorksten et al., 1980
	21%	62.5°C	30 min.	Gibbs, 1978
	64%	72°C	15 sec.	Goldsmith, Dickson, Barnhart, Toledo, & Eitenmiller, 1983
	67–100%	62.5°C	30 min.	Bjorksten et al., 1980
	80%	62.5°C	30 min.	Ford, Law, Marshall, & Reiter, 1977
	84%	56°C	30 min.	Eitenmiller, 1990
	100%	62.5°C	30 min.	Evans et al., 1978
	105%	60°C	30 min.	Evans et al., 1978
	150%	72°C	15 sec.	Goldblum et al., 1984
IgG	0%	73°C	30 min.	Evans et al., 1978
	58%	72°C	15 sec.	Goldsmith, Dickson, et al., 1983
	66%	62.5°C	30 min.	Bjorksten et al., 1980
	66%	62.5°C	30 min.	Evans et al., 1978
	82.8%	60°C	30 min.	Evans et al., 1978
IgM	0%	73°C	15 sec.	Goldsmith, Dickson, et al., 1983
	0%	72°C	30 min.	Evans et al., 1978
	0%	62.5°C	30 min.	Ford et al., 1977
	0%	62.5°C	30 min.	Bjorksten et al., 1980
Lactoferrin	0%	73°C	30 min.	Evans et al., 1978
	43.2%	62.5°C	30 min.	Evans et al., 1978
	72%	56°C	30 min.	Eitenmiller, 1990
	84.3%	62.5°C	30 min.	Ford et al., 1977
	123%	72°C	15 sec.	Goldblum et al., 1984
Lysozyme	0%	73°C	30 min.	Evans et al., 1978
	Almost all destroyed	73°C	Approx. 15–20 min.	Ford et al., 1977
	46%	> 90°C	30 min.	Gibbs, 1978
	76.3%	62.5°C	30 min.	Evans et al., 1978
	77%	62.5°C	30 min.	Bjorksten et al., 1980
	Stable	62.5°C	30 min.	Ford et al., 1977
	115.6%	60°C	30 min.	Evans et al., 1978
	132%	56°C	30 min.	Eitenmiller, 1990
	393%	72°C	15 sec.	Goldblum et al., 1984

Table 13-1 Effects of Time and Temperature on Milk Components During Pasteurization (continued)

	% Retention (Range)	*Temperature*	*Duration*	*Reference*
Cellular components				
Leukocytes	Number decreased; 0% functionality at both temperatures	56°C 72°C	30 min. 15 sec.	Lawrence, 2001 Lawrence, 2001
Lymphocytes	Number decreased; 0% functionality at both temperatures	56°C 72°C	15 sec. 30 min.	Lawrence, 2001 Lawrence, 2001
Enzymes, growth factors, etc.				
Alpha-1-antitrypsin	61.8%	73°C	30 min.	Evans et al., 1978
Lipoprotein lipase	Completely destroyed	62.5°C	30 min.	Henderson et al., 1998
Bile salt stimulated lipase	Completely destroyed	> 55°C	Not specified	Wardell et al., 1984
	0%	62.5°C	30 min.	Henderson et al., 1998
Esterase	Completely destroyed	> 55°C	Not specified	Wardell et al., 1984
Transforming growth factor-alpha	93.9%	56.5°C	30 min.	McPherson & Wagner, 2001
Transforming growth factor-ß2	99%	56.5°C	30 min.	McPherson & Wagner, 2001
Whey:casein ratio	Whey decreased relative to fat	62.5°C	30 min.	Goes et al., 2002
Nutrients				
Fatty acids	100%	62.5°C	30 min.	Fidler et al., 2001
	94%	62.5°C	30 min.	Lepri, Del Bubba, Maggini, Donzelli, Galvan 1997
Vitamin A	103%	62.5°C	30 min.	Van Zoeren-Grobben, Schrijver, van den Berg, & Berger, 1987
Folic acid	65%	62.5°C	30 min.	Goldsmith, Eitenmiller, Toledo, & Barnhart, 1983
	69%	62.5°C	30 min.	Van Zoeren-Grobben et al., 1987
	72%	56°C	30 min.	Eitenmiller, 1990
	84%	62.5°C	30 min.	Donnelly-Vanderloo, O'Connor & Shoukri, 1994
	95%	72°C	15 sec.	Goldblum et al., 1984

Table 13-1 Effects of Time and Temperature on Milk Components During Pasteurization (continued)

	% Retention (Range)	*Temperature*	*Duration*	*Reference*
Vitamin B1	65%	62.5°C	30 min.	Goldsmith, Eitenmiller, et al., 1983
	85%	72°C	15 sec.	Goldblum et al., 1984
Vitamin B2	77%	72°C	15 sec.	Goldblum et al., 1984
	94%	62.5°C	30 min.	Van Zoeren-Grobben et al., 1987
Biotin (B complex)	110%	62.5°C	30 min.	Goldsmith, Eitenmiller, et al., 1983
	102%	72°C	15 sec.	Goldsmith, Eitenmiller, et al., 1983
Niacin (B complex)	100%	72°C	15 sec.	Goldsmith, Eitenmiller, et al., 1983
	106%	62.5°C	30 min.	Goldsmith, Eitenmiller, et al., 1983
Pantothenic acid	93%	62.5°C	30 min.	Goldsmith, Eitenmiller, et al., 1983
(B complex)	98%	72°C	15 sec.	Goldsmith, Eitenmiller, et al., 1983
Vitamin B6	85%	62.5°C	30 min.	Van Zoeren-Grobben et al., 1987
	93%	72°C	15 sec.	Goldblum et al., 1984
Vitamin C	64%	62.5°C	30 min.	Van Zoeren-Grobben et al., 1987
	94%	72°C	15 sec.	Goldblum et al., 1984
Vitamin D	103%	62.5°C	30 min.	Van Zoeren-Grobben et al., 1987
Vitamin E	106%	62.5°C	30 min.	Van Zoeren-Grobben et al., 1987
Zinc	Redistribution of zinc binding pattern	62.5°C	30 min.	Goes et al., 2002

Source: Arnold, 2005. Used with permission of the author.

that the nutrients in human milk remain relatively stable at the temperature variables. The enzymes are the most heat sensitive. Immune components are also compromised but are not destroyed completely. While the concentrations of various beneficial components may be decreased, the remaining portions still have protective activity, although this activity may be somewhat compromised (Silvestre, Ruiz, Martinez-Costa, Plaza, & Lopez, 2008). In this study, the bactericidal capacity of untreated milk (control refrigerated for 3 hours from time of expression to time of analysis), and milk pasteurized at low temperatures (63°C/30 minutes) and high temperatures (75°C/15 seconds) against an inoculum of *Escherichia coli* was measured. Colony counts of the control group were reduced by 70.1%, in the low temperature group by 52.27%, and in the high temperature group by 36.39%. This study demonstrates that the usual rule of thumb is applicable: the higher the temperature of treatment, the greater the loss of milk components. It should also be noted that in this same study, refrigeration only of samples for 72 hours reduced the bactericidal capacity to 26.61% when compared to controls, indicating that longer storage times for human milk may not be beneficial. On the other hand, no protective components are found in infant formulas (cow's milk based, soy based) or in any other food product. It would appear that processed and stored donor milk thus retains an advantage over formulas despite the losses of bactericidal capacity. Safety of donor milk is paramount. The small losses in composition still make for a high quality product that is safe even for immunocompromised sick or preterm infants.

Once pasteurized, a random sample of milk is selected from the batch and cultured to determine whether there is bacterial growth. No milk is dispensed unless the bacteria growth is zero, indicating that the pasteurization process was successful. After chilling and labeling with its own individual batch identification number, the pasteurized milk is frozen and held until the results of the bacterial tests are known. The milk is then deemed safe to dispense. Some milk banks use infrared equipment to analyze the nutrient content of the pasteurized milk, and this content is also noted on the label for the batch. It indicates the number of grams of protein per 100 cc of donor milk as well as the number of grams of carbohydrate and fat present and allows neonatologists to better estimate the amount of fortification that is required for an individual infant.

Once milk is cleared for distribution, dispensing is authorized by a prescription. Milk banks ship milk frozen so that it will arrive within 24 hours of receipt of the prescription. Milk banks have shipped milk within countries in which they are located and on occasion to other countries as well. For example, according to the map on its Web site, the eleven milk banks[1] belonging to the Human Milk Banking Association of North America (HMBANA) dispensed milk to hospitals in 34 states and 3 Canadian provinces in 2007 (see also pp. 354–355). Distribution is not limited to hospitals alone; outpatient recipients also receive banked donor milk. Instructions for thawing and storage accompany each shipment of donor milk.

In some countries, milk banks are part of the healthcare system, and milk from the milk bank is provided as part of the hospitalization of a newborn who does not have access to his own mother's milk. When the milk bank system is outside the healthcare service sector, as in the United States,

---

[1] The Human Milk Banking Association of North America (HMBANA), as of now is comprised of 10 milk banks—1 in Canada and 9 within the United States. Changes in the number of existing milk banks can be expected as new milk banks are established. Contacts for these milk banks and associated Web sites can be accessed through http://www.hmbana.org.

processing fees are charged on a per-ounce basis to defray processing costs. This processing fee enables the milk bank to cover some of the expenses incurred for labor, utilities, donor screening, and shipping. This processing fee is sometimes covered by insurers or HMOs, but the physician must argue each case individually. For a major U.S. carrier like Blue Cross Blue Shield, for example, different plans exist in different states and multiple plans are found in each state, so what is covered for one family may not be covered for another even though the carrier's name seems the same. Medicaid also covers the processing fee in some states, but not uniformly in all 50 states. Often milk banks will have to write off significant chunks of income if a family is unable to pay the processing fee.

HMBANA milk banks follow well-established milk banking procedures that are laid out in *Guidelines for the Establishment and Operation of a Donor Human Milk Bank* (HMBANA, 2007). This document is reviewed and revised every 1 to 2 years to remain current with new research and issues that arise. HMBANA also publishes a guide to starting a donor human milk bank (Flatau & Brady, 2006) and many milk banks serve as mentors for start-up donor milk bank personnel, training them in donor intake methods and pasteurization techniques. In the United Kingdom, Australia, and other countries, milk banking associations have established similar guidelines for operation. In some countries, the Health Ministry dictates the policies and procedures for donor milk banking.

BENEFITS OF USING BANKED DONOR HUMAN MILK

Some infants still require human milk for their survival, despite the advent of manufactured human milk substitutes. When a mother chooses not to breastfeed her own infant for one or more of a variety of reasons, or when a mother is unable to provide her own milk, donated human milk can make the difference between her infant's health and survival or morbidity and mortality. Historically, human milk has also been used around the world for feeding the elderly, as well as treating various types of diseases and conditions (Baumslag, 1987). However, in the United States, infants receive the bulk of the amount distributed each year.

Even in an age of manufactured human milk substitutes in the form of formula, we have seen that there is a growing body of scientific literature about the shortcomings and even hazards of using these substitutes, including the long-term deficits involved in misprogramming development of the human body even in parts of the world with clean water, literate mothers, and clean utensils (see also Chapter 2 in this book). In developing countries, use of these human milk substitutes is associated with increased morbidity and mortality due to malnutrition, wasting, starvation, and diarrhea. While we cannot say with absolute certainty that banked donor milk will have the optimal outcomes expected from fresh mother's milk, either expressed or breastfed directly, donor milk remains species specific and proven to be highly digestible, bioavailable, and bioactive. Benefits of using banked donor milk accrue directly to the recipient, as well as the recipient's family and society as a whole.

The Benefits to the Recipient

The benefits of donor milk are similar to those for breastfeeding/human milk in general, including species specificity; ease of digestion; promotion of growth, maturation, and development of organ systems; and immunological benefits. All are related to the unique composition of human milk and the dual and synergistic functions of many milk components (see Arnold, 2002b).

Species Specificity

Occasional reference to the theoretically worrisome potential for a graft-versus-host reaction to donor milk by the recipient when fresh milk is used have appeared in the literature (AAP, 1980; Xanthou, 1987). Young animals fed fresh milk containing live white blood cells from a *different species* exhibit this type of reaction. However, this has not been shown to occur in humans when human milk is given to humans (Xanthou, 1987). The success of wet nursing throughout human history would also appear to negate the graft-versus-host theory in the case of donor milk banking. Current milk banking practice includes pasteurization of all milk prior to dispensing. Thus, there are no live cells in the final product and therefore no potential for a graft-versus-host reaction.

Ease of Digestion

Donor milk is advantageous to premature infants and infants and children with certain digestive and metabolic conditions because it is easy to digest and creates minimal metabolic stress to organs and tissues. There is very little gastric residual left when infants are fed banked human milk, making it the ideal postsurgical feeding after gastrointestinal surgery for gastroschisis repair, necrotizing enterocolitis, or Hirschsprung's disease (Rangecroft, de

San Lazaro, & Scott, 1978; Riddell, 1989; Springer, 1997). Despite the loss of the milk's digestive enzymes that complement the baby's digestive enzymes during pasteurization (Henderson, Fay, & Hamosh, 1998; Wardell, Wright, Bardsley, & D'Souza, 1984), donor milk remains very digestible.

Promotion of Growth, Maturation, and Development of Organ Systems

Many components of human milk are heat stable at the temperatures used during pasteurization (Fidler, Sauerwald, Demmelmair, & Koletzko, 2001; Goes, Torres, Donangelo, & Trugo, 2002; McPherson & Wagner, 2001). The nutrient composition is rarely affected. Growth factors and essential fatty acids that enhance neurological development in the infant are also heat stable. For premature infants who have been deprived of the full complement of developmental factors in utero, the presence of these factors in donor milk is highly advantageous. These components do not occur in formulas. When infants and children have suffered tissue damage (e.g., damage to the mucosal epithelial lining of the digestive tract as a result of allergies to formulas), donor milk allows healing and maturation of the tissues and enzyme systems so that foods can be tolerated as the child heals and matures.

The unique nutrients and growth factors in human milk are implicated in the improved developmental outcome of infants who are fed human milk (Lucas, Morley, Cole, Lister, & Leeson-Payne, 1992). These advantages are particularly strong in premature infants, as shown in a meta-analysis of published studies (Anderson, Johnstone, & Remley, 1999). The essential fatty acids found naturally in human milk, arachidonic acid, and docosahexaenoic acid are not affected by pasteurization (Luukkainen, Salo, & Nikkari, 1995) and may promote better visual acuity by promoting better development of neurological synapses and impulse conduction. Finnish neonatologists have concluded that the use of banked donor milk is preferable to formula because it is a good (and natural) source of these long-chain polyunsaturated fatty acids (Luukkainen, et al., 1995). However, a more recent article has shown that infants who are fed their own mother's milk unpasteurized (raw) have better fat absorption and gained more in knee-heel length than infants who are fed their own mother's milk pasteurized (Andersson, Savman, Blackberg, & Hernell, 2007). This would make sense, since the enzymes responsible for assisting the infant to digest fat are extremely sensitive to heat. Banked donor milk would almost certainly have the similar issues.

Immunological Benefits

Lucas and Cole (1990) documented a reduction in the incidence of necrotizing enterocolitis in premature infants fed donor milk. Donor milk is an ideal way to acquire many of the immune factors that are not present in formulas or other animal milks. Although some of these properties are partially affected by the processing that occurs with donor milk, there is still enough retained to provide benefit to the recipient.

Benefits for the Recipient's Family

For the family of the recipient, one major benefit is that the infant's discomfort and pain are relieved. Many parents report that the infant on donor milk is less fussy and spends less time being uncomfortable and complaining about being in pain, even in situations where the infant is known to have a fatal condition. For parents, this easing of infant discomfort relieves some of their own anguish and stress. Other parents of recipients find that the availability of donor milk offers a sense of security; if a mother's own milk supply runs low, there is appropriate backup for her own milk supply.

Benefits to Society

In a larger community setting, the availability and frequent use of donor milk speaks volumes about the importance of human milk/breastfeeding to the health and well-being of infants. This is very positive public press for the benefits of breastfeeding and the medical necessity of providing human milk to fragile infants. Considerable cost savings can also be accrued by insurance companies, hospitals, and families when donor milk is used, as it prevents expenditures for long-term sequelae further down the road (Arnold, 2002a; Wight, 2001).

SETTING PRIORITIES FOR CLINICAL USE OF BANKED DONOR MILK

In the World Health Organization's hierarchy of feeding choices, a mother's own milk is always the first choice for feeding infants. Donor milk is the second choice when mother's own milk is unavailable and is usually preferred to formula use (F. Savage, personal communication, October 5, 1992). Donor milk may be used to supplement a mother's supply. Donor milk is primarily used when an infant is ill or has some medical condition where the use of banked donor milk is beneficial. Donor milk may be provided for certain maternal conditions in which breastfeeding by the biological mother would be contraindicated. Examples of such conditions include HIV-positive status of the mother or a mother undergoing chemotherapy treatments. Donor milk may also be used when the mother is healthy and the baby is adopted, or in cases where the mother dies, and the baby is healthy. Other uses include buying time until a diagnosis is made. Donor milk will first do no harm and so may become part or all of a solution to a problem. The use of banked donor human milk is meant to be temporary, although the definition of temporary may vary according to the needs of the individual recipient and national standards as well as availability.

In order to meet the increasing demands for donor milk from a disparate population of individuals, the HMBANA milk banks have developed a list prioritizing uses. In a case of short supply, milk banks first collaborate to see if a shortage in one geographic area can be covered by another milk bank. If a short supply continues, individuals with the lowest priority are denied access to donor milk so that those with the highest priority will continue to receive it. A prioritization list may be found in the guidelines (HMBANA, 2007).

Milk banks in Europe and Scandinavia reserve their donor milk primarily for use by premature infants. Banked donor milk is routinely used as first feedings in many NICUs when a mother's own milk is unavailable (Arnold, 1991, 1999). In 1986, approximately 72% of donor milk dispensed in the United States went to infants in neonatal intensive care units (NICUs), 23% to infants in the home, and 2% to patients in pediatric units of hospitals (Arnold, 1988). In 1994, a survey of seven HMBANA milk banks was conducted. Findings of this survey indicated that the distribution pattern had shifted, with only 40% going to premature or ill infants in the NICU and the balance going to older infants (Arnold, 1997b).

In 2007 only 22% average went to preterm infants (M. Tagge, personal communication, August 12, 2008), although there may be wide variability from one milk bank to another. At the Triangle Lactation Center and Mother's Milk Bank in Raleigh, North Carolina, where 70–80% of mothers of preterm infants express their milk, the donor milk bank is a psychologically reassuring entity. Mothers may be more successful in producing milk if they know that the option of donor milk is available as backup if their own milk supplies falter (M. Tully, personal communication, September 21, 1993).

CLINICAL USES IN PRETERM INFANTS

The clinical uses of banked donor human milk may be arbitrarily divided into nutritional, medicinal, therapeutic, and preventive uses. However, in practice, donor milk may serve several purposes for the same recipient. For example, a preterm infant receives *nourishment* when fed donor human milk. The infant also receives *therapy* in the form of immune substances and growth factors, and disease, e.g., necrotizing enterocolitis (NEC), diabetes, cancers, etc., is potentially *prevented*. The younger the recipient, the more significant the role of nutrition; in an adult recipient, the role of donor milk may be almost exclusively therapeutic or medicinal.

Studies looking at donor milk use in the preterm population have been sporadic. There is still disagreement among neonatologists in the United States about the benefits for the preterm infant, and this controversy was given new energy with the publication of a 2005 study by Schanler, Lau, Hurst, and O'Brian Smith (2005). This study examined short-term outcomes in preterm infants who were randomized to diets of donor milk (DM) or preterm formula (PF) as a supplement to mother's own milk (MM) and found no short-term advantages to donor milk use. However, others have been quick to point out that there were major methodological problems with this study and that no definitive conclusions can be reached on the basis of this study. (Bertino et al., 2006; Lee, 2006; Wight, 2006). First, there were no pure donor milk groups. Each of the groups was fed mother's own milk as approximately 50% of their enteral intake, and 21% of the donor milk-fed infants were switched to preterm formula. There were also significant differences between the groups in terms of maternal demographics and the amount of skin-to-skin contact that the mothers and babies reported in each group. Better statistical methods would have shown different results according to Lee (2006), and there are strong arguments against the research model used, the intent to treat, which the researchers defined in a nonstandard way. However, it is interesting to note that even Schanler's data show a nearly twofold increase in NEC in the preterm formula-supplemented group compared to MM alone and MM + DM even though the sample size of these groups exposed to formula is too small to reach statistical significance.

Compelling support for donor milk use in the NICU comes from two systematic reviews (Boyd, Quigley, & Brocklehurst, 2007; McGuire & Anthony, 2003). In the McGuire and Anthony review, the incidence of NEC was three times less likely in the donor milk-fed groups than in the preterm formula-fed groups, and the incidence of confirmed NEC was four times less. Boyd et al. found a similar reduction in NEC. However, both authors point out that despite the lower risk of NEC, the research studies meeting the inclusion criteria for the review were all done in the 1970s and 1980s, well before changes were made to formulas and well before the advent of fortification and the routine administration of steroids that might have changed the potential impact of donor milk feeding on the risk of NEC (McGuire & Anthony, 2003). In fact, the donor milk in the Schanler et al. (2005) study was all fortified with cow's-milk-based fortifiers. Could this in itself have been a confounding variable? A recent article by Chan, Lee, and Rechtman (2007) comparing the antibacterial activity of human milk fortified with standard bovine-based fortifiers or a human milk-based fortifier showed that the bovine-based fortifier almost totally inhibited the antibacterial activity of the human milk while the human milk-based fortifier had little effect on the antibacterial activity of the milk. Based on this information, it is clear that new studies need to be done where feeding groups are kept uncontaminated with formula or bovine-based fortifiers and where confounding variables such as skin-to-skin holding behaviors are taken into account.

Despite the conflicting evidence for better short-term outcomes in infants fed donor milk, there is some evidence from long-term outcome research studies that donor milk is beneficial. Many of these outcome results have been demonstrated (Lucas, Morley, Cole, & Gore, 1994; Singhal, Cole, & Lucas, 2001; Singhal et al., 2002; Singhal, Cole, Fewtrell, & Lucas, 2004) in Lucas's long-term study described more fully on p. 19. Bishop, Dahlenburg, Fewtrell, Morley, and Lucas (1996) found better bone mineralization at age 5 in those who, as preterm infants, had been fed MM + DM compared to those who were fed MM + PF. Increasing human milk consumption was associated with better bone mineralization in preterm infants, even when compared to children of similar size who were born at term. For other studies that have emerged from the original cohort, see **Table 13-2**.

OTHER NEONATAL AND PEDIATRIC USES

Newborn nurseries may offer banked donor milk to supplement healthy, term infants while still in the hospital. Physicians will choose to supplement rather than risk kernicterus, seizures, or other harmful outcomes. Most often this supplementation is done with formula because it is readily available and the mother may be unable to quickly express the desired volume during the colostral phase of lactation. Banked donor milk is the ideal milk for supplementing when mother's own milk is unavailable since it preserves the human milk-fed environment of the baby's GI tract (ABM, 2002). It is also preferred

Table 13-2 Long-Term Outcomes in Donor Milk-Fed Preterm Infants—Lucas's Cohort

Comparison Groups	*Outcomes*	*Study*
DM* vs. SF** (All babies of mothers who chose not to provide own milk)	At 18 months of age, infants fed sole diet of DM had 9-point advantage on psychodevelopmental tests and 14-point advantage in small-for-gestational age subgroup; trend seen in mental developmental index advantage; no disadvantage when compared to PF-fed infants.	Lucas, Morley, Cole, & Gore, 1994
DM (either alone or as supplement to MM) vs. PF vs. standard formula (SF)	Lower mean arterial blood pressure in 13- to 16-year-olds assigned DM (± MM). Proportion of DM (± MM) inversely related to blood pressure; protection from later cardiovascular disease by early diet.	Singhal et al., 2001
DM (± MM) vs. PF vs. SF	Consumption of DM (± MM) resulted in lower levels of leptin relative to fat mass in 13- to 16-year-olds; demonstrates early influence of diet on obesity (lower leptin levels with less-nutrient-rich diet of HM).	Singhal et al., 2002
DM (± MM) vs. PF vs. SF	DM group of 13- to 16-year-olds had lower C-reactive protein levels (indicative of inflammatory process in athero-sclerosis); DM had lower LDL to HDL ratio; reduction in risk for atherosclerosis by early diet.	Singhal et al., 2004

*Donor milk was drip milk collected in a breast shell from the contralateral breast while the donor was nursing on the other side. This milk is notorious for being low in fat (see Arnold, 1997a; Gibbs, Fisher, Bhattacharya, Goddard, & Baum, 1977; Lucas, Gibbs, & Baum, 1978). In Lucas et al. (1994), the drip milk used was lower in protein and energy content than either formula or MM.

**DM = donor milk; MM = mother's own milk; PF = preterm formula; SF = standard formula

over formulas by the World Health Organization (see **Table 13-3**). It may be that only 1 or 2 ounces is needed, and then the mother takes over. But the baby's gut pH is preserved, establishment of beneficial gut flora is not disrupted, the baby is not exposed to a cow's milk protein antigen, etc.

Other pediatric uses of banked donor human milk include cases of malabsorption and feeding intolerances (Asquith, Pedrotti, Stevenson, & Sunshine, 1987). (See **Box 13-4**.) Malabsorption is also a well-recognized complication

Table 13-3 WHO Hierarchy of Feeding Choices for the Preterm Infant

Best	Mother's own expressed milk	Helps bonding
		Helps establish lactation
		Good balance of nutrients (may need supplemental Ca, P, protein, vitamin D)
		Prevents infection
		Easily digested
		Species specific
	Pasteurized donor milk	Easily digested
		Protective against infection
		Species specific
		Long-term outcomes good
		Less metabolic stress
		May need supplementation with protein, Ca, P, vitamins
	Preterm formula	Correct nutrients? Not necessarily easily digestible
		No anti-infective properties; more severe infections
		Increase in allergies
		Rapid growth—more obesity?
	Standard formula (term)	Wrong balance of nutrients
		No anti-infective properties
Worst		Less optimal growth and development

Source: Arnold, 2002b. Used with permission from Jones and Bartlett Publishers.

of neonatal surgical short gut. Banked milk is beneficial following surgery to repair damage from NEC and to repair congenital anomalies of the gastrointestinal tract, such as gastroschisis, tracheoesophageal fistulas, intestinal atresia, intestinal obstruction, anorectal abnormalities, and diaphragmatic hernias (Brink, 1977; Rangecroft et al., 1978; Riddell, 1989). Historically, donor milk has also been used to control an outbreak of diarrhea in a NICU when antibiotics failed to stem the infection (Svirsky-Gross, 1958).

Infants who fail to thrive on manufactured formulas benefit from the use of donor milk, which helps them heal, gain weight, and gradually wean to foods they can tolerate without adverse effects (Arnold, 1995a). Subtle,

Box 13-4 Lacie's Story

Lacie was born in April 1981. Her mother tried to breastfeed her but was told she should not do so because of her own health problems (degenerative disc disease, kidney problems requiring dialysis, environmental allergies) and the medications she was taking for them. When she discovered that Lacie became violently ill from various formulas, the hunt was on to try to find a food on which Lacie could survive. Over 200 different foods and animal milks were tried in the first few months of life, including goat's milk, "milk" from sugar cane juice, and the milk of an African elephant. But Lacie's body rejected all foods including vitamins, starches, synthetic formulas, and intravenous feedings. The family medical records indicate that there might be a genetic component to this, as several ancestors had died in infancy of similar symptoms 60–70 years earlier when they were weaned from the breast.

Lacie's persistent allergies caused high fevers and bloody diarrhea. Additionally, Lacie suffered from malabsorption problems due to the scarring of her stomach and the lining of her gut from all the allergic reactions. By 3 months of age she had shrunk to 5 pounds! Banked donor human milk was introduced at this point and a steady diet of it begun. Her family and physicians continued to hope she would grow out of it.

At 16 months of age, Lacie weighed 25 pounds and the milk from about 50 donors was required to meet her daily intake needs. Frequently, the family was on the verge of running out of milk, but through heroic efforts of her parents, milk banks and private donations kept the freezers full. Donations came from all 50 states and 18 different countries over the years. By 20 months of age, daily consumption had increased to approximately 150 ounces per day, and by 2 years of age, she was consuming approximately 200 ounces a day, frequently with enzymes added to help improve digestion and absorption.

Food trials were initiated to try to test for foods other than human milk that Lacie could tolerate. During one such trial at age 2, she was given 3 teaspoons of cow's milk over a 24-hour period. This trial generated gastrointestinal bleeding that lasted for 2 weeks and necessitated transfusions of 5 pints of blood.

At 3 months shy of her third birthday, Lacie weighed 35 pounds and was 38 inches tall. On her third birthday, she was requiring 300 ounces of milk a day to survive and weighed 39 pounds and was 39 inches tall. She was in the 95th percentile for growth trajectory and mental development. Growth factors and other components of human milk that promote growth and cellular proliferation were held responsible. One negative physical side effect of this constant diet of human milk was that all her teeth had to be capped as they deteriorated from the continuous bathing in human milk sugars. At age 3, the Worcester (Massachusetts) Regional Milk Bank was providing about 60% of the volume of milk that Lacie needed. The entire cost of the milk shipped by the milk bank was forgiven by the hospital, and the shipper, Federal Express, deemed Lacie a medical emergency and began to ship all milk to her free of charge.

Food trials continued every 6 to 8 weeks, with each one resulting in a weight drop and GI bleeding that took weeks to resolve. Other reactions during food trials included drops in blood pressure, labored breathing, kidney malfunction, and rashes. A diagnosis at the time was disaccharide malfunction, a genetic disorder where carbohydrate-digesting enzymes are lacking. At age 5, a new diagnosis of hypergammaglobulinanemia was determined. This condition is characterized by an immune system that recognizes any food other than human milk as something foreign against which the body must mount an allergic or immune response—a case of an immune system that is too sensitive, perhaps in reaction to all the different foods to which she was exposed at a very young age. Doctors continued to be hopeful that she would one day outgrow the condition, but at age 8, this had not yet happened. Research drugs to suppress her immune system were tried, sometimes in combinations of up to 36 different medications. Food trials were attempted during these medicated periods, but repercussions and side effects were severe, with nausea, vomiting, bloody diarrhea, respiratory distress, and anaphylaxis. Additionally, suppressing her immune system for food trials made her vulnerable to many different infections, and after one such food trial, 27 different infections were diagnosed.

In 1991, as Lacie's 10th birthday approached, she was extremely ill, and the doctors told her she might die—depressing news for all concerned. She continued to have infection after infection. Antibiotic treatment caused ulcers in her stomach. Reflux and asthma created a severe cough that caused her to faint or aspirate. The coughing caused multiple tears in her esophagus and trachea, and even the donated milk burned. Biopsies continued to show either little or no enzymatic activity to all starches, sugars, and some proteins and fats.

Box 13-4 Lacie's Story (continued)

She did survive, however, and with the onset of puberty, some things began to change. At 13 she ate her first school lunch. (Prior to this she had to eat her human milk popsicles in the school nurse's office.) At 5'7" she weighed 130 pounds. At this point she no longer tolerated frozen milk, but could rely on smaller amounts of fresh donor milk daily along with three different research medications and cromolyn. When things were going well, Lacie could eat almost anything in moderation on a rotation diet that did not expose her to any one food too frequently. At age 18 she continued to require about 80 ounces of fresh donated milk on a daily basis and steak was her favorite food. One donor provided milk continuously for over 7 years.

Lacie's development did not suffer from this constant diet of human milk. She is an extremely bright and intelligent young woman who completed her senior year in high school while simultaneously being a freshman at the local community college, choosing to graduate with her friends who had been extremely protective and supportive of her throughout school when she could not eat with other children or participate in birthday parties. She was inducted into Phi Beta Kappa after her first semester of college with a 3.75 grade point average. She was involved with 4-H throughout high school, was a state 4-H officer, and won numerous prizes for projects at state fairs. She was elected as a class officer and to student council, played in a band, volunteered for literacy groups, tutored children, participated in quiz bowls, wrote articles for the local paper, swam, and played soccer. In the summer of 1998 Lacie traveled with her 4-H group as an officer and went to 12 states. Almost everywhere she went there was a local donor who could help with a fresh supply of milk. During the summer of 1999, she traveled to Mexico for a graduation trip and managed to take a milk supply with her and then have more shipped midweek. Her biggest success story was learning to fly. At age 13, the FAA gave her special permission to take flying lessons. She completed ground school at age 13, second in her class. She continues to take lessons.

This young woman would not be alive today were it not for thousands of volunteer donors who supplied their milk. Medical science is learning more about her condition because she is alive. Furthermore, Lacie has not been harmed by the milk, despite the fact that it has all been given either unpasteurized or unfrozen. The opposite is true. She has thrived on it. Some have jokingly suggested that her intelligence comes from the fact that all those donors "pumped their brains out!"

Sources: Arnold, 2005, Used with permission of the author; Campbell, 1996; Ciampa, 1984a, 1984b; M. Erickson, personal communications, 1981–1996; Fink, 1984; Fischer, 1983, Gates & Buckley, 1984; Jacobs, 1989a, 1989b; Kardon, 1982; P. Smith, personal communications, 1994–2004; Supernovich, 1984; Torriero, 1982.

sometimes unrecognized, feeding intolerances may lead to failure to thrive or slow weight gain. Other feeding intolerances and allergies are more obvious, as indicated by gastrointestinal bleeding, projectile vomiting, wheezing, and rashes. Donor milk has been used in a number of cases where gastrointestinal bleeding was severe. In one case, within 24 hours of starting exclusive donor milk feedings, bleeding ceased and the infant began to show improvement (M. Tully, personal communication, April 10, 1996).

Donor milk has also been used in infants with the following conditions: cardiac problems (A. Radcliffe, personal communication, January 23, 1995); chronic renal failure (Anderson & Arnold, 1993); bronchopulmonary dysplasia (Buchter & Wright, 1996); a glycolytic pathway defect (Arnold,

1995b); intractable diarrhea (Asquith, et al., 1987; Rinaldi, Brierley, & Bekker, 2009); gastroenteritis and ulcerative colitis (Asquith et al., 1987); infantile botulism (Asquith et al., 1987); allergies to bovine proteins (Asquith et al., 1987); and IgA deficiency (Asquith et al., 1987; Tully, 1990). It has also been noted by Jeppesen, Hasselbalch, Ersboll, Heilmann, and Valerius (2003) that in infants born to HIV-positive mothers, the thymus, an organ of importance to the development of cell-mediated immunity in the infant, is larger at 4 months of age in infants exclusively fed pasteurized donor human milk when compared to infants who were exclusively formula-fed.

Adult and Innovative Uses

Merhav, Wright, Mieles, and Van Thiel (1995) used donor milk to supply IgA to adult liver transplant patients who were IgA deficient. Donor milk has also been used in patients with immunodepressed states related to bone marrow transplants or leukemia therapy (Asquith et al., 1987). Wiggins and Arnold (1998) describe the use of donor milk in the case of a young adult male with episodes of severe gastroesophageal reflux.

Based on laboratory research conducted by Hakansson, Zhivotovsky, Orrenius, Sabharwal, and Svanborg (1995) and by Svensson, Duringer, Hallgren, Mossberg, Hakansson, and Svanborg (2002), an isolate from human milk, human alpha-lactalbumin made lethal to tumor cells (HAMLET), is now being used in in vivo research on human skin papilloma cells and human glioblastoma cells (Fischer, Gustafsson, Mossberg, Gronli, Mork, Bjerkvig, et al., 2004; Gustafsson, Leijonhufvud, Aronsson, Mossberg, & Svanborg, 2004). Through a process of programmed cell death called apoptosis, the folding molecule kills cancer cells of different types in tissue culture while leaving healthy cells intact. The molecule also survives heat treatment. While lacking definitive proof of efficacy of donor milk from clinical trials, some cancer patients are nevertheless using banked donor milk as complementary and alternative medicine to improve quality of life and to provide hope of a cure or remission (Rough, Sakamoto, Fee, & Hollenbeck, 2009). (See **Box 13-5**.) Banked donor milk has also been used as hospice care in infants, children, and adults who are dying to provide them with amelioration of symptoms and a better quality of life remaining. (See **Box 13-6**.)

Innovative uses have also been explored by some. Donor milk is a metabolically ideal feeding medium for severely burned infants and children. Complications from stress ulcers are fewer when elemental formulas (e.g.,

Box 13-5 Stephanie's Story

Stephanie was diagnosed at 2 months of age with liver cancer. Her mother was also diagnosed with cancer, and the placenta was traced as being the source of the cancerous cells. Both Stephanie and her mother had to undergo chemotherapy, and breastfeeding had to be discontinued. Doctors had virtually no hope for Stephanie's survival. Stephanie did not tolerate the chemotherapy well at all, and all the formulas that were given were also not tolerated. Stephanie lost a lot of weight. Someone finally suggested that banked donor human milk be tried, without real hope that it would help. Much to everyone's surprise, Stephanie began to gain weight on the donor milk, and she had many fewer complications from the chemotherapy while she was being fed donor milk. At the end of the course of chemotherapy, surgery was performed and most of her liver was removed, leaving healthy liver and the hope that it would regenerate into a full-size liver as Stephanie grew. At the age of 6, Stephanie was a healthy little girl developing normally, and neither she nor her mother had had any recurrences of cancer.

Source: Arnold, 2005. Used with permission of the author.

Box 13-6 Edward's Story

While he was in his mid-20s, Edward was stabbed multiple times while walking with his girlfriend, whom he protected from the attacker. He lost a significant amount of blood, and he suffered severe brain damage, lapsing into a permanent, vegetative state. When life support was disconnected at the request of his family, he continued to live for several months. He was fed an adult formula through a tube and suffered severe diarrhea. Despite frequent turning by the nursing home staff, he also developed massive bedsores. His mother, a lactation consultant, requested that banked donor milk be added to his feeding tube as well as applied to his bedsores. The bedsores resolved, and his diarrhea lessened. His mother reported that his last days were more comfortable with donor milk as palliative care.

Source: Arnold, 2005. Used with permission of the author.

formulas that have fats, proteins, and carbohydrates broken down into their simplest elements) are added to the diet of burn victims (Young, Motil, & Burke, 1981). However, elemental formulas are hyperosmolar, formulated for adults, and not meant for long-term pediatric use (Brady, Rickard, Fitzgerald, & Lemons, 1986). Burn victims have an increased metabolism and therefore greater energy requirements, but they do not utilize glucose efficiently. They also have a higher rate of sepsis and would benefit from more immune factors (Young et al., 1981). Human milk provides lactose as a more easily metabolized source of energy, immunoglobulins and other bacteriostatic protection, and growth factors for wound healing. Unpublished research from a milk bank in Mexico demonstrates that using donor milk as a topical agent in burn dressings is advantageous in cutting healing time by about 50% from traditional burn dressings (E. Bustos, personal communication, October 12, 1992).

There are reports of using human milk in eye conditions such as conjunctivitis (CDC, 1982), and as nourishment in AIDS patients who are already suffering from malabsorption syndromes (R. Lawrence, personal communication, March 17, 2000). The uses of donor milk are limited only by the prescriber's imagination and knowledge of physiology.

SUMMARY

Access to banked donor milk *does* make a difference in the health and well-being of individuals, even in situations where the condition is known to be terminal. My journey in donor milk banking over the last 30 years has been an effort to improve and ensure access for patients who need it, and to prevent the sort of occurrences that are given in **Boxes 13-7** and **13-8**. For this to happen, ethical, evidence-based practices are needed from physicians and nurses, donors and milk bank personnel, recipients, and government entities (Arnold, 2006). Parents who desire access to donor milk need to have barriers to access removed, and donor milk banking should be integrated into the healthcare system fully. Milk banking can be a vital contribution to the nation's public health, one individual at a time.

Box 13-7 Katy's Story

Katy was born in 1987 with severe feeding intolerance as well as true allergies to some formulas. After a number of months of trying to find the right formula and failing and not knowing what else to try, her physician admitted her to a large teaching hospital, where she was placed on total parenteral nutrition. This type of nutrition has limited usefulness and is meant to be temporary because long-term use can cause severe liver damage, causing the liver to shut down and cease functioning in some cases. Katy's case was presented at pediatric grand rounds, and a suggestion to try banked donor milk was fielded. The hospital was reluctant to have the donor milk brought into the hospital because of liability issues—in 1987, worries about HIV in human milk were prevalent and research had not yet been done to allay fears about donor milk. It took 3 weeks for the hospital and the milk bank to negotiate through all the red tape. The day the milk finally arrived, Katy died. She was 7 months old.

Source: Arnold, 2005. Used with permission of the author.

Box 13-8 John's Story

John is a gentleman in his 40s with the diagnosis of severe allergies and sinus problems related to a deficiency of immunoglobulin A (IgA), a major protective factor produced by the normal immune system. His wife contacted the International Society for Research on Human Milk and Lactation to see if there were any clinical trials being conducted in the use of human milk to treat his condition, knowing that human milk is an excellent source of IgA. Her inquiry was posted to the e-mail list. I responded to her e-mail by saying that there were no trials going on to my knowledge, but that they could access banked donor milk in the United States. I explained that it would require a physician's prescription, and then continued to describe the processing and screening that occurs prior to dispensing. She and her husband then discussed it with their physician. Following is an excerpt from her e-mail to me of what happened (used with their permission).

> Our physician thought this [using human milk] was a great idea and feels anytime you can help someone using natural products rather than drugs, it is a good thing. He was very supportive. He was however, opposed to using milk bank milk. We know, as does he, that everything is done to prevent any disease transmission, but he still feels that it is taking a risk that is not necessary. I then asked what his opinion was of me inducing lactation to provide breast-milk for my husband. We have been happily married for 22 years and are child-hood [sic] sweethearts. Our physician was very supportive of THIS idea, and asked me to keep him informed of our results.
>
> We are starting to work on this "project" but since our youngest child is 12 years old, our progress to produce any measurable milk will likely be slow. We would love to participate in any research regarding this. Please let me know of anything you hear of. I must admit, this situation is a bit strange and unusual and trying to induce [lactation] in basic secrecy from our family is difficult and frustrating. I wish we were participating in an official research project, then maybe our family could be informed . . .

Source: Arnold, 2005. Used with permission of the author.

REFERENCES

Academy of Breastfeeding Medicine (ABM). (2002). *Protocol No. 3: Hospital guidelines for the use of supplementary feedings in the healthy term breastfed neonate.* Retrieved June 24, 2009, from http://www.bfmed.org/Resources/Protocols.aspx

American Academy of Pediatrics, Committee on Nutrition (AAP). (1980). Human milk banking. *Pediatrics, 65*(4), 854–857.

Anderson, A., & Arnold, L. D. W. (1993). Use of donor breastmilk in the nutrition management of chronic renal failure: Three case histories. *Journal of Human Lactation, 9*(4), 263–264.

Anderson, J., Johnstone, B., & Remley, D. (1999). Breast-feeding and cognitive development: A meta-analysis. *American Journal of Clinical Nutrition, 70*(4), 525–535.

Andersson, Y., Savman, K., Blackberg, L., & Hernell, O. (2007). Pasteurization of mother's own milk reduces fat absorption and growth in preterm infants. *Acta Paediatrica, 96*(10), 1445–1449.

Arnold, L. D. W. (1988). Milk bank survey—Preliminary report of findings and discussion. *HMBANA Newsletter, 3*, 7–9.

Arnold, L. D. W. (1991). The statistical state of human milk banking and what's in the future. *Journal of Human Lactation, 7*(1), 25–27.

Arnold, L. D. W. (1995a). Use of donor human milk in the management of failure to thrive: Case histories. *Journal of Human Lactation, 11*(2), 137–140.

Arnold, L. D. W. (1995b). Use of donor milk in the treatment of metabolic disorders: Glycolytic pathway defects. *Journal of Human Lactation, 11*(1), 51–53.

Arnold, L. D. W. (1997a). A brief look at drip milk and its relation to donor human milk banking. *Journal of Human Lactation, 13*(4), 323–324.

Arnold, L. D. W. (1997b). How North American milk banks operate: Results of a survey. Part 2. *Journal of Human Lactation, 13*(3), 243–246.

Arnold, L. D. W. (1999). Donor milk banking in Scandinavia. *Journal of Human Lactation, 15*(1), 55–59.

Arnold, L. D. W. (2002a). The cost-effectiveness of using banked donor milk in the neonatal intensive care unit: Prevention of necrotizing enterocolitis. *Journal of Human Lactation, 18*(2), 172–177.

Arnold, L. D. W. (2002b). Using banked donor milk in clinical settings. In K. Cadwell (Ed.), *Reclaiming breastfeeding for the United States: Protection, promotion, and support* (pp. 161–178). Sudbury, MA: Jones and Bartlett.

Arnold, L. D. W. (2005). *Donor human milk banking: Creating public health policy in the 21st century*. Doctoral dissertation, Union Institute and University. [UMI Number 3162984]

Arnold, L. D. W. (2006). The ethics of donor human milk banking. *Breastfeeding Medicine, 1*(1), 3–13.

Asquith, M., Pedrotti, P., Stevenson, D., & Sunshine, P. (1987). Clinical uses, collection, and banking of human milk. *Clinics in Perinatology, 14*(1), 173–85.

Azema, E., & Callahan, S. (2003). Breast milk donors in France: A portrait of the typical donor and the utility of milk banking in the French breastfeeding context. *Journal of Human Lactation, 19*(2), 199–202.

Baumslag, N. (1987). Breastfeeding: Cultural practices and variations. In D. B. Jelliffe & E. F. P. Jelliffe (Eds.), *Advances in international maternal and child health: Vol. 7* (pp. 36–50). Oxford: Clarendon Press.

Bertino, E., Giuliani, F., Tonetto, P., Fabris, P., Profeti, C., Magnani, C., et al. (2006). Randomized, controlled trial of breastfeeding versus formula feeding in extremely low birth weight infants [Letter to the editor]. *Pediatrics, 117*(3), 985–986.

Bishop, N., Dahlenburg, S., Fewtrell, M., Morley, R., & Lucas, A. (1996). Early diet of preterm infants and bone mineralization at age five years. *Acta Paediatrica, 85*(2), 230–236.

Bjorksten, B., Burman, L., de Chateau, P., Fredrikzon, B., Gothefors, L., & Hernell, O. (1980). Collecting and banking human milk: To heat or not to heat? *British Medical Journal, 281*(6243), 765–769.

Boyd, C., Quigley, M., & Brocklehurst, P. (2007). Donor breast milk versus infant formula for preterm infants: Systematic review and meta-analysis. *Archives Disease in Childhood, Fetal Neonatal Edition, 92*(3), F169–F175.

Brady, M., Rickard, K., Fitzgerald, J., & Lemons, J. (1986). Specialized formulas and feedings for infants with malabsorption or formula intolerance. *Journal of the American Dietetic Association, 86*(2), 191–200.

Brink, S. (1977). The successful use of human breast milk in a premature infant with the surgical short gut syndrome. *American Journal of Disease in Childhood, 131*(4), 471.

Buchter, S., & Wright, L. (1996, March). *Use of donor milk for the treatment of severe formula intolerance in a preterm infant with chronic lung disease and failure to thrive: A case presen-*

tation. Paper presented at the annual meeting of the Human Milk Banking Association of North America, Raleigh, NC.

Campbell, P. (1996). Milkmen from the sky. *Woman Pilot, 4*, 26–28.

Centers for Disease Control (CDC). (1982). Acute hemorrhagic conjunctivitis—American Samoa. *Morbidity and Mortality Weekly Review, 31*(3), 21–22.

Chan, G., Lee, M., & Rechtman, D. (2007). Effects of a human milk-derived human milk fortifier on the antibacterial actions of human milk. *Breastfeeding Medicine, 2*(4), 205–208.

Ciampa, G. (1984a, January 31). Human milk still Lacie's lifeline: She'll visit city for third birthday. *Worcester Telegram*.

Ciampa, G. (1984b, April 18). Lacie passes milestone in food allergy fight. *Worcester Telegram*, pp. 1A, 19A.

Donnelly-Vanderloo, M., O'Connor, D., & Shoukri, M. (1994). Impact of pasteurization and procedures commonly used to rethermalize stored human milk on folate content. *Nutrition Research, 14*(9), 1305–1316.

Dworsky, M., Stagno, S., Pass, R., Cassady, G., & Alford, C. (1982). Persistence of cytomegalovirus in human milk after storage. *Journal of Pediatrics, 101*(3), 440–443.

Eglin, R., & Wilkinson A. (1987). HIV infection and pasteurisation of breast milk. *The Lancet, 1*(8541), 1093.

Eitenmiller, R. (1990, October). *An overview of human milk pasteurization*. Paper presented at the annual meeting of the Human Milk Banking Association of North America, Lexington, KY.

Evans, T., Ryley, H., Neale, L., Dodge, J., & Lewarne, V. (1978). Effect of storage and heat on antimicrobial proteins in human milk. *Archives of Disease in Childhood, 53*(3), 239–241.

Fidler, N., Sauerwald, T., Demmelmair, H., & Koletzko, B. (2001). Fat content and fatty acid composition of fresh, pasteurized, or sterilized human milk. In D. Newburg (Ed.), *Bioactive components of human milk* (pp. 485–495). New York: Kluwer Academic/Plenum Publishers.

Fink, J. (1984, April 23). Milk run. *US Magazine*, 12–13.

Fischer, K. (1983, May 27). 'Liquid gold': LV women keep Okla. child alive. *The Express*.

Fischer, W., Gustafsson, L., Mossberg, A., Gronli, J., Mork, S., Bjerkvig, R., et al. (2004). Human alpha-lactalbumin made lethal to tumor cells (HAMLET) kills human glioblastoma cells in brain xenografts by an apoptosis-like mechanism and prolongs survival. *Cancer Research, 64*(6), 2105–2112.

Flatau, G., & Brady, S. (2006). *Starting a donor human milk bank: A practical guide*. Raleigh, NC: HMBANA.

Ford, J., Law, B., Marshall, V., & Reiter, B. (1977). Influence of the heat treatment of human milk on some of its protective constituents. *Journal of Pediatrics, 90*(1), 29–35.

Friis, H., & Andersen, H. (1982). Rate of inactivation of cytomegalovirus in raw banked milk during storage at -20°C and pasteurization. *British Medical Journal, 285*(6355), 1604–1605.

Gates, D., & Buckley, J. (1984, May 14). A happy birthday for Lacie Smith. *Newsweek*.

Gibbs, J. H. (1978). Effect of storage and heat on antimicrobial proteins in human milk. *Archives of Disease in Childhood, 53*(10), 827–828.

Gibbs, J. H., Fisher, C., Bhattacharya, S., Goddard, P., & Baum, J. D. (1977). Drip breast milk: Its composition, collection, and pasteurization. *Early Human Development, 1*(3), 227–245.

Goes, H., Torres, A., Donangelo, C., & Trugo, N. (2002). Nutrient composition of banked human milk in Brazil and influence of processing on zinc distribution in milk fractions. *Nutrition, 18*(7–8), 590–594.

Goldblum, R., Dill, C., Albrecht, T., Alford, E., Garza, C., & Goldman, A. (1984). Rapid high-temperature treatment of human milk. *Journal of Pediatrics, 104*(3), 380–385.

Goldsmith, S., Dickson, J., Barnhart, H., Toledo, R., & Eitenmiller, R. (1983). IgA, IgG, IgM and lactoferrin contents of human milk during early lactation and the effect of processing and storage. *Journal of Food Protection, 46*, 4–7.

Goldsmith, S., Eitenmiller, R., Toledo, R., & Barnhart, H. (1983). Effects of processing and storage on the water soluble vitamin content of human milk. *Journal of Food Science, 48*(3), 994–997.

Gustafsson, L., Leijonhufvud, I., Aronsson, A., Mossberg, A., & Svanborg, C. (2004). Treatment of skin papillomas with topical alpha-lactalbumin-oleic acid. *New England Journal of Medicine, 350*(26), 2663–2672.

Hakansson, A., Zhivotovsky, B., Orrenius, S., Sabharwal, H, & Svanborg, C. (1995). Apoptosis induced by a human milk protein. *Proceedings of the National Academy of Sciences of the United States of America, 92*(17), 8064–8068.

Henderson, T., Fay, T., & Hamosh, M. (1998). Effect of pasteurization on long chain polyunsaturated fatty acid levels and enzyme activities of human milk. *Journal of Pediatrics, 132*(5), 876–878.

Human Milk Banking Association of North America (HMBANA). (2007). *Guidelines for the establishment and operation of a donor human milk bank* (11th ed.). Raleigh, NC: Author.

Jacobs, R. (1989a, August 20). Normal eating trends greatly affecting schoolgirl Lacie. *Daily Ardmoreite*, p. 3A.

Jacobs, R. (1989b, August 20). Vital breast milk supply for child is low. *Daily Ardmoreite*, p. 1A.

Jeppesen, D., Hasselbalch, H., Ersboll, A., Heilmann, C., & Valerius, N. (2003) Thymic size in uninfected infants born to HIV-positive mothers and fed with pasteurized human milk. *Acta Paediatrica, 92*(6), 679–683.

Kardon, F. (1982, December 3). Milk bank donors sustain Lacie. *Worcester Evening Gazette.*

Lawrence, R. (2001). Milk banking: The influence of storage procedures and subsequent processing on immunologic components of human milk. In B. Woodward & H. Draper (Eds.), *Immunological properties of milk*. New York: Kluwer Academic/Plenum Publishers.

Lee, M. (2006). The design and analysis of studies in premature infants using human donor milk or preterm formula as primary nutrition: A critique of Schanler et al. *Breastfeeding Medicine, 1*(2), 88–93.

Lepri, L., Del Bubba, M., Maggini, R., Donzelli, G., & Galvan, P. (1997). Effect of pasteurization and storage on some components of pooled human milk. *Journal of Chromatography B, 704*(1–2), 1–10.

Lucas, A., & Cole, T. (1990). Breast milk and neonatal necrotising enterocolitis. *The Lancet, 336*(8730), 1519–1523.

Lucas, A., Gibbs, J. H., & Baum, J. D. (1978). The biology of human drip breast milk. *Early Human Development, 2*(4), 351–361.

Lucas, A., Morley, R., Cole, T., & Gore, S. (1994). A randomized multicentre study of human milk versus formula and later development in preterm infants. *Archives of Disease in Childhood, 70*(2), F141–F146.

Lucas, A., Morley, R., Cole, T., Lister, G., & Leeson-Payne, C. (1992). Breast milk and subsequent intelligence quotient in children born preterm. *The Lancet, 339*(8788), 261–264.

Luukkainen, P., Salo, M., & Nikkari, T. (1995). The fatty acid composition of banked human milk and infant formulas: The choices of milk for feeding preterm infants. *European Journal of Pediatrics, 154*(4), 316–319.

McGuire, W., & Anthony, M. (2003). Donor human milk versus formula for preventing necrotising enterocolitis in preterm infants: Systematic review. *Archives Disease in Childhood, Fetal Neonatal Edition, 88*(1), F11–F14.

McPherson, R., & Wagner, C. (2001). The effect of pasteurization on transforming growth factor alpha and transforming growth factor beta 2 concentrations in human milk. In D. Newburg (Ed.), *Bioactive components of human milk* (pp. 559–566). New York: Kluwer Academic/Plenum Publishers.

Merhav, H., Wright, H., Mieles, L., & Van Thiel, D. (1995). Treatment of IgA deficiency in liver transplant recipients with human breast milk. *Transplant International, 8*(4), 327–329.

Orloff, S., Wallingford, J., & McDougal, J. (1993). Inactivation of human immunodeficiency virus type I in human milk: Effects of intrinsic factors in human milk and of pasteurization. *Journal of Human Lactation, 9*(1), 13–17.

Osbaldiston, R., & Mingle, L. (2007). Characterization of human milk donors. *Journal of Human Lactation, 23*(4), 350–357.

Pimenteira Thomaz, A., Maia Loureiro, L., da Silva Oliveira, T., Furtado Montenegro, N., Dantas Almeida Júnior, E., Fernando Rodrigues Soriano, C., et al. (2008). The human milk donation experience: Motives, influencing factors, and regular donation. *Journal of Human Lactation, 24*(1), 69–76.

Rangecroft, L., de San Lazaro, C., & Scott, J. (1978). A comparison of the feeding of the postoperative newborn with banked breast-milk or cow's-milk feeds. *Journal of Pediatric Surgery, 13*(1), 11–12.

Riddell, D. (1989, October). *Use of banked human milk for feeding infants with abdominal wall defects.* Paper presented at the annual meeting of the Human Milk Banking Association of North America, Vancouver, British Columbia, Canada.

Rinaldi, M., Brierley, E., & Bekker, A. (2009). Donor breastmilk saved infant lives during an outbreak of rotavirus in South Africa. *Breastfeeding Medicine, 4*(2), 133–134.

Rough, S., Sakamoto, P., Fee, C., & Hollenbeck, C. (2009). Qualitative analysis of cancer patients' experiences using donated human milk. *Journal of Human Lactation, 25*(2), 211–219.

Schanler, R., Lau, C., Hurst, N., & O'Brian Smith, E. (2005). Randomized trial of donor human milk versus preterm formula as substitutes for mothers' own milk in the feeding of extremely premature infants. *Pediatrics, 116*(2), 400–406.

Silvestre, D., Ruiz, P., Martinez-Costa, C., Plaza, A., & Lopez, M. (2008). Effect of pasteurization on the bactericidal capacity of human milk. *Journal of Human Lactation, 24*(4), 371–376.

Singhal, A., Cole, T., Fewtrell, M., & Lucas, A. (2004). Breastmilk feeding and lipoprotein profile in adolescents born preterm: Follow-up of a prospective randomized study. *The Lancet, 363*(9421), 1571–1578.

Singhal, A., Cole, T., & Lucas, A. (2001). Early nutrition in preterm infants and later blood pressure: Two cohorts after randomised trials. *The Lancet, 357*(9254), 413–419.

Singhal, A., Farooqi, I., O'Rahilly, S., Cole, T., Fewtrell, M., & Lucas, A. (2002). Early nutrition and leptin concentrations in later life. *American Journal of Clinical Nutrition, 75*(6), 993–999.

Springer, S. (1997). Human milk banking in Germany. *Journal of Human Lactation, 13*(1), 65–68.

Supernovich, G. (1984, April 22). Officials call for national bank for mother's milk. *Middlesex News.*

Svensson, M., Durniger, C., Hallgren, O., Mossberg, A., & Svanborg, C. (2002). HAMLET—A complex from human milk that induces apoptosis in tumor cells but spares healthy cells. *Advances in Experimental Medicine and Biology, 503*, 125–132.

Svirsky-Gross, S. (1958). Pathogenic strains of coli (0,111) among prematures and the use of human milk in controlling the outbreak of diarrhea. *Annals of Pediatrics, 190*(2), 109–115.

Torriero, E. (1982, August 30). Milk banks saving life of little Oklahoma girl. *The Kansas City Times*, pp. A1, A9.

Tully, M. (1990). Banked human milk in the treatment of IgA deficiency and allergy symptoms. *Journal of Human Lactation, 6*(2), 75.

Tully, M. (1997). Donating human milk as part of the grieving process. *Journal of Human Lactation, 15*(2), 149–151.

Van Zoeren-Grobben, D., Schrijver, J., van den Berg, H., & Berger, H. (1987). Human milk vitamin content after pasteurization, storage, or tube feeding. *Archives of Disease in Childhood, 62*(2), 161–165.

Wallingford, J. (1987, October). *Nutritional and anti-infective consequences of pasteurization of breast milk.* Report presented at the annual meeting of the Human Milk Banking Association of North America, Raleigh, NC.

Wardell, J., Wright, A., Bardsley, W., & D'Souza, S. (1984). Bile salt-stimulated lipase and esterase activity in human milk after collection, storage and heating: Nutritional implications. *Pediatric Research, 18*(4), 382–386.

Wiggins, P., & Arnold, L. D. W. (1998). Clinical case history: Donor milk use for severe gastroesophageal reflux in an adult. *Journal of Human Lactation, 14*(2), 157–158.

Wight, N. (2001). Donor human milk for preterm infants. *Journal of Perinatology, 21*(4), 249–254.

Wight, N. (2006). Donor milk: Down but not out [Letter to the editor]. *Pediatrics, 116*(6), 1610.

Xanthou, M. (1987). Immunology of breast milk. In L. Stern (Ed.), *Feeding the Sick Infant* (pp. 101–117). New York: Raven Press.

Young, T., Martens, P., Taback, S., Sellers, E., Dean, H., Cheang, M., et al. (2002). Type 2 diabetes mellitus in children: Prenatal and early infancy risk factors among native Canadians. *Archives of Pediatric and Adolescent Medicine, 156*(7), 651–656.

Young, V., Motil, K., & Burke, J. (1981). Energy and protein metabolism in relation to requirements of the burned pediatric patient. In R. Suskind (Ed.), *Textbook of pediatric nutrition* (pp. 309–340). New York: Raven Press.

chapter fourteen

U.S. Milk Banking: A Century of Safety

Donor milk banking originates in wet nursing. Even in prehistory, it must have become rapidly apparent to families that infants could only survive if they were given the species-specific milk of another human. If the mother died in childbirth, unfortunately a too common outcome, the infant's survival was ensured only if another woman nursed the baby. Extensive and interesting histories of wet nursing have been written by Fildes (1986, 1988), Golden (1996), and Sussman (1982) and cases also show up in the Bible (see **Box 14-1**).

We know from historical accounts that there have been two consistent concerns about wet nursing—prevention of disease transmission from the wet nurse to the recipient and safety and adequacy of the milk. Elaborate tests for the adequacy of the wet nurse's milk existed in ancient Greece and the Roman Empire and strict rules and regulations for conduct of the wet nurse were also codified as early as the 18th century BC by Hammurabi in his Code of Laws (Fildes, 1986; Lawrence & Lawrence, 2005).

Wet nursing was not without its problems, however. When infants were sent out of their homes to be wet nursed, there was little if any supervision of the wet nurse, and many infants died while in the care of a wet nurse. Causes of death and illness that have been attributed to wet nurses include lack of attention and neglect, rickets, and overlaying (suffocating the infant by rolling over on him in bed) (Fildes, 1986).

Syphilis was a risk for the wet nurse herself. Introduced to Europe in the 1490s, syphilis spread rapidly through both sexual intercourse and breastfeeding. A healthy wet nurse could contract the disease from an infected infant or a healthy infant could be infected by a syphilitic wet nurse. Foundling hospitals of the period were partly to blame for the spread of the

Box 14-1 A Famous Case of Wet Nursing

In the Judeo-Christian tradition, probably the most famous story of a baby who was wet nursed is that of Moses. After his abandonment, Moses' survival hinged on his being found and wet nursed by his biological mother, who was hired by Pharaoh's daughter, thinking she was hiring an ordinary, unrelated wet nurse.

1: And there went a man of the house of Levi, and took to wife a daughter of Levi.
2: And the woman conceived, and bare a son: and when she saw him that he was a goodly child, she hid him three months.
3: And when she could not longer hide him, she took for him an ark of bulrushes, and daubed it with slime and with pitch, and put the child therein; and she laid it in the flags by the river's brink.
4: And his sister stood afar off, to wit what would be done to him.
5: And the daughter of Pharaoh came down to wash herself at the river; and her maidens walked along by the river's side; and when she saw the ark among the flags, she sent her maid to fetch it.
6: And when she had opened it, she saw the child: and, behold, the babe wept. And she had compassion on him, and said, This is one of the Hebrews' children.
7: Then said his sister to Pharaoh's daughter, Shall I go and call to thee a nurse of the Hebrew women, that she may nurse the child for thee?
8: And Pharaoh's daughter said to her, Go. And the maid went and called the child's mother.
9: And Pharaoh's daughter said unto her, Take this child away, and nurse it for me, and I will give thee thy wages. And the woman took the child, and nursed it.
10: And the child grew, and she brought him unto Pharaoh's daughter, and he became her son. And she called his name Moses: and she said, Because I drew him out of the water. (Exodus 2:1–10)

Source: *The Bible*. Authorized King James Version. (1997). New York: Oxford University Press.

disease. Many of the newborn abandoned babies were illegitimate, unwanted, and syphilitic, although the newborns were asymptomatic. The wet nurses in the foundling hospital became infected with syphilis by nursing the foundlings. Syphilis became an occupational hazard of wet nursing (Fildes, 1988). Feeding foundlings without wet nurses led to experiments in dry nursing infants (feeding another animal's milk, either by itself or mixed with cereals, by cup, bottle, or spoon). These experiments met with little success. In 18th-century Europe, for example, foundling hospitals with an infant feeding practice of routine dry nursing had much higher rates of infant mortality than did those hospitals that utilized wet nurses (Fildes, 1988).

Across the Atlantic, wet nursing in colonial America took on many aspects of its European counterparts. When women died from childbirth-related conditions, diseases such as malaria, and other infections, demand was created for wet nurses. Wet nursing definitely was a business, with women negotiating for higher wages if they lived in the country or took the risk of taking care of a sick infant who probably was going to die (Golden, 1996). In the South, many slaves were forced to wet nurse their owner's children, sometimes to the detriment of their own infants.

After the Revolutionary War, period medical treatises on infant care and feeding placed greater weight on maternal nursing. These treatises portrayed the wet nurse as a potential threat. Because most wet nurses in America were poor women, class distinctions arose. Suspicion of poor women meant that sending babies out to be nursed away from their homes occurred less and less often because of lack of trust. Direct supervision of wet nurses was urged by physicians and lay advisors. With closer supervision, the perception of wet nursing as a medical threat or risk increased (Golden, 1996).

Health and behavior continued to be an important factor in the selection of a wet nurse. Physicians, according to medical textbooks of the time, were the best ones to hire the wet nurse for a family. They scrutinized the potential wet nurse's health, her milk, and her children to make sure that they were free of disease. Venereal disease was thought to be spread upward from the lower classes, so as the social class of wet nurses fell, the prospect of the infant contracting a venereal disease from a wet nurse was perceived to increase. Since physical inspection of the wet nurse was beyond the bounds of morality of the time, inspection of the wet nurse's baby for health was used as a substitute. Emotions such as grief, envy, hatred, fear, and jealousy in the wet nurse or the mother were believed to have a negative impact on the quality of the milk (Golden, 1996).

THE EMERGENCE OF MODERN MILK BANKING IN THE UNITED STATES

Studies that examined practices of the late 19th and early 20th centuries showed that infants in the United States or Europe who were breastfed by their own mothers or wet nurses had mortality rates lower than those of artificially (dry-) fed infants (Cunningham, 1981). In the early 20th century, a Boston study of infant mortality showed that bottle-fed babies were six times more likely to die of diarrhea and enteritis in the first year of life than were breastfed babies (Davis, 1913). At the turn of the 20th century, many poor women in urban areas went to work to supplement family incomes, which meant that the duration of breastfeeding in urban areas was greatly shortened. Physicians tried to alter cow's milk that was used as a substitute to make it as good for babies as human milk, but there were few regulations and standards for cow's milk and its handling. The urban cow's milk supply was stored in large, open vats, shipped in railroad cars that were not refrigerated, and was delivered to the city heavily contaminated with pathogens as well as other contaminants and in spoiled condition. Furthermore, it was easily adulterated (Wolf, 2001). More often than not, the milk also came from sick animals. Many cities mounted campaigns to try to teach mothers how to store the milk and care for it properly, and legislative agendas were set to regulate cow's milk collection, storage, and handling, with much resistance from the dairy industry.

Wet nurses also became exceedingly difficult to find during this period. In 1910, a Boston physician, Fritz Talbot, established the Boston Wet Nurse Directory, a home for wet nurses waiting placement in the community. While waiting for a referral from a physician, these mothers would wet nurse the babies in the nearby Massachusetts Infant Asylum (also known later as the Massachusetts Babies Hospital). Talbot oversaw the medical aspects of screening wet nurses and did extensive follow-up with the families in which wet nurses were placed. The directory also required that wet nurses keep their own babies with them during service. The rationale for this innovation was twofold: first, maternity homes felt that single women needed to keep and care for their own babies as part of moral redemption; and second, keeping the baby was a means of maintaining a milk supply when wet nurses were sent to feed and care for sick or premature infants who did not have a strong sucking reflex. This type of social welfare program was extremely costly to maintain, however, and Talbot closed the Wet Nurse Directory in 1925 (Golden, 1996; Talbot, 1911, 1927, 1928).

Doctors were again at the forefront of innovation with the separation of the product from the producer, thus purging the milk of any associated history of the person providing it. Golden refers to this as ". . . commodification—the process by which things come to have economic value . . ." (Golden, 1996, p. 179). Human milk became identified as a therapy. In 1910, the first modern milk bank in the United States opened at the Boston Floating Hospital. Francis Parkman Denny, also a physician at the Massachusetts Infant Asylum, developed a method for collecting milk from mothers in the community. This type of collection enabled more efficient use of the milk because more than one baby could be fed the same mother's milk, since many babies were taking only small amounts of milk. Healthy married women living in the neighborhood of the hospital were referred to the Directory for Mothers' Milk by their obstetricians, hospitals, or community health centers. Mothers supplying the milk underwent a physical exam and were screened for tuberculosis, syphilis, and other contagious diseases. They also had to have healthy infants and clean homes. They were paid for their milk.

Two nurses worked for this new directory, and they visited the mothers in their homes, inspected the homes, and taught the mothers how to express their milk. Sterile collecting bottles and caps were left with each mother, and the expressed milk was collected by the nurses on a daily basis. By keeping in such close contact with the mothers, the nurses could identify potential health problems in the homes of the women producing the milk. The milk was ". . . strained, pooled, then boiled for one minute, allowed to cool, then restrained and bottled" (Talbot, 1927, p. 654). This processed milk went directly to hospitalized infants. Hospitals in other cities quickly followed suit and developed their own milk banks (Golden, 1988, 1996).

By 1929, at least 20 of these human milk banks existed around the country. In some cities, such as Chicago, mothers were carefully screened and were paid for their milk. The Chicago Breast Milk Station also required that mothers collect their milk only in the hospital where the collection procedure could be carefully supervised. Milk thus collected was bottled, pasteurized, and dispensed. The Chicago Board of Health required that the Breast Milk Station furnish milk to a hospital "immediately upon request" with no charge for the milk supplied (Wolf, 2001, p. 153).

In Hartford, Connecticut, the Junior League of Hartford established a human milk station in 1924 within the Visiting Nurse Association, which supervised the collection and distribution of the milk. The League employed a matron who collected milk from mothers in their homes. Mothers were paid 10 cents an ounce for their milk. The milk was collected in the morning, pooled, and pasteurized. The Hartford Board of Health Laboratory also frequently tested the milk to make sure that standards remained high and the milk clean and safe. Orders were filled in the early afternoon. A fee of 30 cents an ounce was charged for the milk, but exceptions were made when families were destitute. A fund for covering the milk in these cases was established to help balance the budget, and no baby who needed the milk was turned away. The Hartford Maternal Milk Station also provided milk to the rest of the state of Connecticut, in essence becoming a regional milk bank. Milk was packed in metal boxes and put on trains for babies in other cities and towns (Runkle, 1997, 2001). Talbot and Denny's Milk Bank in Boston also shipped milk to other parts of New England (Talbot, 1928). In 1927, the Directory for Mothers' Milk collected 174,466 ounces, of which 142,680 ounces were sold and 27,486 ounces were given away to needy families (Talbot, 1928). Other milk banks also shipped milk, and in 1934, processed milk was shipped from Chicago to Ontario, Canada, to help feed the Dionne quintuplets (Arnold, 1994).

There were variations in the collection process. Chapin (1923) reported that the New York City Children's Welfare Federation required all mothers to come to the health station to express their milk so that cleanliness could be monitored and adulteration avoided—a collection process similar to that in Chicago. In Detroit, mothers were given carfare in order to come into the hospital and express, but some exceptions were made for mothers for whom it was too difficult to get to the hospital and who had been deemed reliable. Mothers who expressed at home were paid 10 cents an ounce as opposed to 12 cents an ounce for milk from the mothers whose milk was certified by expression in the hospital. Mothers expressing at home were provided with all the necessary supplies and equipment, including boric acid to wash their breasts before expression (Jones, 1928). In Minneapolis, mothers hand expressed their milk for premature infants and it was then fed by tube until the infant was strong enough to suck and swallow (Sedgwick, 1921).

Expressing milk could be extremely lucrative. One mother in Detroit earned approximately $3,500, enabling her to buy her own home (Golden, 1996). In Hartford, a mother wrote to the Junior League to express her appreciation for making it possible for her to provide milk. With the income she earned (almost $260) she purchased an electric refrigerator, a crib, and other items for her baby, purchases she could not have afforded otherwise. But the mother also comments in her note that providing her milk gave her a feeling of service and altruism, a motivation of modern day milk donors as well (Azema & Callahan, 2003; Pimenteira Thomaz, Maia Loureiro, da Silva Oliveira, Furtado Montenegro, Dantas Almeida, Fernando Rodrigues Soriano, et al., 2008). She had been able to help babies survive (Runkle, 2001).

Methods of quality control of the donated milk were instituted. In Boston, a test for the chloride content of the milk was conducted. This test was conducted without the knowledge of the donor and was for the purpose of checking for adulteration with cow's milk, which contains very high levels of chloride, or water, which would mean the milk had very low levels of chloride. If chloride levels did not match the narrow range of chloride in human milk, the milk was discarded. Talbot reported no cases of cow's milk adulteration, but one case of water dilution (Talbot, 1927). New York City's experience was different in that so many women tried to cheat to boost their incomes that New York was forced to require hospital-based expression (Golden, 1996). Frequent bacteriological testing was also done to make sure that the milk would not make a baby sick.

The establishment of human milk banks had the desired effect on the infant mortality rate. In Hartford, for example, the composite infant mortality rate in 1920 was 95.9 per thousand live births. For minority children, it was 168 per thousand live births. In its first year of operation of the Hartford milk station, the Junior League collected and distributed 25,000 ounces, and the infant mortality rate for infants of American-born parents in the Hartford area had dropped to 41 per thousand live births (Runkle, 2001).

Technology also played a role in the way milk was handled. Improving the shelf life of the milk was important so that a more even supply could be maintained for periods when demand was greater. Applications from the dairy industry were employed. Emerson, working with the Borden Company, experimented with evaporating and drying the milk. This process was not efficient, however, as only small amounts could be processed at one time and milk became rancid and musty after a few months (Emerson, 1922; Smith & Emerson, 1924). Again with the help of the Borden Company, Emerson experimented with freezing and refrigeration. He froze milk in thin sheets by placing it in metal molds and placing the molds on dry ice. The thin wafers were then stored in Mason jars in an ice cream company's freezers (Emerson & Platt, 1933). Emerson also reported the results of a clinical feeding trial of milk stored in this manner and noted that all the premature babies fed this milk grew well (Emerson, 1933). The advent of freezing and refrigeration enabled milk to be stored for much longer periods of time and to be shipped over greater distances, especially if packed in dry ice.

In 1939, MacPherson and Talbot published standards for operating a mothers' milk bank based on the Mothers' Milk Directory in Boston. The first official recognition of donor milk banking from the Committee on Mothers' Milk of the American Academy of Pediatrics came in 1943 with its recommendations for mothers' milk bureaus. This is a much more detailed document than the 1939 MacPherson and Talbot standards. In the foreword, the committee acknowledges that MacPherson and Talbot did such a comprehensive job that "considerable sections" of that document were incorporated into the AAP standards (AAP, 1943, p. 112). However, there are some important additions and distinctions in the AAP version, including recommendations for operation, the health of the staff, donor screening, and the physical plant.

Missing from the AAP document is any recommendation about who orders the milk. There is also no requirement for recipient information, although the appendix contains a generic babies' report form that indicates on a monthly basis how many babies were carried by the mothers' milk bureau, whether they were preterm or not, how many expired during the month, and how many were discharged. If a baby died, the hospital, the diagnosis, and the number of days on mothers' milk were to be noted. Records were also to be kept of the names of physicians ordering the service (AAP, 1943, p. 127).

This omission is of interest. It is Golden's premise that as milk became a commodity in the guise of therapeutic merchandise, the interest in the producers of the product shifted to the consumers of the product, those fragile babies who were being saved from certain death. "Once infants became the focus, new questions arose. Should a woman sell or should she donate a commodity that could keep an infant alive?" (Golden, 1996, p. 200). World War II raised further questions about the sale of milk. As donating blood was seen to be a patriotic duty, it was also thought by some to be a patriotic duty to provide one's milk free of charge (Golden, 1996).

Golden notes that the numbers of milk banks increased during the Depression, perhaps because of the need for women to earn extra income. However, as opportunities for employment increased during and after World War II, many milk banks closed. By 1955 only seven remained open. One of the last to close was the Directory for Mothers' Milk in Boston, which finally shut down operations in 1962. By then the demographics of the donors had changed from poor women to middle class women. By the 1970s, however, only one milk bank was still paying donors (Langerak & Arnold, 1991).

The Impact of Milk Banks on the Development of Services

In the early 1970s, rapid advances in neonatal intensive care technology led to the increased survival of smaller and smaller infants who had to be fed. Formulas available at the time were standard formulas meant for term, healthy newborns, and it was understood that these formulas were more difficult for the immature preterm infant to metabolize. Despite the fact that human milk did not contain enough calcium and phosphorus for the premature infants' needs, there was widespread recognition that human milk provided special properties that improved survival and decreased complications in preterm infants. Milk banking became popular once again, and many hospitals established milk banks in house. While the exact number is unknown, Asquith (1982) lists 27 milk banks in her manual of protocols and procedures for donor milk banking, four of which were kitchen milk banks that were started by dedicated women in their homes in response to a community need.

The milk dispensed by kitchen milk banks was collected with only donor screening for clean houses and reports from physicians that the donor was healthy. Sometimes results of blood tests conducted during pregnancy were considered, but usually not. Milk was stored in freezers in the home of the milk bank coordinator, usually in the dining room or kitchen, and dispensed from there when there was a need for it. Bacteria counts were not done. Despite these relaxed standards of milk banking, there are no reports in the literature of any cases of disease transmission from kitchen milk banks, although the lack of reporting does not mean such instances never occurred.

Even in hospital-based milk banks, there were no uniform policies or procedures for milk banking. Different milk banks screened donors for different things. The oldest continuously operating milk bank, founded in 1947 in Wilmington, Delaware, sent a person (the volunteer coordinator) out to the home of the donor to inspect its cleanliness as recently as the early 1990s. The Wilmington Milk Bank donors were paid 20 cents an ounce for their milk. Amish donors were the primary group to accept payment as it contributed to the family's cash income. Other donors considered their milk a charitable donation (Langerak & Arnold, 1991).

Milk that met certain bacterial standards could be dispensed raw (unpasteurized) in some milk banks, while in others all milk was pasteurized. The bacterial standards also varied from milk bank to milk bank. Pasteurizing of milk (when it occurred) also differed, according to the milk bank. The Wilmington Milk Bank autoclaved all of its milk for 5 minutes at 212°F (Langerak & Arnold, 1991). Hawaii Mothers' Milk Bank pasteurized all its milk; the Central Massachusetts Regional Milk Bank (Worcester, Massachusetts) dispensed only raw milk and discarded milk that contained too many colony-forming units of bacteria. Reports of bacterial outbreaks in nurseries where single donors were the cause are few, but they do exist (Donowitz, Marsik, Fisher, & Wenzel, 1981; Ryder, Crosby-Ritchie, McDonough, & Hall, 1977). Usually, the precautions of screening and pasteurization are lacking in these cases.

Noting that donor human milk banking had come back into favor, the American Academy of Pediatrics issued another statement in 1980, this time from the Committee on Nutrition. This statement raised questions about the nutritional adequacy for premature infants of pooled donor milk when the donors are nursing term and older babies. They also raised issues of safety and the theoretical possibility of a graft-versus-host reaction in the baby if live white blood cells from an unrelated donor were passed to the baby. However, they did not go so far as to say that all milk should be pasteurized, and continued to give the option of feeding raw donor milk. The following three methods for supplying a premature infant with human milk are delineated:

(1) collection of a mother's milk for her own infant; (2) collection of milk from a specific donor for a specific baby; and (3) collection of pooled donor milk. The advantages of pooling donor milk were a more uniform nutrient content and dilution of any drugs or toxins which might be present in the milk. ". . . [B]acteriologically safe milk from a donor seems a reasonable alternative . . ." (AAP, 1980, p. 856).

In 1982 the National Institutes of Child Health and Development (NICHD) held a workshop called "Breast Milk Banking: Current Status and Future Needs," at Elkridge, Maryland, August 30–September 2. Asquith (1982) noted in her introduction that the content of her manual had been modified to conform to the recommendations that came from this workshop. However, as with the 1980 AAP statement, collection and storage of a mother's milk for her own infant is discussed in the same document with donor milk, an issue that has created great confusion in the research literature. It is sometimes unclear whether the milk that is banked is maternal milk (MM) or donor milk (DM).

When making recommendations about donor screening, the NICHD draft stated that all donors should be screened for ". . . acute illness and chronic infections, such as tuberculosis, syphilis, hepatitis, recurrent herpes simplex, and cytomegalovirus. . . . The medication history should be reviewed with careful attention given to current and past intakes of prescription and nonprescription drugs, oral contraceptives, large doses of nutrients, illicit drugs, alcohol, caffeine, and nicotine" (NICHD, 1982, p. 6). Diet of the donor should also be considered, with special concern paid to women on weight reduction and vegetarian diets. Because of lack of screening methods for environmental toxins, milk banks were simply supposed to be aware of potential problems and choose donors carefully through geographic and employment histories (NICHD, 1982, p. 8). Payment to donors for their milk was not recommended. Purchase of milk was seen to increase the likelihood of adulteration and perhaps put the donor's infant's health at risk. Confidentiality of donors was stressed.

In discussing heat treatment options for milk, NICHD stated that *if* heat treatment is used, it should be done using what is known as Holder pasteurization (62.5°C for 30 minutes), but also mentions that a ". . . promising alternative to this pasteurization procedure may be a short time/high temperature technique. This approach appears to provide good bacterial reduction and improved retention of key milk components. The dairy industry has had the most experience with these techniques. Milk bank personnel should consult individuals familiar with the operation of this equipment" (p. 13).

New in this NICHD draft is a statement on the indications for use of banked human milk, that only infants and children under 2 years of age should be recipients of donor milk. Use in older children and adults "is not recommended unless the intended use has been reviewed and approved by the local Institutional Review Board" (NICHD, 1982, p. 16). All milk dispensed was to be done so under a physician's supervision and order. Follow-up of recipients as to weight gain, feeding intolerance, morbidity, and mortality were also to be kept.

Establishing relationships with local, state, and national laboratories and public health facilities was also strongly recommended, and local hospitals and medical associations were mentioned as allies in assisting milk banks with third-party billing and payment. NICHD also acknowledged that most milk banks operated in isolation and recommended a national milk banking organization that could serve as a clearinghouse for information, encourage research on processing of milk as well as clinical uses, maintain guidelines for operations of milk banks, and assist in the formation of new milk banks (p. 18).

The formation of a national organization occurred in 1985 when a number of milk bank coordinators met in Washington, DC, and formed the Human Milk Banking Association of North America (HMBANA) (see **Box 14-2**). There was widespread agreement among those attending this organizational meeting that the time had come to standardize operations among milk banks so that a physician who was ordering milk could be guaranteed the same uniform quality and safety no matter which milk bank he/she ordered from. The goals of HMBANA were to:

- Provide a forum for networking among experts in the field on issues relating to human milk banking
- Provide information to the medical community on the benefits and appropriate uses of banked human milk
- Develop guidelines for milk banking practices in North America
- Communicate among member milk banks to assure adequate supplies for all patients
- Encourage research into the unique properties of human milk and its uses
- Act as a liaison between member institutions and government regulatory agencies (HMBANA, 1990)

In the mid- to late 1980s, milk banking once again declined in North America, this time because of the development of special formulas for

Box 14-2 My Association with HMBANA: A Personal Story

In 1985, when the meeting to form HMBANA took place in Washington, DC, I was the Assistant Director of the Hawaii Mothers' Milk Bank and attended this meeting as that milk bank's representative. All through graduate school, as I worked on my master's degree in public health, I worked with others to develop the first set of guidelines for HMBANA based on the recommendations of representatives from the FDA and the CDC. I also wrote a newsletter for HMBANA and worked on various committees. In 1990, after I had completed my master's and was moving from Hawaii to Connecticut, I was asked to become the first executive director of HMBANA. Grant funds were not available at the time, so I operated as a volunteer. Some of the highlights of my 8-1/2-year tenure as the volunteer executive director were incorporation of HMBANA and acquiring nonprofit status for the organization; participation in the 1993 CDC expert panel looking at handling of tissue and organ transplants to prevent HIV transmission (CDC, 1994); publication of three editions of *Recommendations for Collection, Storage and Handling of a Mother's Milk for Her Own Infant in the Hospital Setting* (Arnold 1993a, 1993b, 1999) as a fund-raising mechanism; publication of annual reports; shepherding the publication of a quarterly column in the *Journal of Human Lactation*, either as author or as editor; funding of several small grant proposals; seeking and achieving representation of donor milk banking on the U.S. Breastfeeding Committee (and its first inception as the National Breastfeeding Leadership Round Table); and annual revisions of the guidelines. I left this position in December 1998 and have focused my milk banking interests and energies since then in the public policy arena through the National Commission on Donor Milk Banking and the American Breastfeeding Institute.

preterm infants and also because of concerns about viral transmission, particularly the human immunodeficiency viruses, which were emerging as a threat. Milk banks closed overnight when HIV was first reported in human milk, partly because of fear of transmission and partly because of the added cost of having to serum screen all donors. The development of goals for HMBANA was intended to address some of these concerns. One of the organizational goals of HMBANA was to formulate standards for donor milk banking operations. However, there was little progress made until 1987 when representatives of the Centers for Disease Control (CDC) and the Food and Drug Administration's (FDA's) Food Safety and Applied Nutrition Division and Consumer Safety Office attended the annual meeting of HMBANA. (This division of the FDA is also responsible for all special nutritional products, which means that they monitor all formulas for nutritional quality as well as safety.) The representatives of the FDA were interested in donor milk banking because donor milk was being shipped across state lines from milk banks to recipients. The CDC was interested because of the potential for disease transmission. The two representatives presented papers concerning the importance of viral screening of donors and the effects of pasteurization on milk components. In candid moments, the message from the government officials was that if HMBANA did not develop guidelines, the government would do it, and HMBANA would have no voice in the policy development. Whether this would have actually happened or not is unknown. In any case, HMBANA was urged to develop basic standards that all milk banks would follow, and that these standards would include donor screening by thorough health history as well as serologic testing, bacteriologic quality control of the milk, and pasteurization of all milk to be dispensed. The guidelines were to be broad enough to accommodate the needs and differences of various milk banks, but all should comply. To reinforce their point, the FDA and CDC also conducted research using the current method of pasteurization. They analyzed nutrient and immunoglobulin content using current methodologies in one study (Eitenmiller, 1990) and proved that HIV was destroyed by pasteurization (Orloff, Wallingford, & McDougal, 1993; see also Eglin & Wilkinson, 1987).

The first edition of HMBANA's *Guidelines for the Establishment and Operation of a Donor Human Milk Bank* was finally published in 1990. The expertise of the CDC and the FDA was used, and a member of the Infectious Disease Committee of the American Academy of Pediatrics also contributed to the development of the guidelines. It was understood that the guidelines were voluntary, but that they set a standard for operation below which milk banks should not fall. While some milk banks instituted changes before the guidelines were finalized, others continued to operate as if guidelines had never been discussed, and there was some resistance to instituting the required changes. It was feared that the added cost of having to assume the burden of serological testing might drive some milk banks out of business. That was not the goal of HMBANA. Similar attitudes were encountered by the government in regard to blood testing and excluding high-risk blood donors (Starr, 1998).

The reaction of the kitchen milk banks was mixed. The Eastern Pennsylvania Milk Bank stopped collecting milk and shipped all its milk to other milk banks, and the milk bank in Naperville, Illinois, closed because of liability issues. Milk for Life in the Albany, New York, area stayed open despite strong words of discouragement. The Wilmington Milk Bank continued to pay some of its donors and refused to institute serum screening of donors, stating that they had never had a case of disease transmission and that autoclaving the milk was more than adequate to destroy any pathogens.

Simultaneously with the development of the first edition of the HMBANA guidelines, there was growing resistance to the use of banked donor milk among neonatologists. First, there was the issue of disease transmission by emerging viruses. Second, during the same time period, the formula companies began marketing to neonatologists their new high-calorie formulas specifically designed for the greater protein, energy, calcium, and phosphorus requirements of the premature infant. **Table 14-1** shows the trends in donor milk banking from 1986, the first year any statistics were kept by HMBANA, through 2007 (Arnold, 2004, 2005; M. Tagge, personal communication, August 12, 2008). These figures include the one remaining Canadian milk bank that is a part of HMBANA. The trend in the 1990s became one of fewer milk banks that operated on a more regional basis. Milk banks shipped frozen pasteurized milk routinely to recipients across state lines, and donors from out of state were accepted by some milk banks, especially when there was a need that could not be met by local donors. There was also a shift in the type of usage seen over time, with less volume being dispensed to premature infants and more going to older infants and children as well as a growing number of adults (Arnold, 1997). In the early 21st century the trend has been for more milk banks and for larger volumes of milk dispensed.

HMBANA is a nonprofit (501[c][3]) organization whose voting members are nonprofit milk banks. Since 1999, HMBANA has continued to update the guidelines on an annual or semiannual basis, fine-tuning them to narrow the range of temperatures allowed for pasteurization. Serum screening recommendations have been updated to include hepatitis C and human T-cell leukemia virus (HTLV). The health history was updated to match more of the questions from the American Association of Blood Banks and now includes questions about where people lived and during what years to rule out the possibility of transmission of the heat-resistant prion that is the cause of mad cow disease and Creutzfeldt-Jakob syndrome. The guidelines became mandatory in 2001 for any HMBANA-association milk bank.

Looking Into the Future: The Next Hundred Years

In 2010 the 100th anniversary of donor human milk banking in the United States will be celebrated with an international conference in Boston, the U.S. origin of donor milk banking. It would be fitting to examine not only what the last hundred years has brought but also what needs to be done in the next hundred years to ensure that donor milk banking is fully integrated into the U.S. healthcare system.

In order to ensure that donor human milk banking becomes a fully integrated and essential component in the health care of the preterm and sick

Table 14-1 Annual Statistics: Milk Dispensed by HMBANA Milk Banks (rounded to the nearest 100 ounces or nearest whole liter)

Year	*Ounces (Liters)*	*Milk Banks*
1986	266,000 (7,988)	14
1989	177,000 (5,315)	8
1991–1992	133,700 (4,015)	9
1992–1993	144,200 (4,330)	8
1993–1994	163,000 (4,895)	8
1994–1995	182,400 (5,477)	8
1995–1996*	203,500 (6,111)	8
1996–1997*	180,100 (5,408)	8
1997–1998	280,000 (8,408)	7
1999	322,700 (9,691)	7
2000	410,100 (12,315)	6
2001	511,700 (15,366)	5
2002*	497,380 (14,921)	5
2003	515,660 (15,470)	6
2004	580,800 (17,423)	8
2005	745,300 (22,359)	9
2006	> 875,000 (> 26,250)	10**
2007	1,166,300 (34,990)	11

* Figures incomplete or missing for one milk bank.
** Unclear when one new milk bank began operations and actually distributed milk.

Source: Arnold, 2004, 2005, used with permission of Jones and Bartlett Publishers and the author; M. Tagge, personal communication, August 12, 2008.

infant and child population, the current status of donor milk banking in the United States needs to change. The case study presented in my doctoral dissertation developed a strategic plan for donor milk banking where none has existed before. The policy statement is directed to non-governmental organizations involved in setting breastfeeding and maternal child health policy, governmental agencies involved in nutrition and maternal and child health policy and regulation, health professional organizations that set standards for maternal and childhealthcare providers, and public health organizations involved with education and establishment of health policy for the United

States. The strategic plan is included in **Appendix 14-1**. It is encouraging to note that individual milk banks in the United States have begun to publish more and to employ some of the strategies outlined in the strategic plan, such as social marketing principles (P. Sakamoto, personal communication, January 30, 2009). Only when donor milk banking comes out of the closet and becomes less of a well-kept secret and more mainstream will more preterm and sick infants have access to it.

EMERGENCE OF COMMERCIAL ENTITIES

Researchers over the years have tried to fortify human milk by using components extracted from human milk or by manipulating the milk in some way (Hylmo, Polberger, Axelsson, Jakobsson, & Raiha, 1984; Polberger et al., 1999). These efforts were on a small scale and usually went no further than the study that used the milk thus fortified. Now a for-profit company funded by venture capital investors (Prolacta Biosciences) provides both a fortifier that is made entirely out of human milk components and a higher calorie, ready-to-feed donor milk product. Neo20 and Prolact20 is donor milk that is formulated to provide 20 calories per ounce and 1.2 grams of protein per 100 cc of milk. Minerals essential for bone mineralization have been added to the latter. The fortifiers, ProlactPlus H2MF, come in four different formulations to add varying amounts of protein to 100 cc of human milk, depending on the individual infant's needs.

Donor milk is provided to the company through the not-for-profit National Milk Bank, which provides incentives to hospitals to enroll donors. Prolacta Bioscience is registered with the Food and Drug Administration and the Department of Homeland Security as a food manufacturer. Its products with added mineral content are regulated as infant formulas by the Center for Food Safety and Applied Nutrition. In addition, Prolacta Bioscience complies with regulations for tissue banks in both California and New York. According to its Web site, the FDA and the California Department of Health have conducted multiple site visits and found no violations to cite (Prolacta Biosciences, 2008).

U.S. POLICY SUPPORTING THE USE OF BANKED DONOR MILK

Arnold (2008) has outlined the U.S. health policy statements that would lend themselves to the incorporation of banked donor milk as a source of therapeutic nutrition for infants. There are many documents and policies already in existence where donor milk banking could be incorporated. However, lacking explicit inclusion becomes a barrier for donor milk banking. Many of the policies focus exclusively on breastfeeding to the exclusion of this important donated resource. In other cases, the policies themselves have not been implemented, and lack of implementation becomes a deterrent to improving access to donor milk. Many potential recipients and their families thus find themselves unable to access donor milk, either in the NICU or in an outpatient setting.

Perhaps the most encouraging sign, however, is the increase in mention of donor milk banking specifically in policy statements coming from the American Academy of Pediatrics (AAP) and the Academy of Breastfeeding Medicine (ABM). In the 2005 statement, "Breastfeeding and the Use of Human Milk," the Workgroup on Breastfeeding of the AAP states that:

> Hospitals and physicians should recommend human milk for the premature and other high-risk infants either by direct breastfeeding and/or using the mother's own expressed milk. . . . Banked human milk may be a suitable feeding alternative for infants whose mothers are unable or unwilling to provide their own milk. Human milk banks in North America adhere to national guidelines for quality control of screening and testing of donors and pasteurize all milk before distribution. . . . Fresh human milk from unscreened donors is not recommended because of the risk of transmission of infectious agents (AAP, 2005, p. 500).

In its clinical protocol on supplementation, ABM (2002) states that, "If the volume of mother's own colostrum does not meet her infant's feeding requirements, pasteurized donor human milk is preferable to other supplements" (p. 2).

These statements establish a standard of practice; in the absence of the mother's own milk, banked donor human milk is *the first* acceptable alternative. When donor milk is not used or at least not considered for use, a standard of practice has not been met, and quality of care suffers.

SUMMARY

There have been several overarching themes in this chapter. The primary theme is the need for prevention of disease transmission from the women providing the milk to the infant being fed. Provision of a safe product has been in place since the earliest human history and is no less a concern today when we are faced with disease-causing viruses and prions that have no treatment or cure. Second, progress in this field seems to have been made only when there is interaction of government agencies (and sometimes commercial interests) with the suppliers of human milk. The need for oversight and quality control has existed for a long time and is even more important today with the threat of new emergent diseases. Finally, there is the business nature of supplying human milk. In the United States, it is only in recent history that volunteerism has been relied on so heavily, yet costs are incurred and must be paid by someone.

REFERENCES

Academy of Breastfeeding Medicine (ABM). (2002). *Protocol No. 3: Hospital guidelines for the use of supplementary feedings in the healthy term breastfed neonate.* Retrieved June 24, 2009, from http://www.bfmed.org/Resources/Protocols.aspx

American Academy of Pediatrics, Committee on Mother's Milk (AAP). (1943). Recommended standards for the operation of mothers' milk bureaus. *Journal of Pediatrics, 23*, 112–128.

American Academy of Pediatrics, Committee on Nutrition (AAP). (1980). Human milk banking. *Pediatrics, 65*(4), 854–857.

American Academy of Pediatrics, Section on Breastfeeding (AAP). (2005). Breastfeeding and the use of human milk. *Pediatrics, 115*(2), 496–506.

Arnold, L. D. W. (1993a). *Recommendations for collection, storage and handling of a mother's milk for her own infant in the hospital setting.* West Hartford, CT: HMBANA.

Arnold, L. D. W. (1993b). *Recommendations for collection, storage and handling of a mother's milk for her own infant in the hospital setting* (2nd ed.). West Hartford, CT: HMBANA.

Arnold, L. D. W. (1994). Donor human milk for premature infants: The famous case of the Dionne quintuplets. *Journal of Human Lactation, 10*(4), 271–272.

Arnold, L. D. W. (1997). How North American donor milk banks operate: Results of a survey, Part 2. *Journal of Human Lactation, 13*(3), 243–246.

Arnold, L. D. W. (1999). *Recommendations for collection, storage and handling of a mother's milk for her own infant in the hospital setting* (3rd ed.). East Sandwich, MA: HMBANA.

Arnold, L. D. W. (2004). Donor human milk banking. In J. Riordan (Ed.), *Breastfeeding and human lactation* (3rd ed., pp. 411–436). Sudbury, MA: Jones and Bartlett.

Arnold, L. D. W. (2005). *Donor human milk banking: Creating public health policy in the 21st century.* Doctoral dissertation, Union Institute and University. [UMI Number 3162984]

Arnold, L. D. W. (2008). U.S. health policy and access to banked donor human milk. *Breastfeeding Medicine, 3*(4), 221–229.

Asquith, M. T. (1982). *Organizing a distributing human milk bank: Human milk banking protocols and procedures.* San Jose, CA: The Institute for Medical Research.

Azema, E., & Callahan, S. (2003). Breast milk donors in France: A portrait of the typical donor and the utility of milk banking in the French breastfeeding context. *Journal of Human Lactation, 19*(2), 199–202.

Centers for Disease Control and Prevention (CDC). (1994). Guidelines for preventing transmission of human immunodeficiency virus through transplantation of human tissue and organs. *Morbidity and Mortality Weekly Report, 43*(RR-8), 1–17.

Chapin, H. D. (1923). The operation of a breast milk bank dairy. *Journal of the American Medical Association, 81*(3), 200–202.

Cunningham, A. S. (1981). Breast-feeding and morbidity in industrialized countries: An update. In D. Jelliffe & E. Jelliffe (Eds.), *Advances in International Maternal and Child Health, Vol. 1*. New York: Oxford University Press.

Davis, W. E. (1913). Statistical comparison of the mortality of breast-fed and bottle-fed infants. *American Journal of Diseases in Childhood, 5*(3), 234–247.

Donowitz, L. G., Marsik, F. J., Fisher, K. A., & Wenzel, R. P. (1981). Contaminated breast milk: A source of *Klebsiella* bacteremia in a newborn intensive care unit. *Reviews of Infectious Diseases, 3*(4), 716–720.

Eglin, R. P., & Wilkinson, A. R. (1987). HIV infection and pasteurisation of breast milk. *The Lancet, 1*(8541), 1093.

Eitenmiller, R. (1990, October 15). *An overview of human milk pasteurization*. Presentation at the annual meeting of the Human Milk Banking Association of North America, Lexington, KY.

Emerson, P. W. (1922). The collection and the preservation of human milk: Preliminary report. *Journal of the American Medical Association, 78*(9), 641–642.

Emerson, P. W. (1933). The preservation of human milk. VII. The feeding to premature babies of human milk preserved by freezing. *New England Journal of Medicine, 209*, 893–905.

Emerson, P. W., & Platt, W. (1933). The preservation of human milk. VI. A preliminary note on the freezing process. *Journal of Pediatrics, 2*(1933), 472–477.

Fildes, V. (1986). *Breasts, bottles and babies: A history of infant feeding*. Edinburgh, Scotland: Edinburgh University Press.

Fildes, V. (1988). *Wet nursing: A history from antiquity to the present*. New York: Basil Blackwell, Inc.

Golden, J. (1988). From wet nurse directory to milk bank: The delivery of human milk in Boston, 1909–1927. *Bulletin of the History of Medicine, 62*(4), 589–605.

Golden, J. (1996). *A social history of wet nursing in America: From breast to bottle*. New York: Cambridge University Press.

Human Milk Banking Association of North America (HMBANA). (1990). *Guidelines for the establishment and operation of a human milk bank*. (L. D. W. Arnold & M. Tully, Eds.). West Hartford, CT: Author.

Hylmo, P., Polberger, S., Axelsson, I., Jakobsson, I., & Raiha, N. (1984). Preparation of fat and protein from banked human milk: Its use in feeding very-low-birth-weight infants. In A. Williams & J. Baum (Eds.), *Human milk banking: Vol. 5. Nestle Nutrition Workshop Series* (pp. 55–61). New York: Vevey/Raven Press.

Jones, K. (1928, March). The mothers milk bureau of Detroit. *Public Health Nurse,* 142–143.

Langerak, E. R., & Arnold, L. D. W. (1991). The Mother's Milk Bank of Wilmington, Delaware: History and highlights. *Journal of Human Lactation, 7*(4), 197–198.

Lawrence, R. A., & Lawrence, R. M. (1999). *Breastfeeding: A guide for the medical profession* (5th ed.). St. Louis, MO: Mosby.

MacPherson, C. H., & Talbot, F. B. (1939). Standards for directories for mother's milk. *Journal of Pediatrics, 15*(3), 461–468.

National Institute of Child Health and Development. (1982, August 2–September 30). *Guidelines for banking human milk*. Unpublished draft of workshop presentation, Breast milk banking: Current status and future needs, Elkridge, MD.

Orloff, S. L., Wallingford, J. C., & McDougal, J. S. (1993). Inactivation of human immunodeficiency virus type I in human milk: Effects of intrinsic factors in human milk and of pasteurization. *Journal of Human Lactation, 9*(1), 13–17.

Pimenteira Thomaz, A., Maia Loureiro, L., da Silva Oliveira, T., Furtado Montenegro, N., Dantas Almeida Júnior, E., Fernando Rodrigues Soriano, C., et al. (2008). The human milk donation experience: Motives, influencing factors, and regular donation. *Journal of Human Lactation, 24*(1), 69–76.

Polberger, S., Raiha, N., Juvonen, P., Moro, G., Minoli, I., & Warm, A. (1999). Individualized protein fortification of human milk for preterm infants: Comparison of ultrafiltrated human milk protein and a bovine whey fortifier. *Journal of Pediatric Gastroenterology and Nutrition, 29*(3), 332–338.

Prolacta Biosciences. (2008). *Homepage.* Retrieved June 24, 2009, from http://www.prolacta.com

Runkle, J. (1997). *Hartford's maternal milk station.* Unpublished master's thesis, Trinity College, Hartford, CT.

Runkle, J. (2001, September). Looking back—JLH nourishes infants in 1920's Hartford. *League Lines,* pp. 1, 9–11.

Ryder, R. W., Crosby-Ritchie, A., McDonough, B., & Hall, W. J. (1977). Human milk contaminated with *Salmonella kottbus*: A cause of nosocomial illness in infants. *Journal of the American Medical Association, 238*(14), 1533–1534.

Sedgwick, J. P. (1921). A preliminary report of the study of breastfeeding in Minneapolis. *American Journal of Diseases in Childhood, 21*(5), 455–464.

Smith, L. W., & Emerson, P. W. (1924). Notes on the experimental production of dried breast milk. *Boston Medical and Surgical Journal, 191*, 938–940.

Starr, D. (1998). *Blood: An epic history of medicine and commerce.* New York: Alfred A. Knopf, Inc.

Sussman, G. D. (1982). *Selling mothers' milk: The wet-nursing business in France, 1715–1914.* Chicago: University of Illinois Press.

Talbot, F. B. (1911). A directory for wet nurses: Its experiences for twelve months. *Journal of the American Medical Association, 56*(23), 1715–1717.

Talbot, F. B. (1927). Directory for wet nurses. *Boston Medical and Surgical Journal, 196*(16), 653–654.

Talbot, F. B. (1928). An organization for supplying human milk. *New England Journal of Medicine, 199*(13), 610–611, 640–641.

The Bible. Authorized King James Version. (1997). New York: Oxford University Press.

Wolf, J. H. (2001). *Don't kill your baby: Public health and the decline of breastfeeding in the 19th and 20th centuries.* Columbus, OH: Ohio State University Press.

APPENDIX 14-1

Protecting, Promoting, and Supporting Donor Human Milk Banking in the United States: A Strategic Plan for the 21st Century

Donor milk banking serves a small but medically needy population that has a right to the highest attainable level of health according to the International Covenant on Economic, Social and Cultural Rights (United Nations, 1966). Analysis of the history, ethics, quality control, and policies relating to donor milk banking in the United States, as well as comparisons with international models, reveal that donor milk banking should be an integral part of public health, yet currently it is not. The same analysis lays blame at the feet of everyone who has a role to play in donor milk banking, from government agencies, to the milk banking industry itself, to parents of recipients, to physicians, and to insurers.

In the United States, this important public health service is frequently ignored, misunderstood, and underutilized. In order to bring donor milk banking into the 21st century as an integral part of public health policy, national, state, and local agencies and nongovernmental organizations (including health professional organizations) need to work in a collaborative manner to develop policy and provide education. Both the public (i.e., consumers) as well as the gatekeepers involved in the clinical uses of donor milk need a new awareness of the service. Gatekeepers also need to be involved in conducting research and collecting data. Efforts to resolve and break down barriers to donor milk usage must involve a public/private partnership to succeed. Agencies and organizations need to address these gaps and shortcomings.

To assist in these efforts I have developed this policy paper, a "Strategic Plan," as a road map and plan of action. Issues that routinely arise with regard to donor milk banking are related to issues of quality and access. For this reason the two goals of the Strategic Plan are related to the principles of quality and access, and address issues of policy, education, and research. Goal I relates primarily to access; Goal II relates primarily to quality.

This Strategic Plan is patterned after the United States Breastfeeding Committee (USBC)'s Strategic Plan (2001) for protecting, promoting, and supporting breastfeeding in the United States. After participating in the development of the USBC's strategic plan, I found that the format was easily adapted to issues relating to donor milk banking. Two of the objectives of the USBC's plan are directly applicable to donor milk banking, and I have utilized many of the concepts in them extensively as the backbone of this Strategic Plan. This is the first time such a strategic plan has been developed for donor milk banking.

GOAL I: ASSURE ACCESS TO BANKED DONOR HUMAN MILK FOR ALL APPROPRIATE INFANTS, CHILDREN, AND ADULTS

Goal Statement

Donated human milk has been used in the United States to nourish and treat infants and children with special medical needs since the early 1900s. All infants and children with identified medical needs should be entitled to access to donor milk of the highest quality and safety.

Objective I.A:

Identify and disseminate evidence-based best practices and policies relating to donor human milk banking throughout the healthcare system.

Strategy I.A.1:
Develop a national donor human milk banking policy statement grounded on a foundation of evidence-based practice. This statement will address safety, quality, and access and aim to eliminate disparities in care and include all babies whether full term or preterm.

Activities:

a) Fund and convene a national donor milk banking committee to draft an evidence-based policy statement that will be disseminated to lawmakers, policymakers, governmental agencies and officials, and nongovernmental organizations for universal adoption.
b) Encourage institutions, including third party payers, hospitals, healthcare agencies, health professional organizations, and others to adopt these policies.
c) Encourage health professional associations, institutions, organizations, and agencies to develop and implement practice guidelines congruent with the donor milk banking policy statement.
d) Disseminate the donor milk banking policy statement to the general public and governmental agencies through governmental and nongovernmen-

tal channels using the media, Internet sites, newsletters, bulletins, electronic mailing lists, meetings, and conferences.

Strategy I.A.2:
Ensure that every facility providing maternity and pediatric healthcare services will offer effective evidence-based donor milk banking services.

Activities:

a) Encourage healthcare systems and hospitals with maternity and pediatric healthcare services to promote best practices within their organizations that foster implementation of the Baby-Friendly Hospital Initiative.
b) Encourage the U.S. Department of Health and Human Services to issue a statement urging all maternity care and pediatric healthcare facilities to provide effective, evidence-based donor milk banking information and practices as part of the Baby-Friendly Hospital Initiative.
c) Encourage the utilization of measurable pediatric outcomes for facilities providing donor milk banking services and encourage healthcare accrediting agencies to include these outcomes in their evaluations.
d) Inform hospital administrators, members of Congress, health management companies, and third party payers about best donor milk banking practices and their inclusion in the Baby-Friendly Hospital Initiative.

Objective I.B:

Educate all healthcare providers and payers about the benefits and clinical uses of banked donor human milk.

Strategy I.B.1:
Establish minimum standards of knowledge about the benefits and clinical uses of banked donor human milk in curricula and textbooks.

Activities:

a) Disseminate to organizations responsible for health professional education programs information relating to the risks of informal sharing of human milk as well as the benefits and clinical uses of banked donor human milk.
b) Urge organizations responsible for accreditation of health professional education programs to require the use of relevant evidence-based curricula that include donor human milk banking.
c) Ensure the development and dissemination of evidence-based curricula relating to donor human milk banking for use in the training and education of health professionals.

Strategy I.B.2:
Encourage healthcare plans and other provider organizations to educate their providers, administrators, managers, and consumers about the importance of donor human milk banking as part of nutrition, therapy, and palliative care for infants, children, and adults with demonstrated medical needs.

Activities:

a) Establish continuing education offerings (e.g., CME, CEU, and CERP) and staff development programs relating to donor milk banking.
b) Foster the integration of education about donor milk banking into conferences, meetings, and written literature that are accessed by staff at top levels of management companies and hospital administrators.

Objective I.C:

Ensure that all infants, children, and adults who are identified with a medical need for donor milk have access to adequate supplies of donor milk in the hospital and in the community.

Strategy I.C.1:
Comprehensive and seamless donor milk programs should be encouraged between hospitals and communities.

Activities:

a) Ensure that all women delivering infants have access to information about becoming a human milk donor.
b) Facilitate community development of distributing milk banks and depots to help eliminate disparities in access to banked donor human milk.
c) Ensure that all medically identified infants, children, and adults have access to donor milk as needed.
d) Develop and disseminate a valid and reliable screening tool that identifies potential donor milk recipients.

Strategy I.C.2:
Encourage third party payers to adequately reimburse for donor human milk for medically identified recipients.

Activities:

a) Create a task force to study the cost savings and cost benefits of utilizing donor milk compared to standard care, factoring in costs of all long term sequelae caused by formula usage.
b) Encourage federally funded programs and all other third party payers to pay for the use of banked donor human milk when it is medically required.

Objective I.D:

Ensure routine collection, coordination, and reporting of data relating to donor human milk recipient outcomes by milk banks and healthcare systems.

Strategy I.D.1:
Collect timely data on collection of donor milk, processing of donor milk, distribution of donor milk, and recipient health outcomes with timely publication of such data.

Activities:

a) Encourage milk banks and depots to explore and implement ongoing collection of statistics relating to donor screening, donor demographics, collection of milk, bacterial contamination of milk, environmental contaminants, drug information, and distribution of milk (how much dispensed, how much discarded, etc.).
b) Encourage healthcare systems and milk banks to explore and implement methods for collection of recipient outcomes in an ongoing fashion, including (where applicable) birth weight, diagnosis, blood work and other diagnostic tests results, volume used and how long the recipient was on banked milk, type of donor milk received (e.g., preterm vs. term vs. late lactation), and other foods/medications the recipient received.
c) Encourage distribution of this data to employers and insurers through dissemination to Health Plan Employer Data Information Systems (HEDIS), Consumer Assessment of Health Plans (CAHPS), and appropriate branches of the government, such as FDA, CDC, USDA, and DHHS for potential inclusion in national databases.

Strategy I.D.2:
Encourage funding for clinical, programmatic, epidemiologic, and other types of research on donor milk uses and donor milk banking.

Activities:

a) Contact governmental and private funding agencies and encourage funding of donor milk banking research.
b) Encourage the inclusion of evidence-based donor milk banking practices into databases such as the Cochrane database.
c) Encourage the expansion of donor milk banking research to include issues such as cost-effectiveness, cost/benefit analysis, and emerging medical concerns.
d) Convene a technical meeting comparing the cost/benefit of donor milk banking and the cost of using human milk substitutes.

GOAL II: ENSURE THAT ALL FEDERAL AND STATE LAWS AND POLICIES RELATING TO INFANT FEEDING RECOGNIZE AND SUPPORT THE IMPORTANCE AND USE OF BANKED DONOR HUMAN MILK

Goal Statement:

Lawmakers and policy makers will recognize the vital role and importance of donor human milk banking to the health and well-being of infants and children with special medical and healthcare needs.

Objective II.A:

Ensure that all lawmakers, policy makers, and government officials at federal, state, and local levels are aware of the importance of banked donor human milk to select populations of infants, children, and adults with special medical needs.

Strategy II.A.1:
Inform lawmakers, policy makers, and government officials at all levels of government and related nongovernmental organizations (such as the Academy of Breastfeeding Medicine, the American Academy of Family Physicians, the American Academy of Pediatrics, the American Dietetic Association, the American Nursing Association, and the American Public Health Association, etc.) to consider donor human milk banking when addressing any policy or practice that has an impact on infant and young child nutrition and health.

Activities:

a) Identify donor milk banking issues that require action by lawmakers, policy makers, and governmental agencies and their officials, such as the Centers for Disease Control and Protection, the Food and Drug Administration, the Department of Health and Human Services, and the U.S. Department of Agriculture.
b) Identify and train advocates for donor human milk banking to inform lawmakers, policy makers, and governmental agencies and officials.
c) Develop legislative fact sheets for lawmakers, policy makers, and government and nongovernment agencies, especially those involved with underserved and special populations.
d) Establish a database of legislation, policies, regulations, and legal precedents with implications for donor milk banking.
e) Establish liaisons with the American Bar Association and other legal organizations and law schools to educate and work with attorneys and

judges in supporting donor human milk banking and the mother's right to access a quality product for her infant or child.

f) Establish national quality control standards and regulations for donor human milk banking to ensure that recipients receive a safe product of optimal nutritional and immunological quality.

REFERENCES

United Nations (UN). (1966). *International covenant on economic, social and cultural rights.* Retrieved June 24, 2009, from http://www2.ohchr.org/english/law/cescr.htm

United States Breastfeeding Committee (USBC). (2001). *Breastfeeding in the United States: A national agenda.* Rockville, MD: U.S. Department of Health and Human Services, Health Resources and Services Administration, Maternal and Child Health Bureau.

chapter fifteen

International Practices and Policies in Donor Human Milk Banking

Donor human milk banks exist around the world in different permutations, but all exist for the same purpose—to improve the chances of survival for the smallest babies, those born prematurely, and for those babies born with conditions and anomalies that make survival difficult. The first section of this chapter gives examples of how milk banks have come into being in different parts of the world and how they operate, including the role, if any, that government plays in promotion and protection of donor milk banks. The second section of the chapter deals with international policies related to human rights and health that ground donor milk banking.

INTERNATIONAL MODELS AND PRACTICES

In India, with an increase in urbanization and movement of nuclear families into the cities, there has been a loss of extended family support as well as an increased exposure to formulas, both of which have contributed heavily to the decline in breastfeeding rates, especially in the urban slums. Mothers in these slums also have a higher risk of premature delivery because of poor sanitation and poor nutrition, making their babies even more vulnerable. Survival of these babies depends on a supply of human milk. Specialists believe that milk banking in India would, therefore, serve two purposes. First, it would reduce infection rates in hospitalized premature and sick babies and establish a foundation of better health for preventing future illness, and second, it would have a positive influence on the community as well as medical staff in emphasizing the importance and efficacy of human milk and breastfeeding (Fernandez & Savargaonkar, 1989; Mehta & Subramanian, 1990).

Yet there are questions about the feasibility of establishing milk banks in countries where economic resources for health care are already stretched or lacking. The cost of operating a milk bank requires significant financial resources, especially if milk banking is practiced as it is in the United States or Europe (Mehta & Subramanian, 1990). On the other hand, Fernandez argues that the cost of establishing a sophisticated human milk bank is negligible when compared with the cost of establishing a neonatal intensive care unit. Furthermore, simpler forms of milk banking could meet the needs of a developing country just as well (Fernandez & Savargaonkar, 1989). For example, infrastructure problems, such as lack of a consistent power source or lack of materials for doing accurate and complete donor screening serologies, might mean that milk would have to be collected only in the hospital where adequate supervision of milk expression could occur. The major difficulties cited as barriers for establishing a milk bank patterned after western models include lack of suitable trained staff, difficulties in maintaining milk at a constant cold temperature (due to power outages and voltage fluctuations), low education and socioeconomic status of potential donors, and lack of resources to provide routine bacteriological screening of the milk (Narayanan, Prakash, & Gujral, 1982).

Despite these challenges, milk banks have been established in India. Where they once utilized milk fresh (Narayanan et al., 1982), pasteurization has become routine because of the rising incidence of AIDS in India. Use of constant-temperature water baths similar to those used in the United States have been deemed more economical in India than the large commercial human milk pasteurizers used in places like the United Kingdom (Fernandez, Mondkar, & Nanavati, 1993).

China also has shown interest in the establishment of donor milk banking. During my first visit to China in 1996, with a delegation of breastfeeding management and health policy experts, many hospitals that had achieved Baby-Friendly Hospital status had small in-house milk banks that pasteurized milk collected from the mothers while they were still in the hospital. Use of donor milk was seen as an extension of step 6 of the Ten Steps to Successful Breastfeeding (i.e., to "give newborn infants no food or drink other than breastmilk, unless medically indicated" [UNICEF/WHO, 1989]). This milk was then processed and dispensed to healthy newborns whose mothers were too ill to nurse immediately or who had insufficient milk to meet the infants' needs in the first 5–7 days of life. Yet in pediatric hospitals, donor milk banking was unheard of and formulas were used extensively. In Hangzhou, for instance, the Zhejiang Medical University operated two hospitals across the street from each other. One hospital is a maternity hospital, the other a pediatric hospital. The pediatric hospital was unaware that there was a small milk bank across the street (Arnold, 1996). At that time, babies in intensive care in the Zhejiang Maternity Hospital also did not receive donor milk despite the presence of the nearby milk bank, most likely due to a mistranslation of step 6 that led neonatologists to believe that formula was the *only* medically indicated feeding for all preterm infants. Many of these infants appeared to be fed the so-called follow-on formulas intended for older, healthier babies rather than preterm formulas. By 2001, on a return visit to China, there was an increased demand for information about donor milk banking, its clinical uses, and how to dispense it. The Ministry of Health had also incorporated guidelines for establishment and operation of donor milk banks into its policies based on a copy of the HMBANA guidelines that I had presented to the Ministry of Health in 1996.

Milk banks are also beginning to spring up in the Philippines, where one senator called for milk banks to be established in more hospitals with maternity services through the Expanded Breastfeeding Act of 2007. As of October 2007, there were two donor milk banks in the Philippines, one at the Philippine Children's Medical Center and the other at Philippine General Hospital in Manila (Dumlao, 2007).

Australia has seen milk banks come and go. A number of milk banks were active prior to the publication of a case report from Australia of HIV transmission through breastfeeding in a mother who had become HIV positive from a blood transfusion in the immediate postpartum period (Ziegler, Cooper, Johnson, & Gold, 1985). The Australian government closed all donor milk banks. People were beginning to talk about opening a milk bank again in 1998 when I visited Australia, and the Pediatric Society Nutrition Committee was looking at HMBANA's guidelines to see if they would be appropriate as a model for reopening donor milk banking services. The first contemporary milk bank opened in Western Australia in 2006, 20 years after previous milk banks had been closed.

The Perron Rotary Express Milk Bank utilizes a hazard analysis critical control point methodology for quality control of donor milk banking. This protocol is commonly used in manufacturing of food and medicinal products to ensure the safety of the product and is very applicable to the donor milk banking process (Hartmann, Pang, Keil, Hartmann, & Simmer, 2007). As Hartmann and colleagues state:

> Without internationally or nationally recognized guidelines for the operation of human milk banks, individual banks must develop their own quality standards. Currently the existing legislation in Australia does not specifically recognise human milk as either a food, or to have a therapeutic purpose. Therefore, like many human milk banks, government does not formally regulate Australian human milk banks under specific legislation. Human milk banks operating in Australia must therefore, be committed to the highest standard of self-regulation that is practically and scientifically warranted. (Hartmann et al., 2007, p. 669)

The continent of Africa presents problems for specialists in public health who are working in the area of child survival. HIV and AIDS are epidemic and high mortality rates from AIDS exist in nearly every country on the continent, but especially in the sub-Saharan region. Add to that a lack of economic development and inadequate infrastructure as well as tribalism and all its incendiary politics, and we have a situation that many would deem hopeless for improving child survival. Some statistics for infant mortality in sub-Saharan Africa are given in **Box 15-1** by Dr. Peter McCormick, who has written a first-person account of the milk banks he has established in Cameroon. Despite lack of resources in Cameroon, milk banking has become quite a successful enterprise on a shoestring budget because McCormick has put a great deal of effort into getting buy-in from local healthcare providers and hospital administrators. He has demonstrated that milk banking can be modified and adapted to fit the needs of the African milieu in an economical way.

According to P. Reimers (personal communication, July 12, 2008), milk banks in South Africa were operational until the mid-1980s when they closed because of fears of the risk of transmission of HIV through human milk. Now they are being redeveloped in response to the AIDS crisis and the increasing number of infants who are orphaned or abandoned because of AIDS who would benefit from human milk. In KwaZulu Natal, approximately 40% of pregnant women attending public health clinics are HIV positive. "Many of these women are severely depressed and traumatized and abandon their newborn babies. The estimated number of orphans in the country is said to be around 2.1 million" (P. Reimers, personal communication, July 12, 2008). In 2001, Professor Anna Coutsoudis, with the help of UNICEF, set up the iThemba Lethu Breastmilk Bank in KwaZulu Natal to meet the needs of some of these orphaned and abandoned infants who are

Box 15-1 Breastmilk Banking in Sub-Saharan Africa: The First-Person Experience of Dr. Peter McCormick

The needs of the newborn are the same in Africa as anywhere else. The situation there is, however, very bad. Neonatal mortality in West Africa is the worst in the world. Forty percent of the under-5-year mortality rate is made up of babies under 1 year old (UNICEF, 2005). This situation is not improving (Lawn, Cousens, et al., 2005). Maternal mortality is many times worse than in the developed world (Harrison, 1997). Exclusive breastfeeding is uncommon (Thaper & Sanderson, 2004). Maternity units are often dirty, ill-equipped, and are hotbeds of infection (Zaidi, Huskins, et al., 2005). Maternal malnutrition is common and is the major contributor to intrauterine malnutrition and small-for-dates infants (Black, Allen, Bhutta, et al.). Women in many communities are still treated as second-class citizens with no executive power to make decisions for themselves or their babies (Harrison, 1997). The HIV/AIDS pandemic has compounded the misery and mortality of mothers and babies (Newell, Coovadia, et al., 2004). Ninety-nine percent of neonatal deaths occur in the developing world (Lawn et al., 2005).

It was not difficult to observe the parlous state of antenatal, intrapartum, and perinatal care in the two sub-Saharan countries in which the author has served as a children's physician (the Gambia and Cameroon). Literature searches readily confirm the clinical impressions. It was easy to observe that early and exclusive breastfeeding was not thought important; that the addition of glucose-water, tea, pap, and anything that a traditional healer might advise the mother, was commonplace, and that kangaroo mother care was unheard of.

Mothers are often sick or febrile at the time of parturition. Many do not lactate readily. Maternal anemia is common; antepartum hemorrhage and eclampsia are common. Some mothers abscond, abandoning their infants to hospital care. Some mothers die. There was thus a need to provide breastmilk for babies whose mothers, for whatever reason, were unable to breastfeed their own newborns.

It was our plan to set up a program for the provision of breastmilk for needy, sick, and preterm babies. We would endeavor to do this during the time the mother and baby were still in hospital; during this time it would be the responsible pediatrician's duty to offer the best nutrition possible for the baby. To fail to do this would be to violate the convention on the rights of the child (United Nations, 1989), to predispose the deprived infant to early infection and mortality (Wills, Han, et al., 1982), and to be derelict in our duty. We must find a way to bridge the gap between birth and the successful establishment of breastfeeding. And if the mother absconds or dies, how do we manage the long-term nutrition of her orphan? We look for surrogate mothers, caring aunts, and even grandmothers. We know that a nonlactating breast will start to lactate if the bonding is beautiful. We know that a suckling baby at the breast will stimulate a dormant pituitary to secrete the hormones that cause breastmilk production and letdown. We have witnessed it. Staff are aware of this plan.

There were constraints to the program. Hospital staff and administrators had never heard of breastmilk banks and were largely unaware of the importance of early and exclusive breastfeeding; they needed to be educated. Mothers needed to be educated; fathers needed to understand; donating mothers needed to be convinced of the need to remove some of their milk for babies other than their own. Hospital laboratories were needed to perform simple bacteriological screening of donated milk. A staff member would be required to perform pasteurization of donated milk. A small, dedicated space for the pasteurizing staff member would be needed. Simple apparatus would be needed, and the program would have to be sustainable and self-perpetuating. A breastmilk banking team would need to be agreed upon and put in place.

All these issues were addressed. Maternity and pediatric staff, administrators and laboratory technicians were introduced to the idea, and all were agreeable and indeed enthusiastic. The source of donated milk would come from healthy mothers attending infant welfare clinics (IWCs) at the hospitals. The clinic nurse would address all mothers, many of them breastfeeding whilst listening and awaiting their turn. In general, 50% agree to donate. A gentle inducement in the form of a cup of a soft drink and a cookie helped!

A questionnaire was devised, which sought to identify potential donors whose milk would or would not be acceptable. Samples from each donation were incubated overnight on blood agar (Wright & Feeney, 1998). All donated milk found to be bacteriologically clear was then mixed together. Simple pasteurization

(*continues*)

Box 15-1 Breastmilk Banking in Sub-Saharan Africa: The First-Person Experience of Dr. Peter McCormick (continued)

apparatus designed by the United Kingdom Association of Milk Banks (UKAMB) for the very purpose of establishing small-scale breastmilk banks (Single Bottle Pasteuriser, n.d.) were purchased in the UK at a price readily affordable by the small trust founded by the author. These were shipped to the recipient hospitals, again at low cost. Inexpensive plastic bottles were purchased, along with sterile laboratory sample containers. Glass bottles, which once held breakfast conserves at a local U.K. hotel, were collected, washed, and sterilized. Electric kettles were found to be more convenient than the standard method of heating water over bottled gas stoves. Glass petri dishes were purchased and everything packed into the same small container. Much of this equipment is reusable and sturdy. The total cost of all items, including shipping, is about $1000 U.S. at the time of writing. A precise protocol for the expression of donor milk was drawn up. Hand hygiene of attendant nurse and donating mother was stressed to be of the utmost importance. A precise protocol for the pasteurization process was also prepared and taught.

Everyone involved was assured that the HIV virus is destroyed by the pasteurization process (Eglin & Wilkinson, 1987); this is to say that raising the donated milk to 60° Centigrade and maintaining this for 30 minutes is all that is required. Thermosensitive stickers applied to the bottles of newly pasteurized milk provide proof that the correct temperature has been maintained.

We have now established breastmilk banks in five Cameroonian hospitals. Others are interested. There have been inquiries about our work from other African countries. There have been no religious or cultural objections to the program in Cameroon. Experience in the Gambia was different. There are six tribes there, and no mother would permit her baby to receive milk from a mother of a tribe different to her own.

How much milk do we collect? It is a matter of simple arithmetic: one IWC of 40 mothers and babies; half of them will donate an average of 100 cc; i.e., 2 L per week; 100 L per year. Five IWCs, each with about the same numbers attending, means 500 L per year.

This is a worthwhile, low-cost, low-tech, small-scale, lifesaving project, tailored to the needs of the resource-poor world.

Peter McCormick, MBChB, DCH, DTM & H
Volunteer Children's Physician, Cameroon
Founder, Beryl Thyer Memorial Africa Trust, UK [http://www.berylthyertrust.com]
Address for correspondence: pa_mccormick@yahoo.com

References

Black, R., Allen, L., Bhutta, Z., Caulfield, L. E., de Onis, M., Ezzati, M., et al. (2008). Maternal and child undernutrition: Global and regional exposures and health consequences. *The Lancet*, *371*(9608), 243–260.

Eglin, R., & Wilkinson, A. (1987). HIV infection and pasteurization of breast milk. *The Lancet*, *1*(8541), 1093.

Harrison, K. (1997). The importance of the educated healthy woman in Africa. *The Lancet*, *349*(9052), 644–647.

Lawn, J., Cousens, S., Zupan, J., & Lancet Neonatal Survival Steering Team. (2005). Four million neonatal deaths: When? Where? Why? *The Lancet*, *365*(9462), 891–900.

Newell, M-L., Coovadia, H., Cortina-Borja, M., Rollins, N., Gaillard, P., Dabis, F., et al. (2004). Mortality of infected and uninfected infants born to HIV-infected mothers in Africa: A pooled analysis. *The Lancet*, *364*(9441), 1236–1243.

Single Bottle Pasteuriser. (n.d.). Hampshire, UK: ACE Intermed. Retrieved June 23, 2009, from http://www.ace-intermed.com/sbp.htm

Thaper, N., & Sanderson, I. (2004). Diarrhoea in children: An interface between developing and developed countries. *The Lancet*, *363*(9409), 641–653.

UNICEF. (2005). *The State of the World's Children 2005—Childhood under threat*. Retrieved June 23, 2009, from http://www.unicef.org/publications/files/SOWC_2005_(English).pdf

Box 15-1 Breastmilk Banking in Sub-Saharan Africa: The First-Person Experience of Dr. Peter McCormick (continued)

United Nations (UN). (1989). *Convention on the rights of the child.* Retrieved June 23, 2009, from http://www2.ohchr.org/english/law/crc.htm [especially articles 3 and 24].

Wills, M., Han, V., Harris, D., & Baum, J. (1982). Short-time low-temperature pasteurisation of human milk. *Early Human Development, 7*(1), 71–80.

Wright, K., & Feeney, A. (1998). The bacteriological screening of donated human milk: Laboratory experience of British Paediatric Association's published guidelines. *Journal of Infection, 36*(1), 23–27.

Zaidi, A., Huskins, W., Thaver, D., Bhutta, Z., Abbas, Z., & Goldmann, D. (2005). Hospital acquired neonatal infections in developing countries. *The Lancet, 365*(9465), 1175–1188.

nutritionally vulnerable and have lowered immune function. Reimers reports that within days of beginning donated human milk feedings, HIV-associated dermatitis begins to improve, and diarrhea also improves. While on donor milk, babies have fewer infections and gain weight consistently. If placed back on formula due to a shortage of milk, dermatitis reappears almost immediately, and often diarrhea does, also. A number of infants have come from hospitals where they have been fed formula and show signs of failure to thrive. Once on donor milk, they gain weight and begin to thrive.

Milk banks are now scattered around the country of South Africa, with one example in Johannesburg that pairs a private hospital with a public hospital (see http://www.sabr.org.za for more information about the South African Breastmilk Reserve and its operations and statistics). The private hospital collects and pasteurizes donor milk and then shares the excess with the government hospital. All the provinces have recently received funding from the Fuchs Foundation for Milk Banking, which will allow for expansion of services. In March 2008, the Human Milk Banking Association of South Africa was formed with goals similar to other milk banking associations of education and development and dissemination of best practices (P. Reimers, personal communication, July 12, 2008).

Donor milk banking is a common practice in much of Europe. The first modern human milk bank was founded in Vienna, Austria, in 1909, with the first milk bank in Germany being founded in 1919 (Springer, 1997, 2000). In 1952, the German Democratic Republic (the former East Germany) decreed that every city with a population over 55,000 was required to have its own milk bank. Donors were rewarded with additional food coupons until 1958. Both East and West Germany had a great interest in donor milk banking until the early 1970s, when aggressive marketing of specialty milks in West Germany resulted in closure of all West German milk banks. In East Germany, pediatricians showed support for maintaining milk banks, largely because the economy dictated that specialty milks from the formula companies could not be afforded. Donor milk banks flourished, and by 1989 there were 60 human milk banks in East Germany, which collected and dispensed approximately 200,000 liters of donor milk a year.

With German reunification in 1990, many of these milk banks closed, again for reasons of economy. Springer points out that this attempt to economize may have actually been more costly in the long run, as increases in the costs of treating cases of preventable necrotizing enterocolitis (NEC) most likely exceeded the savings achieved by closing milk banks (Springer, 1997). In 1994, the remaining 18 milk banks dispensed 15,000 liters of milk, and in 1998, the remaining 15 milk banks (9 of them regional) supplied 8000 liters (266,400 ounces) of donor milk (Springer, 1997, 2000; see also Arnold, 2001).

There are no guidelines similar to those of HMBANA in Germany. However, a 1991 statement by the Nutrition Commission of the German Pediatric Society makes reference to regulations relating to human milk banks from as early as 1941 and revised in 1975 (Springer, 1997). This lays the legal foundation for donor milk banking in Germany. Pediatric support comes from the Nutrition Commission, which states:

> From a pediatric point of view these regulations should be maintained for the following reasons:
>
> Donor milk is needed as an important option for the care and treatment of premature and sick newborns and babies. Its use in pediatrics has a primarily preventive and therapeutic character, particularly with immature newborns and in cases of serious intestinal illness in infancy such as NEC, Morbus Hirschsprung, intractable diarrhea and cow's milk protein intolerance. (As translated by Springer, 1997, p. 66)

Even as late as 1997, some milk banks in Germany were still providing fresh donor milk to premature infants, although pasteurized and lyophilized milk could also be supplied. In Leipzig, one of the largest milk banks in the country, a member of the Children's Hospital driving pool picks up milk on a daily basis from donors. Each incoming bottle of milk is tested for bacteria and milk is not pooled. Bottles containing $>10^5$ CFU (colony-forming units)/ml are not used. Milk is used fresh within 72 hours of collection for premature infants and pediatric patients who have undergone gastrointestinal surgery. Neonatal intensive care units that use the fresh milk report an incidence rate for NEC of 0.2%. The Leipzig milk bank repeats blood work on donors every 2 months, including HIV testing. This practice and monthly group meetings of donors to answer questions and provide lactation support means that donors are carefully selected and supervised, allowing physicians to feel comfortable using a fresh product. Community acceptance of donor milk banking in Leipzig is high and has resulted in some families having a third generation of women providing donated milk (Springer, 1997).

Other European countries have also developed standards for milk banking practices. In France, for example, standards for operation are incorporated into public health law (Ministère des Affaires Sociales et de l'Intégration, 1992). These laws and regulations dictate donor-screening procedures, pasteurization methods, and bacteriological standards (Arnold, 1994b; Arnold & Courdent, 1994). The first milk bank opened in Paris in 1947, but these regulations did not come fully into place until it was discovered that the French national blood bank had knowingly released contaminated blood. At that point, the Ministry of Health took over regulation of all tissue banks, including milk banks (Tully, 2001). Donor screening tests are conducted when the donor first enrolls and are repeated every 3 months (Circulaire No. 589, Ministère de la Santé et de l'Action Humanitaire, November 24, 1992, as cited in Arnold & Courdent, 1994). By law, there can be no direct donation of unscreened, unprocessed milk to a recipient (Circulaire DGS/2A/2B No. 233, Ministère des Affaires Sociales et de l'Emploi, 1987, as cited in Arnold & Courdent, 1994). Therefore, all 18 milk banks in France pasteurize the donated milk.

One milk bank in France stands out from the rest. It is the only one that is not housed in a hospital. Instead it is housed in a Red Cross blood bank. The Lactarium Docteur Raymond Fourcade in Marmande in the southwest of France does follow the regulations of the French government, except that it pays donors a subsidy for their milk. In 1994, this amounted to approximately $8.00 (U.S.) per liter. In 1994, this milk bank collected and dispensed approximately 40,000 liters of milk from the 13 provinces surrounding it, a radius of about 220 miles, necessitating a large network of collectors (Arnold, 1994b). As milk comes in to the milk bank, individual donor pools are created and tested for bacteria. Acceptable prepasteurization bacteria counts are $<10^6$ CFU/ml of aerobic bacteria and $<10^4$ CFU/ml of *Staphylococcus aureus*, a normal skin flora. If milk is deemed acceptable and has not been fraudulently diluted, it is pasteurized and then lyophilized, a method of freeze drying under vacuum. The dry extract contains no more than 1% water and allows for extended periods of room temperature storage, up to 18 months. Shipping milk in this form would theoretically reduce shipping costs as well; however, the milk bank also ships the mineral water with which the parents are supposed to reconstitute the lyophilized milk powder (Arnold, 1994b). This is the only milk bank that appears to be lyophilizing milk on a large scale.

The French government has fixed the price of donor milk, with a premium placed on the lyophilized milk. Recipients pay nothing, however, because the milk must be prescribed and is therefore covered under social security and the national healthcare plan.

An Association des Lactariums de France was created in 1981. Its goals are to:

- Promote breastfeeding and the donation of excess milk
- Coordinate research on donor milk, including bacteriology, immunology and biochemistry
- Refine different treatment techniques for donor milk
- Centralize information on milk donations and the needs of different milk banks around the country (Arnold & Courdent, 1994)

Great Britain also has a milk banking association, the United Kingdom Association of Milk Banks (UKAMB) and a long history of milk banking beginning in 1935 with the premature birth of a natural set of quadruplets in Cambridgeshire. The matron of Queen Charlotte's Hospital in London arranged to have sterilized human milk flown to the quads twice a day. Their births followed closely on the heels of the birth of the Dionne quintuplets in Canada, about whom there was much publicity, including the fact that they had been fed milk from a milk bank in the United States (Arnold, 1994a). An eccentric benefactor paid for the matron at Queen Charlotte's to visit the Boston milk bank, where she studied its operations. The benefactor also paid for the processing equipment and donated several thousand pounds towards the operation of the first official milk bank in England in 1939 (Weaver & Williams, 1997).

UKAMB publications about how to establish and operate a milk bank were authored by personnel representing several different milk banks (Balmer & Wharton, 1992; Baum, 1982; Williamson, Hewett, Finucane, & Gamsu, 1978; Williams et al., 1985). In 1981, the Department of Health and

Social Security published the report of a Working Party on Human Milk Banks set up by the Committee on Medical Aspects of Food Policy (DHSS, 1981). By 1993, it was widely recognized that these guidelines and standards for operation needed updating, considering the advent of new viruses such as HIV. At that time, a symposium on milk banking was held in Birmingham and the UKAMB was formed. A working party was formed to create guidelines that would be applicable to Britain, and different models were examined. The working party represented different areas of expertise, including microbiology, pediatrics, midwifery, epidemiology, nutrition, and physiology. When the guidelines were complete, the British Pediatric Association, now called the Royal College of Paediatrics and Child Health, endorsed them and agreed to publish them, indicating the importance that pediatricians place on the use of expressed human milk (Balmer, 1995). This working relationship between milk banking and the Royal College of Paediatrics and Child Health exists to this day, with guidelines now in review for the fourth edition. Similar to guidelines in the United States, although government representatives have participated in the development of these latter guidelines, they are not officially sanctioned by the British health authorities.

Bacteriologic standards for U.K. milk banks currently state (UKAMB, 2003) that prepasteurization bacteria counts must not exceed 10^5 CFU/ml. A minimum (57°C) and maximum (63°C) temperature are given for pasteurization, with milk being held for 30 minutes at either temperature. Milk may be dispensed fresh frozen or pasteurized frozen, but not stored for longer than 3 months.

Donor milk banks have existed for many years in Scandinavian countries. In Finland, a system of collection was established in the 1930s (Siimes & Hallman, 1979). Milk banks in Finland appear to be primarily research oriented (K. Cadwell, personal communication, September 9, 1997). In Sweden and Denmark, milk banks in existence today were established in the 1940s (Arnold, 1999). In Denmark, the Ministry of Health has rules for the four existing milk banks, and hospital infection control departments enforce these rules, but there are no national standards. The largest milk bank in Hvidovre, outside of Copenhagen, takes milk from mothers who are referred to them from the health visitors who visit all new mothers and babies on the Island of Sjaelland. A full-time milk-man is employed to collect the milk on a once-a-week schedule. Mothers are paid by the liter for milk that meets the bacteriological criteria of the milk bank. This income is tax free (about $24.00 [U.S.] per liter in 1999). Milk is pasteurized in a specially designed pasteurizer and then analyzed for protein, fat, carbohydrate, and calorie content. Nutritional labels specifying the amounts of each are attached to every bottle. This enables milk to be fortified individually according to the needs of the recipient infant (Arnold, 1999). Hospitals using the milk from the Hvidovre milk bank are charged a fee for the milk, which amounts to approximately $4.00 (U.S.) per ounce, which has reduced demand somewhat (K. Michaelsen, personal communication, October 14, 2003).

In Sweden, there appear to be no national guidelines. As of 1999, there were three milk banks in Sweden. In Göteborg, the emphasis is on a clean product rather than a sterile one, hence pasteurization is done in an open system rather than in closed bottles. Quality control, such as checking post-pasteurization bacteria counts, is only done several times a year to check methods. This milk bank also uses infrared analysis for nutrient content and labels each bottle accordingly. Donors are paid (about $21.00 [U.S.] per liter in 1999). Outpatient recipients are charged a small fee for the milk (about 90¢ [U.S.] per ounce). If a hospital outside the county orders milk, however, it is charged a considerably higher fee ($18.20 [U.S.] per ounce in 1999 (Arnold, 1999).

Norway currently has 13 milk banks located in and operated by hospitals with level III NICUs (Grovslien & Gronn, 2009). In 2002 the Norwegian National Board of Health published guidelines for donor milk bank operations. Only one milk bank pasteurizes all its milk; the others continue to dispense raw milk to premature infants, a practice that is deemed reasonable by the government in a country that has very low HIV and hepatitis rates and where retesting of donors is frequent. The Rikshospitalet milk bank in Oslo, a regional referral center serving approximately 20% of the preterm infants in the country, dispenses raw milk, testing each 500 ml container for bacteria. The cleanest milk ($<10^4$ CFU/ml) is reserved for the smallest preterm infants. Milk containing pathogens or $>10^5$ CFU/ml is destroyed. Donors are paid 150 NOK per liter (approximately $20 U.S.), but compensation is not uniform across all milk banks in Norway. Guidelines stipulate that payment for the milk cannot be given but that reasonable compensation for expenses incurred (travel, parking fees, etc.) may be given. Minimal enteral feeding is started on the first day of life with either mother's own milk or banked milk (Grovslien & Gronn, 2009).

Other European countries that currently have milk banks include:

- Bulgaria: The Human Milk Bank in Sofia, Bulgaria, was founded in 1989 and is funded and staffed by the Municipality of Sofia (V. Sotirova, personal communication, March 12, 2003).

- The Czech Republic: Thirteen small milk banks are operated under Ministry of Health standards. The first was established in 1958. Donors are paid in tax-free income (Jones, 2003).
- Greece: Donors at this milk bank are primarily mothers in the first week postpartum and still in the hospital. Milk thus collected is primarily colostrum and transitional milk. As reported by Zachou (1996, in Arnold, 2002, p. 170) preterm infants fed this milk grow very well. The establishment of the milk bank is seen as a positive factor in promoting breastfeeding (Jones, 2003).
- Italy: Guidelines were established in 2002. Twenty milks banks existed as of 2003, mostly in the northern part of the country (Jones, 2003).
- Poland: See Penc (1996).
- Spain: The first milk bank was established in 2001 on the island of Majorca (Verd Vallespir, Calvo Benito, Saez Torres, & Gaya Puig, 2003).
- Switzerland: The five Swiss milk banks provide donor milk for any baby less than 2 kg at birth who does not have access to his own mother's milk (Jones, 2003).

The first human milk bank in Brazil was founded in 1943 with the main objective to collect and dispense milk to infants with special medical needs. Human milk was thus considered a premium resource because of its pharmacologic characteristics. It was also seen as a more modern and safer alternative to a wet nurse. "Banked human milk was not seen as a competitor for commercial formulas; [rather] it was a safe alternative for situations in which the commercially induced weaning paradigm failed" (Almeida, 2001, p. 85). Between 1943 and 1985, milk banks operated like large-scale dairies. Donors were paid for their milk, perhaps to the detriment of the donors' babies. Donors were encouraged to donate through promises of benefits such as free health care for themselves and their babies (to which they were already entitled) as well as supplies of infant formula. The formula companies supplied the formula given to the donors via the milk banks at the request of the milk bank staff, making it appear as if the milk banks also endorsed formula as good nutrition, a confusing message. These services were already available to poor women through government entitlement programs, but were reportedly misused by milk banks in order to acquire more milk. Breastmilk donors thus came from the poorest of the population, functionally illiterate or barely literate women from the favelas (slums) around large cities, who subsisted by selling their milk. They were given bonuses for volume in excess of the daily expectation, bonuses if they donated on Sundays, and bonuses if they had regular attendance at expression sessions. This targeting of the poor population, it is believed, further jeopardized the health of poor infants who were already at increased risk of infant mortality and morbidity. Formula feeding by the donor mothers was a dangerous choice in the absence of clean water to dilute it, sterile feeding apparatus, and proper dilution instructions. Milk banks also did nothing to help mothers of the recipient infants reestablish or recover their own milk supplies, becoming simply suppliers of a product.

Beginning in 1981, the Brazilian Ministry of Health developed its comprehensive Program to Promote Breastfeeding (Programa Nacional de Incentivo ao Aleitemento Materno) to reduce infant mortality rates. Milk banks were included in this program, but the resulting newly established milk banks lacked uniform standards. There was found to be a general lack of awareness of milk banks in the medical community (Gutierrez & Almeida, 1998). A preliminary meeting was held in 1984 to discuss milk banking. The following conclusions were reached: ". . . that the operational structure of existing HMBs [human milk banks] posed risks to the health of patients receiving their products; that the vast majority actually served to discourage breastfeeding; that there was no legislation to standardize relevant procedures; and that a pilot project was needed to identify alternatives" (Almeida, 2001, p. 92). The largest milk bank, at the Fernandes Figueira Institute, was the first to attempt this program. The result was a public health law that outlined all the necessary steps for establishing and operating a donor milk bank (Gutierrez & Almeida, 1998). The first stage was to improve quality control of the milk, including pasteurization of all milk. The next stage was to begin the process of promoting, protecting, and supporting breastfeeding, with the collection, processing, and distributing of banked milk a secondary priority. One of the ways in which this was achieved was to accept only volunteer nursing mothers as donors. Mothers were urged to continue breastfeeding and were given assistance with counseling and support. The profile of the donors thus changed to more affluent mothers. Contrary to popular belief, this change in donor profile did not reduce the donor milk supply; it actually increased it.

In 1986, The Instituto Fernandes Figueira/Fundaçao Oswaldo Cruz (FIOCRUZ) became the National Reference Center for Human Milk Banks. This reference milk bank does the following:

> (1) Oversees national networking among HMBs, communicating information in the field of milk banking, monitoring the compliance of donor milk banks with the national milk banking guidelines

> regarding quality control of donor milk supplies, organizing periodic conferences to improve milk banking services, and training professionals to work in HMBs; (2) acts as the liaison with the government to comply with the policies of the Ministry of Health; (3) conducts research in the areas of the basic and social sciences as well as the development of quality control methodology to lower processing costs and still maintain a quality product to meet national needs; (4) disseminates information among HMBs; and (5) publishes a biannual bulletin (Gota de Leite) which is distributed to all HMBs. (Gutierrez & Almeida, 1998, p. 333)

Because FIOCRUZ is also an academic center, training is an integral part of the National Reference Center's mission. Continuing education of health professionals in breastfeeding promotion, regional training programs on the legal aspects of marketing of formula, graduate and specialty courses on organizing and operating a milk bank, master's and PhD programs with research opportunities in maternal and child health, provision of technical support to regional departments of health, and training milk bank personnel from other countries have all been part of the comprehensive program operated by FIOCRUZ. The milk banks in Brazil have also served as the foundation for implementing the Baby-Friendly Hospital Initiative in Brazil, acting as training centers for hospital staff (step 2), helping hospitals to create evidence-based breastfeeding policies and practice (step 1), and acting as referral centers for lactation support for individual mothers (step 10) (Almeida, 2001; Gutierrez & Almeida, 1998).

Additionally, FIOCRUZ has become the training center for teams of health professionals from other South American and Caribbean countries. Venezuela has two milk banks fashioned on the Brazilian model, and Brazilian model milk banks also exist in Argentina, Chile, Costa Rica, the Dominican Republic, Mexico, Nicaragua, and Panama (Jones, 2003; Tully, 2001). Support for equipment as well as training has come from UNICEF in many cases.

In 2001, Dr. Almeida's enormous accomplishments in the field of milk banking and breastfeeding promotion and policy were acknowledged internationally with the awarding of the prestigious Sasakawa prize. The statistics to demonstrate the effectiveness of this new paradigm for milk banking are as follows:

- The average duration of breastfeeding increased from 5.5 months in 1989 to 10 months in 1999.
- As of April 2001, Brazil had 182 hospitals with Baby-Friendly designation.

- A network of more than 150 milk banks collects donated milk, gathering more than 218,000 liters of milk during 1999–2000 and providing milk for nearly 300,000 preterm and low-birth-weight babies.
- The provision of banked human milk saved Brazil's Ministry of Health about $540 million per year.
- Trained firefighters or employees of the Human Milk Bank go to the mother's home to pick up milk.
- More than 6000 letter carriers have been trained in the Breastfeeding Friendly Postman Program to share information on breastfeeding with pregnant women and mothers as they go door-to-door delivering mail.
- Legislation regulates the promotion and use of human milk substitutes and complementary foods as well as the use of feeding implements such as nipples, bottles, and pacifiers.

By involving groups such as firefighters and mail carriers in breastfeeding support roles, the government of Brazil underlines the importance of breastfeeding to the entire country (IBFAN, 2001; INFACT Canada, 2001, p. 10).

The experience of a milk bank in a working class low-income area near Brasilia is reported in Almeida and Dorea (2006). The authors analyzed 909 samples of milk from 195 women (ages 15–45 years) who donated 792 liters of milk during the first 11 months of 2002. The primary recipients were infants in the hospital (66.4% were between 1 and 7 days of age) with diagnoses of respiratory distress, prematurity, metabolic distress, and jaundice. Full-term infants also benefited from donor milk in the hospital when their mother's own milk was unavailable. All donors hand expressed their milk, which resulted in slightly lower energy content of their milk when compared with other forms of expression (529 ± 85 kcal/L compared with European donors who pumped with an average of 730 kcal/L; mean total lipids 22.7 g/L compared with European donors with 30 g/L). Almost all the milk samples (99.2%) met hygienic standards for clinical use.

Cultural issues also impact the way donor milk banking is practiced. Even when healthcare providers accept the use of donor milk, opposition may exist from both donors and parents of recipients. Among Africans, it is widely believed that diseases and personality traits can be transferred through human milk. I encountered similar beliefs in a nursing school in Moscow in 1997 when I was told that it would be impossible to have donor milk banks because the personalities and genes of the donors would get transmitted to the recipients. In a survey conducted in Nigeria, 70% of mothers were unwilling to accept donated human milk for their infants because of these fears and because of sociocultural and religious beliefs (Ighogboja, Olarewaju, Odumodu, & Okuonghae,1995). The other 30% of mothers surveyed would accept donor milk only if it came from a close relative. Similar reasons would prevent 40% of women from donating milk. In Zimbabwe, the idea of expressing milk and heating it for mothers who were HIV positive met with resistance due to cultural beliefs that expression was a confession of adultery or perhaps could lead to accusations of witchcraft. Beliefs also existed that one could be contaminated by touching milk or even entering a home where milk had been placed in a container (Israel-Ballard et al., 2006). Once focus group participants were educated, however, these beliefs were seen as minor obstacles that could be overcome in a population by appropriate education. Survival of the babies was a much more important issue.

Narayanan, Prakash, Bala, Verma, and Gujral (1980) noted that some Muslim women objected to their babies receiving milk from Hindu women, although the converse was not true. The Koran treats human milk as altered blood; children suckled by the same woman become blood relations or milk siblings, and they are forbidden to marry each other to avoid the possibility of incest from a consanguineous marriage (Ighogboja et al., 1995; Koçturk, 2003). There are ways of dealing with this issue, and Al-Naqeeb, Azab, Eliwa, and Mohammed (2000) describe a donor milk bank in Kuwait. Wet nursing of full-term babies is an acceptable practice in Kuwait, if or when the wet nurse is well known to the parents of the baby being fed. The solution to establishing a milk bank in a Kuwait neonatal intensive care unit (NICU) was to introduce the mother of the recipient to the donor mother so that their offspring could avoid the potential of a consanguineous marriage. In most cases elsewhere, milk bank donors remain anonymous and donor information is confidential.

INTERNATIONAL HEALTH POLICIES

Policy and practice go hand in hand. When practice reflects sound policy that is evidence-based, great outcomes can be achieved, such as in the case of Brazil, where infant mortality rates were successfully lowered by their breastfeeding promotion, protection, and support campaign (Almeida, 2001). Policy was enacted and enforced in various ways and practices and protocols developed to support the policies. Without sound policies, practice is left to its own devices and a hodgepodge of people doing very different things and giving conflicting information develops. As an example of this, Winikoff and Baer (1980) conducted a study in a New York City hospital looking at practices that supported the establishment of successful breastfeeding. Among the practices they examined were the effects of staff training, and whether educating the midwives and educating the nurses about breastfeeding actually helped mothers to breastfeed and get off to a good start. Surprisingly, training for these two crucial elements of the staff had very little positive impact on breastfeeding. The authors reason that this was because the policies never changed to reflect the staff's training. The new knowledge never got put into practice because everyone had to follow the old, outdated policies.

This can be thought of in a broader sense as well. There are numerous international policy statements on human rights, for example, yet many countries consistently violate these policies. The achievement of optimal health for every individual is a goal of many of these human rights statements, yet a number of countries have extremely high infant mortality rates, children under 5 mortality rates, and maternal mortality rates, all indicators of national health status. The goal is to try to develop practices that will help achieve the goals of optimal health.

Many of the international policies whose goals are the achievement of optimal health for every individual are human rights statements from the United Nations (UN), the World Health Organization (WHO), and the United Nations International Children's Emergency Fund (UNICEF). Arnold (2006) has reviewed these statements for applicability to donor milk banking. Breastfeeding is the foundation for achieving individual as well as population health. These policies can be applied to breastfeeding promotion, protection, and support, and by extension to donor human milk banking.

Human Rights Conventions from the United Nations

Individual national governments have a responsibility to their citizens to take an active role in areas that provide for basic human needs. Individual countries first adopt the UN conventions, then enact them, and then make sure that they are integrated into the behavior of their citizens. When a nation adopts human rights conventions, there is then pressure on its government to be responsible for protecting the rights that have just been adopted. Many countries use these conventions as a basis for legislation and regulation. However, UN conventions do not have the force of law in any country unless that country's legislature specifically enacts them (Bar-Yam, 2003). Bar-Yam (2000, 2003) has synthesized the material and placed breastfeeding and human milk in the UN conventions that address three categories of human rights—women's rights, children's rights, and the right to health and health care (see also Kent, 2006).

In terms of children's rights, UN conventions clearly refer to *all* children and do not distinguish between sick and well children. What may be inferred is that if a child is sick, then there is a responsibility on the part of both the family and government to remedy the situation as much as possible so that the infant/child can attain the highest standard of both physical and mental health. Breastfeeding and the use of human milk, including banked donor milk, thus become a right that preterm and sick infants and children should expect.

In order for this right to be attained by the infant, the mother needs to exercise her right to breastfeed or provide her expressed milk, and she is obligated to do so. But government also has an obligation to both the mother and the baby to protect (e.g., create national legislation to protect families from formula company marketing tactics), promote (e.g., develop and implement national campaigns to inform the public of the benefits of breastfeeding/hazards of formula), and support breastfeeding (e.g., find funding for peer counselor programs that instill self-confidence in breastfeeding mothers and provide assistance when problems arise). In the absence of the mother's expressed milk, governments become obligated to provide human milk in some other way, such as through a milk bank (Bar-Yam, 2003). They do not have to operate the milk bank, but they need to facilitate the development of these services and provide oversight to ensure the safety of the process.

Table 15-1 outlines the basic premises of the human rights conventions that encourage the use of human milk for fragile infants.

UNICEF Policy Statements Encouraging the Use of Human Milk for Fragile Infants

The WHO and UNICEF policy statements regarding the use of human milk for fragile infants are outlined in **Table 15-2**. Beginning with the GOBI[1] Initiative in 1982 (UNICEF, 1982), the policies mentioned have been consistent in their support of human milk, including, in some instances, explicit support for donor milk banks and the use of banked donor milk.

Over the years, WHO has had a remarkably consistent policy with regard to human milk banking. In 1979, WHO and UNICEF issued a joint resolution on infant and young child feeding that was fully endorsed by the World Health Assembly in 1980. The first alternative when a mother is unable to breastfeed should be human breastmilk, using banked donor milk where appropriate and available (WHO/UNICEF, 1980). In 1992, banked donor milk was included as an acceptable feeding alternative when the biological

[1] GOBI is an acronym standing for Growth, Oral rehydration, Breastfeeding, and Immunization.

Table 15-1 Human Rights Declarations and Conventions from the United Nations

Convention/Declaration (Date)	*Pertinent Article and Content*	*What It Means for Donor Milk Banking*
Universal Declaration of Human Rights (1948)	*Article 25:* Establishes a right to a standard of living (including adequate food) that supports health and well-being of both the family and the individual. Mothers and children are identified as being entitled to special care and assistance.	Individual infants are identified. This means all infants, including preterm, where donor milk has a definite role to play in long-term health.
International Covenant on Economic, Social and Cultural Rights (1967)	*Article 12:* States that all individuals have the right to the "highest attainable standard of physical and mental health."	Countries need to lower infant mortality and ensure the healthy development of the child. Donor milk can do this for specific populations of infants.
Convention on the Elimination of All Forms of Discrimination Against Women (1981)	*Article 5:* Certain groups deserve special protection, including women and children. Maternity is described as a social function that protects society. Pregnant women and mothers should, therefore, be afforded special protection so that they might care for their children in an optimal way. If the interests of the child have top priority, providing them optimal nutrition when they most need it should also be a priority.	Breastfeeding and banked donor milk fit here as needing special protection.
Convention on the Rights of the Child (1989)	*Article 3:* The best interests of the child should always be primary. *Article 18:* Governments should provide assistance to families through institutional and legislative support. *Article 24:* Breastfeeding is addressed directly (section 2e), and is an activity for the whole society. Mothers are not mandated to breastfeed, but governments are mandated to educate all mothers and parents so that they can make informed choices.	*Article 18:* A country has a responsibility for protecting breastfeeding through legislation, including legislation to restrict marketing practices of formula companies. If other forms of infant nutrition are needed, the manufacture of these foods should be regulated for safety and adequacy, e.g., donor milk banking. *Article 24:* Parents also should be educated about the uses of banked donor milk and its benefits, so that they know about this option and can request it if necessary.

See also Arnold, 2006; Bar-Yam, 2000.

Table 15-2 WHO and UNICEF Policy Statements Regarding the Use of Human Milk for Fragile Infants

Policy Statement (Date)	*Major Principles*	*Application to Donor Milk Banking*
UNICEF's GOBI Initiative (1982)	Sets forth the following four principles for child survival: growth, oral rehydration, breast-feeding, and immunization. The act of breastfeeding provides the other three principles.	Banked donor milk provides similar immune protection to preterm or ill infants, species-specific nutrition to foster adequate growth, and has been used medicinally to treat cases of diarrhea and keep babies hydrated.
WHO/UNICEF Baby-Friendly Hospital Initiative and the Fragile Infant (1989)	Based on the Ten Steps to Successful Breastfeeding.	
	Step 1: Have a written breastfeeding policy that is routinely communicated to all healthcare staff.	Develop policies and procedures relating to the use of donor milk when mother's own milk is unavailable.
	Step 2: Train all healthcare staff in skills necessary to implement the policy.	All staff in contact with mothers and sick babies need to be trained in the policies and practices that are developed.
	Step 3: Inform all pregnant women about the benefits and management of breastfeeding.	Parents need to be educated on the benefits and availability of donor milk and how to be a donor if applicable.
	Step 4: Help all mothers initiate breastfeeding within the first hour of birth.	Should include early initiation of banked donor milk feeds if a mother and/or her milk are not available.
	Step 5: Show mothers how to breastfeed and maintain lactation *even if separated from their infants* [italics added].	Educate mothers on how to establish and maintain a milk supply if separated (includes mothers of older nursing babies) and use of donor milk as backup.
	Step 6: Give newborn infants no food or drink unless medically indicated.	Give donor milk preferentially before formula; give formula only for medical reasons. (These reasons are very limited!)
Global Strategy for Infant and Young Child Feeding (2003)	Section 18: Defines what to do in situations where mothers' own milk is unavailable.	Recommends banked donor milk as an option when the infant cannot breastfeed and/or the mother's own expressed milk is unavailable.

See also Arnold, 2006; Bar-Yam, 2000.

mother tests positive for HIV (WHO/UNICEF, 1992). In 1998, banked donor milk was presented as an option in a publication on HIV and infant feeding (WHO, 1998). In 2002 the World Health Assembly unanimously endorsed the *Global Strategy for Infant and Young Child Feeding*, which recommends banked donor milk as an option when the infant cannot breastfeed and/or the mother's own expressed milk is unavailable (section 18, WHO/UNICEF, 2003).

> The vast majority of mothers can and should breastfeed, just as the vast majority of infants can and should be breastfed. Only under exceptional circumstances can a mother's milk be considered unsuitable for her infant. For those few health situations where infants cannot, or should not, be breastfed, the choice of the best alternative—expressed breast milk from an infant's own mother, breast milk from a healthy wet nurse or a human-milk bank, or a breast milk substitute fed with a cup, which is a safer method than a feeding bottle and teat—depends on individual circumstances. (WHO/UNICEF, 2003, p. 10)

What makes this global statement so important is the delineation of responsibilities and obligations that various parties have. Governments, health professional associations, nongovernmental organizations including community-based support groups, commercial enterprises, employers, and other groups all have responsibilities for making the strategy successful.

In May 2008, the World Health Assembly approved Resolution WHA61.20 (WHA, 2008). This biennial progress report on infant and young child nutrition builds on other resolutions and reaffirms them, including ones that recognize the health risks of feeding infant formula, particularly powdered infant formula, which is intrinsically contaminated with *Enterobacter sakazakii*, a cause of meningitis outbreaks and death among infants around the world. Section1(4) states that member states should:

> . . . investigate, as a risk-reduction strategy, the possible use and, in accordance with national regulations, the safe use of donor milk through human milk banks for vulnerable infants, in particular premature, low-birth-weight and immunocompromised infants, and to promote appropriate hygienic measures for storage, conservation and use of human milk.

In Section 2(4), the director-general of WHO is requested to:

> . . . provide support urgently for research on the safe use of expressed and donated breast milk, given the current challenges facing countries in the implementation of safe infant feeding practices, mindful of national rules and regulations and cultural and religious beliefs.

SUMMARY

In the WHA61.20 (WHA, 2008) resolution, achieving food security for infants and children is a major objective. Exclusive breastfeeding for the first 6 months of life supplies a means for infants to achieve food security (adequate nutrition and adequate volume for optimal health). But what about the infant whose mother has difficulty establishing a milk supply, or the infant who is an AIDS orphan and perhaps HIV positive himself? Food security means that this baby should have access to donor milk, because the use of formula is a very *insecure* form of feeding. Maybe the mother cannot afford the formula and dilutes it; maybe there are unsafe pathogens in the water it is mixed with; maybe the composition of formula itself causes illness or allergies in the infant; maybe it has bacteria in it already; maybe some essential element has been left out in a manufacturing error or too much of another element has been added, all to the detriment of the infant. All of these things can happen in a developed country as well as a developing one, and they do happen. Having access to donor human milk is the safety net for achieving food security in an otherwise vulnerable population.

Donor milk banking around the world presents variations on a theme. Where milk banking is most successful there appears to be cooperation between government health authorities and the milk banking industry to establish standards of operation that provide a safe product. The most successful milk banks are those *systems* that recognize and implement an expanded role as promoters and protectors of breastfeeding. Yet with modifications, donor milk banking can fit in almost every society, even those with cultural barriers, infrastructure challenges, and seemingly inadequate economic resources.

REFERENCES

Almeida, J. A. G. (2001). *Breastfeeding: A nature-culture hybrid.* Rio de Janeiro, Brazil: Editora FIOCRUZ.

Almeida, S., & Dorea, J. (2006). Quality control of banked milk in Brasilia, Brazil. *Journal of Human Lactation, 22*(3), 335–339.

Al-Naqeeb, N., Azab, A., Eliwa, M., & Mohammed, B. (2000). The introduction of breast milk donation in a Muslim country. *Journal of Human Lactation, 16*(4), 346–350.

Arnold, L. D. W. (1994a). Donor human milk for premature infants: The famous case of the Dionne quintuplets. *Journal of Human Lactation, 10*(4), 271–272.

Arnold, L. D. W. (1994b). The lactariums of France: Part 1. The Lactarium Docteur Raymond Fourcade in Marmande. *Journal of Human Lactation, 10*(2), 125–126.

Arnold, L. D. W. (1996). Donor milk banking in China: The ultimate step in becoming baby friendly. *Journal of Human Lactation, 12*(4), 319–321.

Arnold, L. D. W. (1999). Donor milk banking in Scandinavia. *Journal of Human Lactation, 15*(1), 55–59.

Arnold, L. D. W. (2001). Trends in donor milk banking in the United States. In D. Newburg (Ed.), *Bioactive components of human milk* (pp. 509–517). New York: Kluwer Academic/Plenum Publishers.

Arnold, L. D. W. (2006). Global health policies that support the use of banked donor human milk: A human rights issue. *International Breastfeeding Journal, 1*(26), 1–8.

Arnold, L. D. W., & Courdent, M. (1994). The lactariums of France, Part 2: How association milk banks operate. *Journal of Human Lactation, 10*(3), 195–196.

Balmer, S. E. (1995). Donor milk banking and guidelines in Britain. *Journal of Human Lactation, 11*(3), 229–231.

Balmer, S. E., & Wharton, B. A. (1992). Human milk banking at Sorrento Maternity Hospital, Birmingham. *Archives of Disease in Childhood, 67*(4), 556–559.

Bar-Yam, N. (2000). *The right to breast: Breastfeeding and human rights.* East Sandwich, MA: Health Education Associates.

Bar-Yam, N. (2003). Breastfeeding and human rights: Is there a right to breastfeeding? Is there a right to be breastfed? *Journal of Human Lactation, 19*(4), 357–361.

Baum, J. D. (1982). Donor breast milk. *Acta Paediatrica Scandinavica, 71*(Suppl. 299), 51–57.

Department of Health and Social Security. (1981). *The Collection and Storage of Human Milk.* London: Her Majesty's Stationery Office.

Dumlao, P. (2007, October 18). *Philippine lawmaker wants 'human milk banks' in hospitals.* Retrieved June 24, 2009, from http://www.allheadlinenews.com/articles/7008869179

Fernandez, A., Mondkar, J., & Nanavati, R. (1993). The establishment of a human milk bank in India. *Journal of Human Lactation, 9*(3), 189–190.

Fernandez, A., & Savargaonkar, R. (1989). Scope of human milk banking. In A. Fernandez, J. Mondkar, R. Savargaonkar, & C. Vaz (Eds.), *Proceedings of International Workshop on Breast Milk Banking for Developing Countries* (pp. 7–15). Bombay, India: Division of Neonatology, Department of Pediatrics, L. T. M. G. Hospital, and L. T. M. M. College, Sion.

Grovslien, A., & Gronn, M. (2009). Donor milk banking and breastfeeding in Norway. *Journal of Human Lactation, 25*(2), 206–210.

Gutierrez, D., & Almeida, J. A. G. (1998). Human milk banks in Brazil. *Journal of Human Lactation, 14*(4), 333–335.

Hartmann, B., Pang, W., Keil, A., Hartmann, P., & Simmer, K. (2007). Best practice guidelines for the operation of a donor human milk bank in an Australian NICU. *Early Human Development, 83*(10), 667–673.

International Baby Food Action Network (IBFAN). (2001). Brazil leads the world in human milk banks. *IBFAN INFO, 3*(4), 5.

Ighogboja, I., Olarewaju, R., Odumodu, C., & Okuonghae, H. (1995). Mother's attitudes towards donated breastmilk in Jos, Nigeria. *Journal of Human Lactation, 11*(2), 93–96.

Infant Feeding Action Coalition (INFACT) Canada. (2001, Summer/Fall). Brazil wins prestigious WHO Sasakawa prize. *INFACT*, p. 10.

Israel-Ballard, K., Maternowska, C., Abrams, B., Morrison, P., Chitibura, L., Chipato, T., et al. (2006). Acceptability of heat treating breast milk to prevent mother-to-child transmission of human immunodeficiency virus in Zimbabwe: A qualitative study. *Journal of Human Lactation, 22*(1), 48–60.

Jones, F. (2003, October). *Milk banking around the world.* Presentation given at the annual meeting of the Human Milk Banking Association of North America, San Jose, CA.

Kent, G. (2006). Child feeding and human rights. *International Breastfeeding Journal, 1*(27). Available at http://www.internationalbreastfeedingjournal.com/content/1/1/27

Kocturk, T. (2003). Foetal development and breastfeeding in early texts of the Islamic tradition. *Acta Paediatrica, 92*(5), 617–620.

Mehta, N., & Siva Subramanian, K. (1990). Human milk banking: Current concepts. *Indian Journal of Pediatrics, 57*(3), 361–374.

Ministère des Affaires Sociales et de l'Intégration. (1992, February). Décret no. 92-174 du 25 février 1992 relatif à la prévention de la transmission de certaines maladies infectieuses [Decree no. 92-174 of 25 February 1992 on prevention of the transmission of certain infectious diseases]. *Journal Officiel de la République Française, 26*, 2929.

Narayanan, I., Prakash, K., Bala, S., Verma, R., & Gujral, V. (1980, September 13). Partial supplementation with expressed breast-milk for prevention of infection in low-birth-weight infants. *The Lancet, 2*(8194), 561–563.

Narayanan, I., Prakash, K., & Gujral, V. (1982). Management of expressed human milk in a developing country—Experiences and practical guidelines. *Journal of Tropical Pediatrics, 28*(1), 25–28.

Penc, B. (1996). Organization and activity of a human milk bank in Poland. *Journal of Human Lactation, 12*(3), 243–246.

Siimes, M., & Hallman, N. (1979). A perspective on human milk banking, 1978. *Journal of Pediatrics, 94*(1), 173–174.

South African Breastmilk Reserve (SABR). (2009). *Homepage*. Retrieved June 24, 2009, from http://www.sabr.org.za

Springer, S. (1997). Human milk banking in Germany. *Journal of Human Lactation, 13*(1), 65–68.

Springer, S. (2000). News about human milk banking in Germany. In B. Koletzko, K. Michaelsen, & O. Hernell (Eds.), *Short and long term effects of breast feeding on child health*, (pp. 441–442). New York: Kluwer Academic/Plenum Publishers.

Tully, M. R. (2001). Excelencia em bancos de leite humano: Uma visao do futuro [Excellence in human milk banking: A vision of the future]—The First International Congress on Human Milk Banking. *Journal of Human Lactation, 17*(1), 51–53.

UNICEF. (1982). *The state of the world's children*. Retrieved June 24, 2009, from http://www.unicef.org/sowc96/1980s.htm

UNICEF/WHO. (1989). *Protecting, promoting and supporting breast-feeding: The special role of maternity services*. Geneva, Switzerland: Author.

United Kingdom Association of Milk Banks (UKAMB). (2003). *Guidelines for the establishment and operation of human milk banks in the UK* (3rd ed.). London: Author.

United Nations (UN). (1948). *Universal declaration of human rights*. Retrieved June 24, 2009, from http://www.un.org/en/documents/udhr/index.shtml

United Nations (UN). (1967). *International covenant on economic, social and cultural rights*. Retrieved June 24, 2009, from http://www2.ohchr.org/english/law/pdf/cescr.pdf

United Nations (UN). (1981). *Convention on elimination of all forms of discrimination against women*. Retrieved June 24, 2009, from http://www2.ohchr.org/english/law/pdf/cedaw.pdf

United Nations (UN). (1989). *Convention on the rights of the child*. Retrieved June 24, 2009, from http://www2.ohchr.org/english/law/pdf/crc.pdf

Verd Vallespir, S., Calvo Benito, T., Saez Torres, C., & Gaya Puig, T. (2003). Recent progress in donor human milk utilization. *Annals of Pediatrics, 58*(3), 281.

Weaver, G., & Williams, A. (1997). A mother's gift: The milk of human kindness. In A. Oakley & J. Ashton (Eds.), *The gift relationship: From human blood to social policy* (2nd ed., pp. 319–332). New York: New Press.

Williams, A., Fisher, C., Greasley, V., Trayler, H., Woolridge, M., & Baum, J. (1985). Human milk banking. *Journal of Tropical Pediatrics, 31*(4), 185–190.

Williamson, S., Hewitt, J., Finucane, E., & Gamsu, H. (1978). Organisation of bank of raw and pasteurised human milk for neonatal intensive care. *British Medical Journal, 1*(6110), 393–396.

Winikoff, B., & Baer, E. (1980). The obstetrician's opportunity: Translating "breast is best" from theory to practice. *American Journal of Obstetrics and Gynecology, 138*(1), 105–117.

World Health Assembly. (2008, May 24). Infant and young child nutrition: Biennial progress report (WHA61.20). Geneva, Switzerland: WHO.

World Health Organization (WHO). (2003). *HIV and infant feeding. A guide for health care managers and supervisors.* Geneva, Switzerland: Author. WHO/FRH/NUT/CHD/98.2. Retrieved June 24, 2009, from http://whqlibdoc.who.int/hq/2003/9241591234.pdf

World Health Organization (WHO)/UNICEF. (1980). Meeting on infant and young child feeding. *Journal of Nurse-Midwifery, 25*(3), 31–38.

World Health Organization (WHO)/UNICEF. (1992). *Consensus statement from the WHO/UNICEF consultation on HIV transmission and breast-feeding.* Geneva, Switzerland: Author.

World Health Organization (WHO)/UNICEF. (2003). *Global strategy for infant and young child feeding.* Geneva, Switzerland: Author.Zachou, T. (1996, March). *Growth in preterm infants fed different types of feedings.* Presentation at the annual meeting of the Human Milk Banking Association of North America, Raleigh, NC.

Zachou, T. (1996, March). *Growth in preterm infants fed different types of feedings.* Presentation at the annual meeting of the Human Milk Banking Association of North America, Raleigh, NC.

Ziegler, J., Cooper, D., Johnson, R., & Gold, J. (1985). Postnatal transmission of AIDS-associated retrovirus from mother to infant. *The Lancet, 1*(8434), 896–898.

chapter sixteen

The Ten Steps for a Baby-Friendly Milk Bank

In the United States and in many other parts of the world, milk banks are focused on their central functions, which include donor intake, pasteurizing milk, and shipping it to recipients—the donor milk banking operations of the individual milk bank. Occasionally, ancillary services such as lactation counseling or electric breast pump rentals may be offered, but are not considered to be the work of the organization. Protection, promotion, and the support of breastfeeding, or industry of donor milk banking are not included in the milk bank's vision.

Brazil has a successful model of donor milk banking that incorporates diverse aspects of public health and of breastfeeding in the expected milk banking functions (see pp. 381–384). The Instituto Fernandes Gigueira/Fundação Oswaldo Cruz and the National Reference Center are actively involved in the breastfeeding management training of health professionals, conducting regional training programs for continuing education, specialty courses, advanced degree programs with research opportunities, and training programs for hospital staff in hospitals that are implementing the Baby-Friendly Hospital Initiative (Almeida, 2001; UNICEF/WHO, 1989).

Milk banks should be working to increase the health of the population by promoting, protecting, and supporting breastfeeding in general. This is a recurrent theme in discussions of the role of milk banks in developing countries; milk banks should function as more than just a distributor of a product. Savage (1989) remarks about milk banks:

> Milk banks need to be considered, not in isolation, but as adjuncts to a comprehensive breast feeding programme . . . Breastfeeding programmes . . . [have] three main components—protection, promotion, and support. A milk bank can protect breast feeding because it can provide an alternate source of milk for those babies whose mother may be temporarily unable to supply enough of [her] own so that dependence on artificial substitutes can be minimised or altogether eliminated. A milk bank can promote breast feeding, because it can provide a tangible demonstration of the institution and staff's confidence that breast milk is necessary for sick and small babies, that it is superior to other milks, and can and will be provided to all babies. However, a milk bank can neither promote nor protect breast feeding if donated milk is used only as a last resort for infants who cannot tolerate artificial feeds. The role of a milk bank to support breast feeding is its most obvious potential function, because it supplies babies with human milk. Yet this is also the function that is the most easily misapplied. Misapplication is particularly likely if the role of a milk bank is seen in the narrow sense of being only a special source of nutriment and protection for vulnerable babies. (pp. 71–72)

Savage has concluded that the misapplication of milk banking occurs when milk banks are used only as a medicinal source of human milk for sick infants, with no attempt on the milk banks' part to assist the mother in (re)establishing her own milk supply. If the availability of donor milk is taken for granted by the hospital staff, then little may be done to help to establish a milk supply, and weaning from donor milk may be directly to formula rather than the biological mother's breast. If donor milk is seen only as nutrition, then it is also more likely to be fed in a bottle—supplanting the mother's breast and milk supply. Mothers may not even be involved in the feeding of human milk if the donor milk is fed by staff. There is a much broader role for milk banks to help with feeding problems, assist in relactation, support mothers of low-birth-weight babies and sick babies, and educate colleagues about the need for a comprehensive package. Almeida (2001, p. 81) reports that "Human milk banks have been one of the most import[ant] strategic elements in public policy favoring breastfeeding in the last two decades in Brazil."

This chapter includes policies and protocols for establishing and operating donor milk banks in the United States that are more in keeping with this broader vision of donor milk banking and its role in protection, promotion, and support of all things related to breastfeeding. We should not be looking to breastfeeding to protect milk banking; it should be the other way around with milk banks leading the way.

ESTABLISHING A COMMUNITY-BASED DONOR HUMAN MILK BANK

The American Breastfeeding Institute (ABI) is a 501c(3) (nonprofit) organization that seeks to improve the health outcomes for all infants in the United States. The overarching goal of the ABI and its National Commission on Donor Milk Banking program is not only to increase the amount of donor milk collected and distributed but also to increase the initiation and duration of breastfeeding and assist communities in meeting the goals established in the Surgeon General's *Blueprint* (DHHS, 2000b) and *Healthy People 2010* objectives (DHHS, 2000a). As part of my work at ABI, I worked with expert panels to develop the 10 steps that are described in this chapter. ABI envisions a network of community-based donor milk banks that provide full lactation services to their donors while simultaneously maintaining the safety and quality of donated banked human milk through appropriate screening procedures and evidence-based storage and handling techniques. In addition, these community milk banks cooperate with each other as part of a larger national organization (such as HMBANA or UKAMB) to ensure the perpetuation of the milk banking industry. The generic policy in **Appendix 16-1** at the end of this chapter has been developed for this purpose. This policy is based on 10 steps, adapted from those that are the basis for the Baby-Friendly Hospital Initiative (UNICEF/WHO, 1989) and designed specifically to address many of the issues that deny mothers access to donor milk for their vulnerable and sick neonates. In the process of acquiring donors, milk banks will be assisting mothers in establishing and maintaining lactation, helping them solve breastfeeding problems that may arise, and encouraging women to breastfeed their own infants for longer durations to meet the national goals for breastfeeding. In addition, milk banks would incorporate education and research purposes, providing education and research funding to the healthcare system in their community, leading to the universal understanding that a donor human milk bank is a community asset. This establishment of community human milk banks meets the needs of potential donors who may be turned away currently because of fluctuations in supply and demand in the current milk banking system.

Additionally, the establishment of a community-based donor human milk bank in a community would assist to:

- Achieve the national targets to increase the proportion of all mothers who breastfeed their babies in the early postpartum/newborn period and onward
- Encourage facilities that provide maternity services to achieve the WHO/UNICEF Baby-Friendly Hospital designation
- Improve access to evidence-based, comprehensive, current, and culturally appropriate lactation care and services for all women
- Increase contributions of human milk to levels more equal to blood bank donations in the community

These goals would be accomplished by the community milk bank's provision of three essential services to the community:

- Coordination of community breastfeeding resources through milk bank participation in existing breastfeeding task forces/coalitions. If such task forces/coalitions are nonexistent, the milk bank should foster their development.
- Development of or participation in resource coordination and information for breastfeeding women in the community such as hot lines, peer counseling, mother-to-mother support groups, and training programs for physicians, nurses, lactation consultants/counselors, and nutritionists/dietitians
- Outreach to healthcare providers and potential donors, screening, collecting, and processing of donated human milk

Defining a Community-Based Donor Human Milk Bank

A community human milk bank is a milk bank established for the dual purpose of supporting mothers' efforts to breastfeed by helping them establish and maintain an ample milk supply and then collecting any excess supply for use as donor milk. The community human milk bank screens donors in a standardized way and collects milk expressed by donors under carefully controlled conditions. Quality control and standardized processing ensure preservation of the maximum unique components in human milk. The use of standard screening procedures and processing techniques ensures the safety as well as quality of donor milk so that no recipient will become ill or be exposed unnecessarily to anything harmful. The policies outlined herein need also to be observed by milk bank depots. In a situation where a milk bank serves a region, collecting and processing milk from contiguous states, the depots feeding milk to the regional milk bank should also fit the definition of a community milk bank in the services they offer to breastfeeding women and healthcare providers in their catchment area.

Beginning in the mid-1980s, the number of donor milk banks in the United States has dwindled dramatically despite a recent resurgence in numbers of HMBANA milk banks and growth in demand for donor milk as seen in the steady increase in the number of ounces dispensed annually (see pp. 354–355). This is in marked contrast to other countries that are either beginning milk banking services for the first time, restarting milk banking services that were halted decades ago, or expanding existing milk banking services dramatically. Growth of milk banking services in these countries is measured by both an increase in the total number of milk banks and an increase in the volume of milk dispensed. Whereas U.S. milk banks calculate volume in terms of *ounces* distributed, milk banks in the rest of the world tally distribution in terms of *liters* dispensed, several orders of magnitude difference. Even in 2007, the latest year for which statistics are currently available, all HMBANA milk banks *combined* did not distribute the amount distributed annually by many *individual* European milk banks. Yet in any given year there are not only potential donors turned away for lack of demand, there are also numerous potential recipients who are denied access to donor milk therapy for lack of prescribers and/or consumer information about the resource of donor milk. A community-based donor milk bank reduces these inadequacies in education, supply, and demand by promoting use of donor milk in local NICUs and educating the community about the need for donors to provide milk. By integrating with hospital-based programs, such as neonatal intensive care units and Baby-Friendly hospitals, donor milk banking becomes an essential public health component and also serves to accomplish goals of the WHA resolution (2008). In the United States, it would also support the 2005 AAP statement on the use of human milk (AAP, 2005) as well as the United States Breastfeeding Committee's strategic plan (USBC, 2001). Only by integration of donor milk banking into communities can we accomplish the seamless provision of human milk to *all* infants while increasing breastfeeding durations beyond the first year of life.

Community-based donor milk banks' implementation of quality control measures for milk collection and processing (such as those of HMBANA or UKAMB, etc.) addresses the concerns of prescribing individuals (Arnold, 2005). The body of research available to support the decision to prescribe donor milk is also small. Supporting milk bank recipient research studies expands the body of knowledge about donor milk banking and the therapeutic uses of banked donor milk, providing physicians with the information they need to be more comfortable making informed decisions about the use of donor milk for and with their patients (Arnold, 2006). By adopting these policies, community human milk banks address the reservations and lack of information about donor milk and help prescribers gain confidence in this important public health resource. An enhanced, reliable supply of quality donor milk allows access for infants in need and will discourage questionable sources such as those found on the Internet.

Organization of a Community Human Milk Bank

Community human milk banks should be organized as not-for-profit entities. They should support the International Code of Marketing of Breast-milk Substitutes (Armstrong & Sokol, 1994; WHO, 1981) and be able to demonstrate that they do not accept funding or in-kind donations from violators of the International Code of Marketing of Breast-milk Substitutes. They should have a board of directors that oversees policy and fiscal responsibility, appoints a licensed physician as medical director to oversee the medical aspects of community human milk banking, and a milk bank coordinator who oversees the day-to-day operations of the milk bank and monitors staff activities. Community human milk banks should maintain policies and procedures that are described in the appendix to this chapter and outlined in **Table 16-1**.

DISCUSSION OF THE POLICIES

Joan is a 34-year-old first-time mother who had breast reduction surgery 2 years ago. She was informed by her surgeon that she would never be able to breastfeed. She became pregnant with triplets and was hospitalized at 23 weeks' gestation to prevent preterm delivery. She was visited by the neonatologist, who, unaware of her previous history of breast surgery, told her how important her milk would be for her triplets. The lactation consultant (LC) who came to see her in the hospital told her that it might be possible for her to produce some milk, and that the only way to know for sure was to give it a try when the babies arrived. The lactation consultant promised to set Joan up with a rental grade breast pump designed for long-term pumping when the babies arrived.

The babies were born at 29 weeks' gestation, each weighing about 2 pounds, and, true to her word, the LC arrived in Joan's room shortly after the birth with an electric breast pump on a trolley and instructions for how to get a similar rental grade pump in the community when Joan was discharged. The LC had already reserved one at a local pharmacy. The LC demonstrated how to use the pump and assisted Joan in trying to pump for the first time with a double kit. Only a few drops of colostrum came out, but that was seen as a hopeful sign that some function remained in her breasts and that Joan would be able to provide some milk for her babies.

After several weeks of pumping eight or more times a day, Joan succeeded in getting an ounce to an ounce and a half combined from both breasts at each pumping session. She was very discouraged and knew that her supply was hindered by the damage from the reduction surgery. She requested that the neonatologist consider using banked donor human milk to supplement what she was bringing in so that the babies would not be exposed to formula and an elevated risk of NEC. The neonatologist said he had never heard of such a thing and that the hospital had no policy about using milk from other women. The LC provided the neonatologist with some research articles about donor milk banking and supported Joan's request. The neonatologist stated that he felt very uncomfortable using milk from women he had never met. Joan thought, "And what about all those dirty cows he has never met?"

Joan continued to provide as much milk as she could for as long as the babies were in the hospital, but she never got more than 1.5 ounces at each session. The babies were supplemented with a preterm formula. Joan's attitude was positive in that she saw her milk as reducing the formula that the babies were getting. One of the triplets developed NEC shortly after the introduction of the formula and died. The other two were finally discharged from the hospital after 3 months in the NICU.

Table 16-1 Summary of Policies for a Community Donor Milk Bank

Every community donor milk bank will complete the following steps:

Step 1: Maintain written policies on the operation of a community-based donor human milk bank that are routinely communicated to all milk bank staff.

Step 2: Train all milk bank staff in skills necessary to implement these policies.

Step 3: Inform all pregnant and postpartum women in the community about donor milk banking and the importance of becoming a donor.

Step 4: Educate healthcare providers about the benefits and use of donor milk for sick or ill patients in the absence of mother's own milk.

Step 5: Assist mothers in becoming donors by providing lactation support services to help them establish and maintain an abundant milk supply for their own infants.

Step 6: Assist mothers in expressing milk in safe, clean ways.

Step 7: Use evidence-based standardized guidelines for the collection, intake, storage, processing, shipping, and dispensing of donor human milk while maintaining confidentiality of the donor.

Step 8: Participate in a standardized quality assurance process and contribute data for system-wide research.

Step 9: Practice in an evidence-based manner compatible with ethical standards and avoid conflicts of interest.

Step 10: Establish working relationships with all members of the community to support and maintain a community donor milk bank.

Although created for purposes of this book, Joan's case is representative of many similar and real experiences of mothers. Mothers of preterm infants whose situations and attitudes mirrored Joan's are in hospitals around the world today. Neonatologists dismiss the idea of using donor milk simply because they do not like the idea or are totally unfamiliar with it. When the gatekeeper needs to prescribe the donor milk, then lack of information and uninformed belief systems are a barrier that mothers and babies face on a daily basis.

How could the development of a community-based human milk bank with a broader scope than simply providing an excellent product erase challenges such as those experienced by Joan? Each one of the 10 steps for community human milk banks works to minimize barriers.

Step 1: Maintain written policies on the operation of a community-based donor human milk bank that are routinely communicated to all milk bank staff.

When evidence-based policies and procedures are developed and implemented, individuals within the organization cannot act in noncompliant ways without jeopardizing their jobs. This places everyone in an organization on the same page and a consistent message is given to the public with whom the individuals in the organization interface. This instills confidence inside the organization and legitimizes it among the public.

Written policies and procedures guide an organization in all its functions and enable consistent, evidence-based practice (WHO, 1998). Updating policies with new evidence-based information as it becomes available protects, promotes, and supports breastfeeding and donor milk banking. When utilizing evidence-based information to justify a policy, studies are examined carefully for the quality of the evidence as well.

Following established evidence-based policies and procedures also protects employees against liability. Policies and procedures establish a standard of practice; it tells employees how things will be done in their institution. We open ourselves up to malpractice claims and community disdain when we behave outside of a policy or standard of practice.

If a milk bank had existed in Joan's community, she and the lactation consultant would have had established policies of the milk bank to provide to the neonatologist. Fears or concerns might have been allayed by the established standards of practice. In addition, the community milk bank and the lactation consultant could have assisted the neonatologist to develop a hospital policy for use of donor milk, including the appropriate uses and the mechanics of thawing and feeding it. Later, other mothers could have then benefited from this foresighted action, and more babies in the community would have been fed human milk per the recommendations of the AAP (2005).

Step 2: Train all milk bank staff in skills necessary to implement these policies.

Having a policy is one thing; knowing how to implement it is another. Staff training in the policies promotes better interfacing between donors, recipients, and prescribers and the organization itself. Training needs to be ongoing and needs to be more than simple memorization of the policy content. Competencies in implementing the policies need to be taught and assessed periodically. With a community human milk bank, which is likely to have only a small number of paid staff and a larger number of volunteers, even the volunteers need training so that they can communicate better with others about the milk bank and what it does. Training in the policies not only guarantees a certain level of quality control, but also is good public relations for the milk bank itself.

In Joan's case, there was no community milk bank, and the public relations aspect of having a local donor milk bank or collection depot was missing. The neonatologist knew nothing about donor milk. Donor milk would have had to be shipped in from several states away. The logistics would have been difficult, but not impossible.

Step 3: Inform all pregnant and postpartum women in the community about donor milk banking and the importance of becoming a donor.

Everyone in the community needs to know about the milk bank. This is a marketing job. Beginning the marketing process starts with pregnant women and their prenatal care providers who should be targeted for information about donor milk banking, in particular about how to become a donor and/or how to get help with a breastfeeding problem from the milk bank.

Marketing begins with networking with other breastfeeding groups in the community and helping on other breastfeeding projects. For example, perhaps a state breastfeeding task force has decided to participate in a fit pregnancy health fair being sponsored by a healthcare system. This is the perfect opportunity for the milk bank to offer to staff the booth in exchange for being able to talk about community resources (the milk bank, among others) for solving breastfeeding problems and to hand out brochures to pregnant women about the possibility of becoming a milk donor. Donor milk banking becomes part of the bigger picture of breastfeeding promotion and support and helps point out to someone who perhaps has not considered breastfeeding at all, how important human milk really is. If the pregnant woman has a preterm infant, she already knows of the importance of becoming a donor through this exposure and can apply that knowledge to having her baby become a recipient if her own supply falters. She also knows that she can get assistance for increasing her supply from the milk bank. Educating physicians and childbirth educators by asking them to cooperate in providing informational brochures to patients is another important aspect of prenatal marketing.

Other tools that can be used to educate postpartum women and their care providers about the community human milk bank and its services are to get hospitals to put informational brochures or magnets in their discharge packets, collaborate with other breastfeeding support groups in the region, and provide in-service training to healthcare providers. Public awareness can also be maintained by frequent articles in the newspaper and press releases about milk bank activities.

If there are no breastfeeding support systems or task forces in the area already, then it is incumbent upon the milk bank to establish them. Overall improvement in services available to mothers will occur, and breastfeeding initiation and duration rates will increase also.

Step 4: Educate healthcare providers about the benefits and use of donor milk for sick or ill patients in the absence of mothers' own milk.

Neonatologists rarely know about the existence of and importance of donor human milk banks. There are two brief studies that have been done about neonatologists' attitudes and knowledge about the use of banked donor human milk. One, by Wight (2003), surveyed neonatologists in the California Association of Neonatology (CAN), and the other, by Harris, Weber, Chezem, and Quinlan (2005), surveyed the members of the Neonatal Pediatric Section of the AAP. The first used a hard copy survey distributed at a CAN conference followed by a mail survey. A response rate of 35.2% was achieved. The second survey utilized an online survey tool and had a response rate of 17%. In the Wight study, a 5-point Likert scale (strongly agree/agree/no opinion/disagree/strongly disagree) was used to assess beliefs about donor milk. In all statements that participants were asked to agree/disagree with, the majority of responses ended up in the neutral column, indicating that responders did not have enough knowledge to either agree or disagree with the statement, let alone strongly agree or disagree. Of the responders, 78% were trained in facilities that did not use donor milk and at the time of the survey worked in facilities that did not use donor milk, again demonstrating the holes in the educational system for healthcare practitioners. Lack of knowledge perpetuates itself. A preponderance of responders (76%) had never prescribed donor milk themselves, and an amazing 47% of pediatric responders had never heard of the San Jose milk bank in their own state! Of the 23.5% of respondents who had prescribed donor milk, the bulk of the use was for prematurity (86.8%), with feeding intolerance following at 50.0%. Transmission of infectious disease was a concern of 66.4% of respondents who had not previously prescribed donor milk. The biggest concerns that those who had prescribed donor milk had about its use were infectious disease transmission (43.5%) and nutritional adequacy (40.5%). Lack of documented benefits came in at 27.5% for the nonprescribers and 37.8% for the prescribers.

In the Harris et al. (2005) study, about 20% of the respondents worked in facilities where donor milk was being prescribed, yet a solid 62% of respondents still had concerns about the transmission of known infectious agents to recipients. About 61% of respondents cited a need for further research, yet 53% indicated they would consider recommending donor milk from a human milk bank for babies in their care despite the lack of research.

As can be seen from these two studies and Joan's case earlier in this chapter, lack of information about the availability, safety, and nutritional adequacy of banked donor milk is a significant barrier to its use. Education within the postpartum care system is extremely important, as many of the providers of such care will be the source of referrals and prescriptions to the milk bank. Physicians and nurse practitioners in neonatology, pediatrics, pediatric gastroenterology, and family practice need to be targeted specifically for education about donor milk banking and its uses and safety.

One way of educating healthcare providers is to do a participatory action research project. In this type of research, the questions in the research tool are aimed at educating at the same time. Thus the questions themselves prompt an examination of previous or current behavior and beliefs and perhaps change in these behaviors and beliefs. Asking the question puts ideas into people's heads.

Q: What do you know about donor human milk banking and its clinical uses?

A: I have never heard of donor milk banking before. What is it?

The researcher explains about donor human milk banking and how other NICUs use donor milk. The research subject thinks, "Hmmm. I should investigate this use for my own NICU to bring it up to speed with other units. If this is a common practice then I am not practicing in an evidence-based way. I should know more about donor milk banking."

Needs assessment surveys also provoke thinking about current practices and whether a change in current practice is warranted.

Step 5: Assist mothers in becoming donors by providing lactation support services to help them establish and maintain an abundant milk supply for their own infants.

In Joan's case, further lactation support might not have increased her milk supply any given her surgical history, and it is doubtful that she would have ever become a donor. However, ongoing encouragement from milk bank staff for the efforts she was making and the amount of milk she was supplying on her own would have been very appropriate. It is discouraging to maintain a positive attitude the way Joan did without a lot of support, especially as the babies grew and their nutritional needs outstripped her supply by larger and larger amounts. Many mothers would have given up very early in the game without the frequent support that Joan received from the LC.

Many mothers in the community find that they do not have that kind of support or do not know where to find it even when they run into breastfeeding problems with a healthy, term infant. For example, a mother has been given a small breast pump in the hospital gift bag when she is discharged. She assumes that she is to use this pump as well as feed the baby, so she pumps after every feeding just to make sure that she has enough milk. Within a few weeks she has an oversupply, the baby is coughing and sputtering when it feeds because of the excess milk and the force with which she lets down her milk, and she has frequent clogs in her breasts from the oversupply and the fact that her breasts are never drained adequately. Now she has a case of mastitis. This mother definitely can be helped by the milk bank counseling her to seek medical care for the mastitis and to continue pumping to prevent milk stasis. Once the mastitis is cleared up, she can be helped to down-regulate her milk supply gradually while donating the excess to the milk bank in an ongoing fashion. Mothers encountering breastfeeding problems sometimes erroneously believe that stopping breastfeeding is the only way to resolve the problem when it may actually cause more problems. Accessible and appropriate breastfeeding support can help prevent untimely weaning caused by breastfeeding problems.

As part of the solution for breastfeeding problems and untimely weaning, milk banks should provide comprehensive lactation services to help not only their donors but also other mothers in the community. A side benefit of this help and support may be that the milk bank acquires another donor. However, the larger benefit is that mothers will be encouraged to breastfeed longer if they can get help with their problems, and communities will be better able to meet the goals for breastfeeding duration and exclusivity. By providing breastfeeding support resources in communities where other sources of assistance are few or poorly publicized, the milk bank may turn the breastfeeding duration statistics around. In communities with more resources, there are always mothers who fall through the cracks who do not get adequate support when they need it. More services, especially those that are proactive in seeking mothers out and anticipating problems, may be what is required.

Even donors with ample milk supplies have breastfeeding problems from time to time. Frequent contact with individual donors by phone can help resolve some of these problems before they become serious enough that the donor has to temporarily cease donating. Frequent contact is also in the best interest of the milk bank itself. Women who feel that their efforts are being appreciated and supported are more likely to continue to donate.

Using evidence-based practice in counseling mothers and donors is also essential, especially when one is trying to work collegially with healthcare providers in the community. Milk bank lactation supporters should also keep physicians/primary care providers apprised of information given to mothers, especially when there is a medical resolution required of a breastfeeding problem. This is also an ideal opportunity to further breastfeeding knowledge among healthcare providers. When gadgets and devices are part of the solution to a breastfeeding problem, lactation supporters and milk bank staff should examine their motives in providing the gadget or device, especially if the mother has to pay for that gadget and the milk bank is profiting from the sale. The staff must determine whether the device is really needed, or if there is another less costly and less interventionist way to resolve the problem. Selling gadgets and devices has the potential to become a conflict of interest that could cause harm to the milk bank's reputation. Lactation care providers in the milk bank should also be very careful not to exceed their scope of practice.

Step 6: Assist mothers in expressing milk in safe, clean ways.

Because milk banks understand about the potential problems that can be encountered when milk is expressed, handled, and stored, they should develop protocols and informational brochures for mothers in the community who wish to collect and store their milk safely. In essence, the milk bank is a bank of information. Sample policies for milk expression can be found in step 7. There are also sample policies for storage and handling of milk for a healthy, term baby in print (Arnold, 2000). These policies need to be carefully differentiated from those developed for hospitalized and sick babies. Guidelines for safe storage and handling of expressed milk are much more stringent for the fragile infant than they are for the healthy, term infant, and storage durations vary.

Donors and nondonors alike should have access through the milk bank to rental grade pumps that can be either rented or loaned. Additionally, spare parts for various models of pumps should be stocked so that mothers do not lose the use of their pumps if something happens to a small part, e.g., a membrane or valve tears or goes down the drain, a flange melts during sterilization, or the family dog chews a hole in the tubing for the kit. Milk banks should make an effort not to be locked into one brand of pump but to select several brands from which mothers can choose.

In Joan's case, she was given thorough instruction in the use of the pump and a method was set up for her to rent one when she was discharged from the hospital. This made it easier for her to access a pump than if she were simply sent home with a list. Knowing how to operate the pump also maximized her efficiency with pumping and ensured that the agency renting the pump would have the pump returned still in working order because it was being used properly.

Step 7: Use evidence-based standardized guidelines for the collection, intake, storage, processing, shipping, and dispensing of donor human milk while maintaining confidentiality of the donor.

Standards of practice for donor milk banking have previously been developed by HMBANA (2008) and are available in print. Other organizations are also developing or revising guidelines, such as the U.K. Association of Milk Banks. These guidelines set a minimum standard of practice to maintain quality and safety of banked donor milk, meaning that if a community milk bank wanted to exceed these standards it certainly could.

Acceptable U.S. standards for donor screening are based on the American Association of Blood Banks (AABB, 2006) guidelines for blood donors with some additions that are specific to donating human milk. As new diseases emerge from ever-mutating bacteria, and new viruses suddenly appear in places where they have not been seen before, guidelines for donor serum screening will change to meet these new concerns. Because blood cannot be pasteurized and still function the way milk can, the blood banking guidelines are going to be very strict as well. It is important for community milk banks to stay in contact with the local blood banks to stay current with their practices. This can be done by either having a blood banking representative sit on the medical advisory board or the board of directors of the milk bank or by having the milk bank medical director maintain contact with the local blood bank medical director. The policies given here are meant to be generic and suitable for expansion to fit the individual community milk bank.

In Joan's case, had the neonatologist known exactly what went into the collection, screening, processing, and dispensing of donor milk, he might have been a bit more enthusiastic about using donor milk to supplement Joan's own supply. Some of his fears would have been allayed. As it is, some mothers, when their requests for donor milk are turned down, will seek milk informally from family members or friends and bring it to the NICU unpasteurized with their own labels on it. The neonatologist and nurses are completely unaware of the arrangement. This has the potential for tragic consequences for the recipient from an unidentified bacteria or virus. This is a much riskier situation than getting donor milk from a milk bank where all precautions have been taken to ensure safety, including pasteurization. When milk banks take the lead in informing neonatologists about their processing protocols, concerns are laid aside. An innovative way of doing this is to hold an open house at the processing facility.

Step 8: Participate in a standardized quality assurance process and contribute data for system-wide research.

Purchasers of care (insurers, employers), accreditation organizations such as The Joint Commission, government agencies involved with the healthcare system, consumers of health care (the public), and healthcare providers all want to be assured of the safety and efficacy of a healthcare service. This assurance comes only with internal and external quality monitoring. Lacking any federal or state oversight of a regulatory nature in the United States (except in California, New York, and Texas), individual milk banks must be responsible for internal monitoring for compliance with policies, protocols, and procedures (Arnold, 2005; Carey, 2003). Quality control begins with the collection of data and statistics that demonstrate where system weaknesses occur and justify the existence of the service.

Reluctance to prescribe donor milk among physicians is highly correlated with concerns about the safety and quality of donated milk as well as a lack of published research, as described previously (pp. 404–405). Current milk banking guidelines do not mandate self-audits for collecting, storing, processing, and distributing milk, nor is there an oversight organization that provides quality assessment and monitoring for individual milk banks. This lack of quality control does not reassure the prescriber, causes perceptions of elevated risk to patients, and creates an environment of mistrust of donor milk (Arnold, 2005). Data collection and publication of statistics therefore becomes even more important to demonstrate safety and efficacy.

In Joan's case, perhaps the neonatologist could have been persuaded to prescribe donor milk if there had been more clinical case reports to show him. Even though the case report is the bottom rung on the evidentiary ladder, at this point so few case reports have been published that prescribers have no body of work to which to refer. Personally, I know of numerous missed opportunities to publish case reports, and many physicians who had prescribed donor milk who had wonderful cases that could have been written up but were not.

Currently, HMBANA data collection consists of the number of cases per year for which donor milk has been prescribed in certain categories of clinical use, and the total number of ounces prescribed annually. This is a good baseline but not enough to demonstrate to a prescriber that due diligence is being used. Data sets that need to be collected include (but are not limited to) the following: How many donors were accepted annually? How many donors were rejected annually? What were the reasons for rejection? How much milk was taken in? How much milk had to be discarded because of high bacteria counts or other issues? What steps were taken to reeducate mothers on collection techniques? Did they work? How much of the discarded milk was retrospectively collected as compared to prospectively collected? How much milk had to be discarded because of ineffective processing? What were the diagnoses of all recipients? What were the outcomes of all recipients? How much milk was distributed to each recipient before it was no longer needed? What is the breakout of ages of recipients? If the infant was healthy and received donor milk, what were the mother conditions that qualified the infant for donor milk?

Statistics of this kind will be beneficial in the long run to public perceptions about donor milk banks and the safety and efficacy of donor milk.

When milk banks apply for funding from other organizations, it is also important to be able to justify the need for the organization through data that has been collected in a systematic way.

Step 9: Practice in an evidence-based manner compatible with ethical standards and avoid conflicts of interest.

In order to promote breastfeeding and help mothers gain confidence in their abilities to produce milk not only for their own infants, but for the infants of other women as well, it is important not to display materials that present conflicting messages and represent a conflict of interest when one is trying to promote human milk as the norm. Breastfeeding is more successful when there are fewer visible signs of commercial influence to undermine a mother's confidence. Funding and supplies for the milk bank's operations must come from governments, grants, and donations that are not connected with any industry that violates the International Code of Marketing of Breast-milk Substitutes (WHO, 1981) in order to remain free of commercial pressure to support the use of formula. Ethically, however, community milk banks and staff should try to not become beholden to any commercial company, in particular one company to the exclusion of a competitor, even when that company is probreastfeeding. Advertising for any commercial company should not be within the job description of the staff of a milk bank.

When dealing ethically with donors and recipients, lactation services must be provided in an evidence-based manner and confidentiality must be respected. Practicing evidence-based breastfeeding management also enhances the credibility of the staff of the milk bank and builds respect for the milk bank's work. Use of non–evidence-based solutions to breastfeeding problems during counseling may negatively impact the health of the infant. Similarly, use of non–evidence-based methods to treat various conditions may introduce pathogens capable of compromising infant health.

All milk bank personnel need to practice within their scope of practice to avoid legal and ethical ramifications. Mothers should be referred to their own healthcare providers when medical problems arise. When medical questions do arise, the medical director of the milk bank is the final authority. Maintaining open lines of communication with healthcare providers is essential to a respectful working relationship within the health care community. In Joan's case, a medical director talking directly to the neonatologist probably would have been an effective strategy in procuring donor milk for Joan's triplets.

Step 10: Establish working relationships with all members of the community to support and maintain a community donor milk bank.

Developing good working relationships within the larger community is a prerequisite to having a successful community donor human milk bank. Milk banks should not envision themselves as isolated members of the healthcare team. They should see themselves as part of the broader interdisciplinary public health picture. This means that boards of directors should have interdisciplinary representation from community agencies, consumers, and the healthcare sector. Other important areas that need to be considered when choosing board members are law, ethics, fund-raising, public relations, service organizations, and language barriers for various ethnic groups.

Cultivating a cadre of community volunteers who come from different walks of life can be a great help. When I was working at Hawaii Mother's Milk Bank, one of my best volunteers was a grandmother, the mother of one of our donors. She was a rather wealthy woman of some social standing in the community and was a member of the board of several charitable organizations. She started out as a volunteer in the hospital and happened to be assigned to us one day to help with a bulk mailing. It turned out she hated to do paper work but loved to wash bottles. All the bottles used in pasteurization had to be washed by hand before they went in the dishwasher. Once they came out of the dishwasher they had to be hand wrapped in a very specific way for autoclaving to sterilize them for the next round of pasteurization. This was a time-consuming process that most of the paid staff disliked doing because we had phone calls to answer and donors to screen and budgets to prepare. Over the years this woman stood at the sink for many hours and never went back to the main part of the hospital as a volunteer. She also turned out to be a fabulous fund-raiser and had numerous contacts with people of means in the community. Her entire Christmas card list went into our fund-raising mailing list, as did many contacts from her other service organizations.

We volunteer because we believe in a cause, not because we want or need reimbursement for our efforts. It is therefore important for the community milk bank to think about ways to honor volunteers and ways to say thank you that are meaningful and keep the volunteers wanting to come back. Volunteers are not just people who collect milk or stand for hours washing bottles. They are also the donors. Donors need special recognition and encouragement to continue donating, and to want to donate again with the next child. It must be wonderful to be the Leipzig milk bank (see pp. 376–377) and have third-generation donors!

SUMMARY

This chapter has been about practice and policy and the need for them to be in place and functioning smoothly for a community human milk bank to be successful. Suggestions have been given in a generic way for policies that are in a 10-step model patterned after the Ten Steps to Successful Breastfeeding, which forms the basis for the Baby-Friendly Hospital Initiative. In order to become a baby-friendly community human milk bank, milk banks must no longer think of themselves as simply the distributors of a product, but interface with the broader breastfeeding community as a critical component, leading the way for improving initiation and duration rates of breastfeeding to meet the national breastfeeding goals.

REFERENCES

Almeida, J. A. G. (2001). *Breastfeeding: A nature-culture hybrid*. Rio de Janeiro, Brazil: Editora FIOCRUZ.

American Academy of Pediatrics, Section on Breastfeeding (AAP). (2005). Breastfeeding and the use of human milk. *Pediatrics, 115*(2), 496–506.

American Association of Blood Banks. (2006). *Standards for blood banks and transfusion services*. Arlington, VA: Author.

Arnold, L. D. W. (2000). *Human milk storage for healthy infants and children*. East Sandwich, MA: Health Education Associates, Inc.

Arnold, L. D. W. (2005). *Donor human milk banking: Creating public health policy in the 21st century*. Doctoral dissertation, Union Institute and University.

Arnold, L. D. W. (2006). The ethics of donor human milk banking. *Breastfeeding Medicine, 1*(1), 3–13.

Armstrong, H. C., & Sokol, E. (1994). *The international code of marketing of breast-milk substitutes: What it means for mothers and babies world-wide*. Raleigh, NC: International Lactation Consultant Association.

Carey, R. G. (2003). *Improving healthcare with control charts*. Milwaukee, WI: Quality Press.

Department of Health and Human Services (DHHS). (2000a). *Healthy People 2010*. Washington, DC: Author.

Department of Health and Human Services (DHHS). Office of Women's Health. (2000b). *HHS blueprint for action on breastfeeding*. Washington, DC: Author.

Harris, H., Weber, M., Chezem, J., & Quinlan, M. (2005). Human milk banking: Neonatologists' opinions and practices. (Abstract No. 30, MWSPR). *Pediatric Research, 58*, 821.

Human Milk Banking Association of North America (HMBANA). (2008). *Guidelines for the establishment and operation of a donor human milk bank*. Raleigh, NC: Author.

Savage, F. (1989). Milk banks and lactation clinics. In A. Fernandez, J. Mondkar, R. Savargaonkar, & C. Vaz. (Eds.), *Proceedings of international workshop on breast milk banking for developing countries* (pp. 70–81, 83). Bombay, India: Division of neonatology, Department of Pediatrics, L. T. M. G. Hospital, and L. T. M. M. College, Sion.

UNICEF/WHO. (1989). *Protecting, promoting and supporting breast-feeding: The special role of maternity services*. Geneva, Switzerland: Author.

United States Breastfeeding Committee (USBC). (2001). *Protecting, promoting, supporting breastfeeding in the United States: A national agenda.* Rockville, MD: U.S. Department of Health and Human Services, Health Resources and Services Administration, Maternal and Child Health Bureau.

Wight, N. (2003). Survey of neonatologists: Use of human milk (Abstract No. P21). *Academy of Breastfeeding Medicine News & Views,* 9, 32–33.

World Health Assembly. (2008, May 24). *Infant and young child nutrition: Biennial progress report* (WHA61.20). Geneva, Switzerland: WHO.

World Health Organization (WHO). (1981). *The international code of marketing of breast-milk substitutes.* Geneva, Switzerland: Author. Retrieved June 25, 2009, from http://www.who.int/nutrition/publications/code_english.pdf

World Health Organization (WHO). (1998). *Evidence for the ten steps to successful breastfeeding* (WHO/CHD/98.9). Geneva, Switzerland: Author.

APPENDIX 16-1

Ten Steps for a Community Human Milk Bank

Community human milk banks require policies and procedures to ensure that operations will be conducted according to certain standards. The 10 steps presented here mirror the Ten Steps to Successful Breastfeeding that are the basis for the Baby-Friendly Hospital Initiative and have been modified from those Steps (UNICEF/WHO, 1989).

SUMMARY OF POLICIES

Every community donor milk bank will complete the following steps:

Step 1: Maintain written policies on the operation of a community-based donor human milk bank that are routinely communicated to all milk bank staff.

Step 2: Train all milk bank staff in skills necessary to implement these policies.

Step 3: Inform all pregnant and postpartum women in the community about donor milk banking and the importance of becoming a donor.

Step 4: Educate healthcare providers about the benefits and use of donor milk for sick or ill patients in the absence of mothers' own milk.

Step 5: Assist mothers in becoming donors by providing lactation support services to help them establish and maintain an abundant milk supply for their own infants.

Step 6: Assist mothers in expressing milk in safe, clean ways.

Step 7: Use evidence-based standardized guidelines for the collection, intake, storage, processing, shipping, and dispensing of donor human milk while maintaining confidentiality of the donor.

Step 8: Participate in a standardized quality assurance process and contribute data for system-wide research.

Step 9: Practice in an evidence-based manner compatible with ethical standards and avoid conflicts of interest.

Step 10: Establish working relationships with all members of the community to support and maintain a community donor milk bank.

DEFINITIONS

Community Human Milk Bank

A not-for-profit organization established for the purpose of screening human milk donors and assisting them in establishing and maintaining a milk supply, collecting their milk, and overseeing the transport of collected milk to a processing facility. The community human milk bank participates in education of the public and healthcare providers about the benefits of donated human milk and its appropriate uses.

Donor Milk

Milk that is voluntarily expressed and given without remuneration to the milk bank by women who have milk supplies in excess of their own infant's needs.

Cleaning of Biologic Equipment

Equipment that is used in the collection of donated milk, such as breast pumps, does not need to be sterilized but is expected to be cleaned in a dishwasher or by hand. If equipment will be washed by hand, a nonsudsing, cationic detergent that is easily rinsed and does not leave a residue on the surfaces of the equipment should be supplied by the milk bank and used by the donor.

Human Milk Preparations

Fresh raw milk: Milk stored continuously at approximately 4°C.

Fresh frozen milk: Fresh raw milk that has been frozen and held at approximately –20°C.

Preterm milk: Milk that is expressed within the first month of lactation by a mother who delivers an infant at or earlier than 36 weeks' gestation.

Prospectively collected milk: Milk that is collected in an ongoing fashion in standard containers provided by the milk bank using standard protocols by donors after they have been screened and enrolled in the community human milk banking program.

Retrospectively collected milk: Milk that has been collected and stored in nonstandard containers prior to the mother enrolling and becoming a milk donor.

KEY PERSONNEL

Community human milk banks shall be governed by the board of directors of the nonprofit organization. The board of directors is responsible for appointing a medical director and a milk bank coordinator.

Medical Director

The medical director shall be a licensed physician who shall oversee the implementation of procedures and protocols and provide consultation with milk bank personnel when questions arise. The medical director will also be the liaison for the milk bank to the medical community.

Milk Bank Coordinator

The person serving as the milk bank coordinator shall have training, experience, and lactation expertise deemed suitable by the medical director and the milk bank board of directors. Clinical duties shall include the planning, development, implementation, and evaluation of the administrative, educational, and clinical lactation services of the milk bank.

Advisory Panel

All community human milk banks shall have a panel of consultants in various specialties whose expertise can be consulted when problems arise. These specialists *must* come from neonatology/pediatrics, lactation, and microbiology/infectious diseases. Additional consultants may be drawn from the following specialties: nursing, immunology, pharmacology, nutrition, public health, obstetrics, pathology, food technology (i.e., dairy industry), law, and marketing.

STEP 1

Maintain written policies on the operation of a community-based donor human milk bank that are routinely communicated to all milk bank staff.

Policy 1.1

Title

Development of a policy manual.

Purpose

To provide guidelines for operation of a community donor milk bank (DMB).

Supportive Data

The World Health Organization (1998) documents the need for written policies to effect change and sustain it. Written policies and the accompanying protocols and procedures act as a road map for the activities of an organization.

Rationale

Written policies and procedures guide an organization and enable consistent, evidence-based practice. Updating policies with new evidence-based information as it becomes available is vital to protecting, promoting, and supporting breastfeeding and donor milk banking. Following established and agreed-upon policies and procedures protects employees against liability.

Scope

The policy applies to all DMB personnel including (but not limited to) the medical director, the milk bank coordinator, staff, and volunteers.

Policy 1.1

The milk bank coordinator should develop a written, evidence-based policy manual that addresses all the steps in this document and protects mothers from the promotion of human milk substitutes.

Elements of the policy manual

Milk bank policies should include (but not be limited to):

Administrative:

- Organization of the milk bank
- Funding sources
- Bookkeeping protocols
- Record-keeping protocols
- Shipping of milk to the central processing facility
- Establishment of working relationships with other organizations in the community
- Training of milk bank staff

Donor related:

- Assistance to mothers in becoming donors
- Assistance to donors with lactation problems
- Standards for donor screening
- Education of donors on collection methods
- Labeling of donated milk
- Procedures for transporting milk
- Acceptance of milk from nonretrospective donors
- Ethical conduct and use of proprietary materials

Equipment related:

- Evidence-based use of gadgets and devices
- Maintenance of electric breast pumps
- Loaning of electric breast pumps to donors
- Standards for storing donated milk

Staff functions:

- Education of pregnant women in the community
- Distribution of educational materials
- Education of healthcare providers
- Education of donors in use of electric breast pumps

Procedure 1.1.1
Write policies that address each of the issues herein.

Procedure 1.1.2
Attach supporting articles and reports to each policy.

Procedure 1.1.3
Place the policy manual in a location that is easily accessible to all staff as a reference during working hours.

Procedure 1.1.4
Communicate the policy regularly to new employees during orientation and training and at other times as determined by the milk bank coordinator.

Procedure 1.1.5
Review the policy manual every 2 years, incorporating new scientific research, using interdisciplinary group processes to revise old policies and create new evidence-based ones.

STEP 2

Train all milk bank staff in skills necessary to implement these policies.

Policies 2.1–2.6

Title

Staff training.

Purpose

To ensure that all staff members are appropriately trained in evidence-based methods for helping mothers and for running the community milk bank.

Supportive Data

Progress towards implementation of policies can occur only through adequate training of staff (DHHS, 2000b; USBC, 2001; WHO, 1998).

Rationale

Adequate training of staff will promote better interfacing with donors and community organizations. Consistent messages will be given with adequate staff training, provided the policies reflect evidence-based practice.

Scope

These policies pertain to all DMB personnel including (but not limited to) the medical director, the milk bank coordinator, staff, and volunteers.

Policy 2.1

The policy should be regularly communicated to new employees during orientation and training as determined by the milk bank coordinator.

Procedure 2.1.1
Current policies and procedures are placed in new employee orientation packets, and employees are trained in these policies as they begin work at the community milk bank.

Policy 2.2

The milk bank coordinator should assess staff training needs and design, implement and evaluate appropriate training.

Policy 2.3

The milk bank coordinator should train all paid staff and volunteers and annually review skills of each person working in/for the milk bank.

Policy 2.4

Competency-based training for milk bank staff should be conducted.

Procedure 2.4.1
Staff shall demonstrate competencies required to maintain quality control of the milk, both during orientation and annually.

Policy 2.5

The milk bank coordinator should assess customer service/interpersonal communication skills of staff members.

Procedure 2.5.1
Training and assessment should include (but not be limited to):

a. Use of devices and gadgets as described in the policy and procedure manual.
b. Use of devices and gadgets as described in the milk bank's code of ethics.
c. Communication skills.
d. Conflicts of interest (including but not limited to: brand name loyalties, free gifts, solicitations by equipment/detail staff and vendors) as mandated by Policy No. 9.

Policy 2.6

The milk bank coordinator should develop job descriptions for all staff positions, including volunteers.

STEP 3

Inform all pregnant and postpartum women in the community about donor milk banking and the importance of becoming a donor.

Policies 3.1–3.2

Title

Prenatal education for women.

Purpose

To educate pregnant women and mothers of newborn infants about the benefits of breastfeeding and human milk and the importance of becoming a milk donor.

Supportive Data

Mothers are very willing to assist other mothers in difficult situations when a baby's nutritional status is at risk. Knowledge of milk banking services in the community is essential for maintaining a good supply of donors. Presence of community milk banking services promotes the importance of breastfeeding.

Rationale

By helping to increase the number of pregnant women who are knowledgeable about the importance of breastfeeding, we can increase the incidence of breastfeeding and help achieve the nation's initiation goals as well as increase the number of donors (DHHS, 2000a; WHO, 1998).

Scope

These policies apply to all DMB personnel including (but not limited to) the medical director, the milk bank coordinator, staff, and volunteers.

Policy 3.1

The milk bank staff should work with breastfeeding support groups, local and state maternal and child health agencies, and hospitals to inform pregnant women about human milk and becoming a donor to a milk bank.

Procedure 3.1.1
Distribute printed materials in obstetric and family practice offices, hospital clinics, and public health clinics informing mothers prenatally about the importance of breastfeeding and how to become a donor.

Procedure 3.1.2
Network with childbirth instructors as well as physicians, midwives, and nurse practitioners, and prepare materials and presentations about donor milk banking.

Procedure 3.1.3
Develop a display and publicity materials suitable for exhibits at health fairs, county fairs, and shopping malls. Participate as an exhibitor during local events.

Policy 3.2

The milk bank staff should work with breastfeeding support groups, local and state maternal and child health agencies, and hospitals to inform *post-partum* women about human milk and becoming a donor to a milk bank.

Procedure 3.2.1
Provide materials in hospital information packets informing new mothers of the opportunity to donate milk and how to go about becoming a donor.

Procedure 3.2.2
Network with NICU staff such as dietitians, nurse practitioners, lactation consultants/counselors, and neonatologists to provide them with information.

Procedure 3.2.3
Collaborate with La Leche League and other mother/baby support groups in the community to recruit donors and milk bank volunteers.

Procedure 3.2.4
Collaborate with WIC and other health agencies that see new mothers to encourage them to become donors and volunteers to the milk bank.

Procedure 3.2.5
Collaborate with lactation consultant associations and breastfeeding task forces.

Procedure 3.2.6
Maintain public awareness of donor milk banking in the community through public service announcements and other media contacts.

STEP 4

Educate healthcare providers about the benefits and use of donor milk for sick or ill patients in the absence of mothers' own milk.

Policy 4.1

Title

Education of health professionals.

Purpose

To educate healthcare providers, especially neonatologists and pediatricians, and other healthcare professionals about community human milk banks. Provide educational opportunities for healthcare organizations, including insurance companies, and mothers regarding the benefits of banked donor milk, its availability, and the prescription process.

Supportive Data

One of the most significant barriers to use of donor milk is the lack of knowledge of healthcare providers. As prescribers, they are the gatekeepers for use of donor milk. As healthcare providers, they also have intimate knowledge of both donors and the donors' infants and can be a useful resource for donor referrals as well as determining the appropriateness of a specific donor (Arnold, 2005).

Rationale

Through education of healthcare providers, including VNA and WIC clinics, the donor base will increase, as will the use of donor milk for sick and ill infants.

Scope

This policy applies to the medical director, the milk bank coordinator, and selected milk bank staff.

Policy 4.1

The milk bank should distribute evidence-based educational materials for healthcare professionals to inform them of the benefits of banked donor milk, its availability, and the prescription process.

Procedure 4.1.1
Present in-service demonstrations/speeches/materials to hospitals and healthcare providers, especially neonatologists and pediatricians, about the benefits of banked donor milk, the possible/potential clinical uses of banked donor milk, and how to access donor milk.

Procedure 4.1.2
Distribute business cards and informational brochures on a regular basis, as a reminder of the availability of donor milk in the community and to assist them in contacting the milk bank and in prescribing donor milk. Distribution should include, but not be limited to:

Physicians (especially those in NICUs, PICUs and pediatric specialties such as gastroenterology)
WIC (nutrition education) clinics

Health departments
Nurse practitioners
Dietitians, especially those in NICUs and PICUs
Family planning centers

STEP 5

Assist mothers in becoming donors by helping them establish and maintain an abundant milk supply for their own infants.

Policies 5.1–5.2

Title

Assisting donors and other mothers with lactation problems.

Purpose

To provide support and assist donors and other mothers with lactation problems. Assisting donors and others in this manner will increase the pool of potential donors and increase the duration of donation.

Supportive Data

Proactive support works best for new mothers. Anticipating periods when problems or questions may arise and addressing them in a proactive and anticipatory manner will help instill confidence in the mother and prolong duration of breastfeeding. Mothers who experience difficulties with breastfeeding may feel that they need to stop breastfeeding. If a knowledgeable support person helps resolve these problems or helps prevent them from occurring in the first place, mothers do not feel the need to stop breastfeeding.

Rationale

Assisting donors in resolving lactation problems promotes breastfeeding success, increases the duration of breastfeeding to better approximate the surgeon general's goals for duration of breastfeeding, and will ensure a continued milk supply and continued donation of clean milk to the milk bank.

Scope

These policies apply to all DMB personnel including (but not limited to) the medical director, the milk bank coordinator, staff, and volunteers.

Policy 5.1

The milk bank should provide lactation services to help donors and other mothers with breastfeeding problems.

Procedure 5.1.1
The milk bank employs certified lactation counselors who practice in an evidence-based manner.

Procedure 5.1.2
The milk bank assures comprehensive lactation counseling services in the community to overcome breastfeeding problems, maintain milk supply, and increase breastfeeding duration.

Procedure 5.1.3
The milk bank staff assures frequent, regular, and proactive contact with donors to prevent breastfeeding problems and to encourage ongoing milk donations.

Procedure 5.1.4
Records are kept of every phone call or other contact, either face-to-face or e-mail, made to/by donors and documented in the donor's file.

Policy 5.2

The milk bank staff should provide evidence-based lactation support services to donors who are having breastfeeding difficulties.

Procedure 5.2.1
If providing direct lactation services, staff of the milk bank should contact donors at a minimum of every 2 weeks to determine the need for support and to encourage donations.

Procedure 5.2.2
Milk bank staff providing direct lactation services should document every contact with donors.

Procedure 5.2.3
Gadgets and devices used to facilitate solutions to breastfeeding problems should be evidence-based and used in accordance with the manufacturer's instructions.

Procedure 5.2.4
Each gadget and device used to resolve breastfeeding problems will have a policy and procedure for its use, and safety and efficacy studies will be attached to each policy (Arnold, 2003; Arnold & Blair, 2007).

Procedure 5.2.5
Milk bank staff will not exceed their scope of practice when helping mothers resolve breastfeeding problems. (See also Policy 9.2)

Procedure 5.2.6
Milk bank staff will refer to the appropriate healthcare provider when a diagnosis is required or when the skills required exceed the staff competencies and scope of practice. (See also Policy 9.3)

STEP 6

Assist mothers in expressing milk in safe, clean ways.

Policy 6.1–6.2

Title

Maintaining a pump depot.

Purpose

To provide each donor with an appropriate method of milk expression, either by teaching them manual expression or by providing an appropriate electric breast pump for expressing their milk. This shows support for their breastfeeding and milk donation.

Supportive Data

Facilitating donation by supplying proper instruction in manual expression techniques or through provision of an efficient electric breast pump will encourage women to continue to breastfeed their own babies longer as well as to continue donating.

Rationale

Many women find that manual expression is a very efficient and effective method of expressing milk. It also provides women with a basic comfort level and knowledge of the feel of their breasts so that they are more apt to recognize changes that might indicate a disease. Access to rental quality pumps will help donors maximize their milk donation. Efficient expression will help to maintain adequate milk supplies and women will breastfeed for longer if they achieve greater success, thus meeting the surgeon general's goals (DHHS, 2000a).

Scope

These policies apply to DMB personnel including the milk bank coordinator, staff, and volunteers.

Policy 6.1

Milk bank staff will all be able to teach mothers the art of manual expression using standard, published protocols.

Policy 6.2

The milk bank will maintain a supply of rental grade electric breast pumps and spare parts to assist donors in supplying their milk to the milk bank.

Procedure 6.2.1
Donors will be provided (by loan, rental, or gift) electric breast pumps for the duration of the donation period to assist them in providing donor milk. Milk banks will set criteria for eligibility of pump loans/donations. No donor shall be denied access to a rental grade pump for inability to pay.

Procedure 6.2.2
Donors will be provided with a demonstration and education on use of the pump, how to assemble and disassemble the kit, and cleaning protocols. A return demonstration is expected.

STEP 7

Use evidence-based, standardized guidelines for the collection, intake, storage, processing, shipping, and dispensing of donor human milk while maintaining confidentiality of the donor.

Policies 7.1–7.12

Title

Standards for donor screening, milk collection, processing, storage and handling, and dispensing of donated milk.

Purpose

To increase the safety of donor milk through the use of standard guidelines for donor milk banking.

Supportive Data

Guidelines for the Establishment and Operation of a Donor Human Milk Bank (HMBANA, 2008) have been developed with input from various experts at the Centers for Disease Control, the Food and Drug Administration, and the Infectious Disease Committee of the American Academy of Pediatrics. The *Guidelines* are reviewed and revised biannually to maintain the highest standards of safety and quality of donor milk. Other countries also have established guidelines and legislation, in some cases to regulate the process of donor milk banking (UKAMB, 2003). Additional resources on the transmission of infectious disease, in particular through organ and tissue transplants, can be found in the most recent edition of the AAP *2006 Red Book on Infectious Disease* (2006) and the CDC (1994). A helpful, practical guide to starting a milk bank can be obtained through HMBANA (Flatau & Brady, 2006).

Rationale

Minimizing the perception of risk of disease transmission is an important factor in getting physicians to prescribe and parents to demand clinical use of banked donor milk. Risk reduction is accomplished by adhering to strict donor screening guidelines as well as storing and handling milk safely. Quality of milk is also better preserved when storage and handling guidelines are strictly followed.

Scope

All DMB personnel including (but not limited to) the medical director, the milk bank coordinator, staff, and volunteers.

Policy 7.1

The milk bank should follow evidence-based standards for donor screening and milk storage and handling to ensure quality control of the milk.

Procedure 7.1.1
Definition of a Donor: Acceptable donors shall be healthy, lactating women who do not use nicotine products. Use of certain medications is acceptable in prospective donors. See the most recent HMBANA *Guidelines* for a current list.

Procedure 7.1.2
Donor Exclusions (based on clinical issues unique to human milk and infants and the American Association of Blood Banks standards, 2006): The

most recent edition of HMBANA *Guidelines* or other evidence-based standards of donor milk banking should be consulted. Exclusions include:

- Receipt of a blood transfusion or blood products, except Rho(D) immune globulin, within the last 12 months
- Receipt of an organ or tissue transplant within the last 12 months
- Ears or other body parts pierced, tattooing, permanent make-up applied with a needle, or an accidental stick with a contaminated needle within the last 12 months[1]
- Regular use of more than 2 ounces of hard liquor or its equivalent in 24 hours (IOM, 1991)
- Regular use of over-the-counter medications or systemic prescriptions
- Regular use of megadose vitamins and/or herbal products used as medication, including vitamin-herb combinations
- Total vegetarians (vegans)
- Use of tobacco products
- Use of illegal drugs
- Chronic infections (e.g., HIV, HTLV, malaria, active TB), a history of hepatitis B or C, or a history of cancer other than nonmelanoma skin cancer or cervical cancer *in situ*
- In the last 12 months had a sexual partner who is at risk for HIV, HTLV, or hepatitis (including anyone with hemophilia or anyone who has used a needle for injection of illegal or nonprescription drugs)
- In the last 12 months had a sexual partner who in the last 12 months has had tattoos, permanent make-up applied with needles, ear or other body parts pierced, or been accidentally stuck with a contaminated needle[1]
- Ever received human pituitary-derived growth hormone, dura mater (brain covering) graft, bovine insulin, or had a family history of Creutzfeldt-Jakob disease
- Since 1990, spent time that adds up to a total of 5 years in Europe (includes Albania, Austria, Belgium, Bosnia-Herzegovina, Bulgaria, Croatia, Czech Republic, Denmark, Finland, France, Germany, Greece, Hungary, Republic of Ireland, Italy, Liechtenstein, Luxembourg, Macedonia, Netherlands, Norway, Poland, Portugal, Romania, Slovak Republic, Slovenia, Spain, Sweden, Switzerland, United Kingdom, and Federated Republic of Yugoslavia
- Incarceration for more than 72 consecutive hours

---

[1] Needle acupuncture with sterile disposable needles shall not disqualify a donor.

- Recent return from service in Iraq or Afghanistan or recent international travel to areas of health concern should be reviewed by the medical director on a case-by-case basis.

Procedure 7.1.3
Temporary Donor Disqualifications: Active donors shall be temporarily disqualified under the following conditions:

- During any infection of any member of the household
- During any acute infection, including clinical mastitis, and monilial and fungal infections of the nipple or breast
- During the 4-week period following a case of rubella or varicella (chicken pox) in the household (starting from when the lesions crust over)
- During a reactivation of latent infection with herpes simplex virus (HSV) or varicella zoster of the breast or thorax (starting from when the lesions crust over)
- During the 12-hour period following consumption of alcohol (hard liquor, beer, wine)
- During the 30 days after the donor herself or anyone with whom she has household contact has received the smallpox vaccine
- During consumption of any over-the-counter or prescription medication, including vitamins, homeopathic remedies, and herbs, at the discretion of the milk bank coordinator

Policy 7.2

The milk bank should implement evidence-based procedures for screening prospective donors, documenting all donor contacts, collecting data on donors, and keeping all donor information confidential according to HIPAA regulations (e.g., individual ID numbers should be kept in a log book under lock and key).

Procedure 7.2.1
Log all phone calls from prospective donors seeking lactation help. Information collected should include whether the phone call led to a donor enrollment; the reasons for rejecting a potential donor; type of information/assistance the donor required; etc.

Procedure 7.2.2
Each donor contact must be documented, including the information given.

Procedure 7.2.3
Conduct initial donor screening to determine preliminary donor eligibility over the phone.

Procedure 7.2.4
Donors shall complete the full screening questionnaire. Donor intake forms should be segregated according to whether the milk has been collected retrospectively, with additional questions about procedures used for the collection of this milk. Personal interviews are encouraged for this process, barring geographical constraints.

Procedure 7.2.5
The milk bank assigns each donor a unique identification/code number to maintain confidentiality. Donor codes are assigned in numerical order of intake of donors. The code book is kept in a locked file according to HIPAA regulations.

Procedure 7.2.6
Donors sign consent forms allowing primary care physicians to share information with the milk bank about the donor's health and her infant's health according to HIPAA regulations. Separate consent forms will be signed for both the donor's healthcare provider and the baby's.

Procedure 7.2.7
Donors acknowledge that, once donated, the milk becomes the property of the milk bank and will

a. be used for research purposes if it does not meet the criteria for clinical use.
b. not be returned to the donor.

Procedure 7.2.8
Complete donor records include, but are not limited to:

Preliminary intake form
Donor intake consent form
Donor screening form
Lab results for serum screening
Pediatrician consent form
Donor's health care provider's consent form
Release of medical information form
Log of donations
Log of contacts
Documentation of lactation support
Documentation of information provided

Policy 7.3

Blood is drawn for serum screening of donors by either a licensed staff member of the milk bank during the screening visit to the milk bank or by other licensed legally qualified individuals (e.g., Red Cross Blood Services, the local blood bank, the hospital laboratory, or an independent regulated [FDA approved] laboratory).

Procedure 7.3.1
All mothers are given a written explanation of why blood testing is important for all donors and asked to read it before consenting and signing permission for a blood test.

Procedure 7.3.2
Serum screening should include at a minimum the following tests:

- HIV-1 and -2
- HTLV
- Hepatitis B
- Hepatitis C
- Syphilis

Additional tests shall be added as conditions warrant.

Procedure 7.3.3
Information about positive blood tests (those confirmed positive on retesting) will be sent to the milk bank coordinator, who will inform the medical director of the milk bank. The medical director will contact the donor's primary care provider.

Policy 7.4

Ongoing prospective donors will be preferred over retrospective donors, but both are acceptable.

Procedure 7.4.1
Milk that has been stored for less than 3 months in a home freezer may be retrospectively collected on a one-time donation basis, provided that the donor meets all screening criteria.

Procedure 7.4.2
Milk from mothers of preterm infants who have died should *always* be accepted to assist with the grieving process. It should only be used clinically if the mother completes the screening process and meets the criteria for a donor.

Procedure 7.4.3
Mothers of infants who have died of SIDS or accidental causes should be allowed to donate to assist with the grieving process.

Policy 7.5

Donors should be given written instructions for expressing milk and adequate supplies for collecting breast milk.

Procedure 7.5.1
Written instructions for prospectively collected milk should include, but not be limited to, the following information:

Before Each Expression

- Wash your hands well for at least 30 seconds with soapy water, using a nail brush on your fingernails. Dry your hands on a clean paper towel.
- Rinse your breasts with warm clear water, blotting them dry with a clean paper towel.
- If using a pump, assemble your clean pump accessory kit after washing your hands.
- Express directly into the bottles provided for you by the milk bank, by screwing them onto the pump collecting kit.
- Use a new collection bottle for each expression, even if you have one that is only partially full.
- Use only coded collection bottles provided by the milk bank. Should you require more bottles, please call the milk bank to request them.
- Keep bottle lids clean while you are pumping. Place face down on a clean paper towel.

While Expressing

- Pumping effectiveness may be increased by pausing in the middle of your pumping session, doing gentle breast massage for a few minutes, then resuming pumping.
- When doing breast massage, be careful not to touch your nipples.
- If manually expressing, collect the milk in a clean bowl before pouring it into the containers provided.
- It is not necessary to fill a collecting bottle; however, do not overfill the bottle. Fill collecting bottles only to the 4-oz. line (fill in appropriate number depending on the container used) to allow for expansion of the milk during freezing.

- Change bottles if necessary, adding new ones as they become full.
- Do not reopen a collecting bottle to add more milk. Use a bottle only once.

After Expression

- Pour manually expressed milk into the sterile bottles provided.
- Unscrew the bottle of milk from the pump accessory kit and place the lid on it.
- Dry off the bottle if any milk has spilled onto the sides of the bottle.
- Mark the date of expression with a waterproof marker on the preprinted label with your donor ID number on the container.

Freezing Instructions

- Place the collected milk in the freezer immediately after collection.
- Place containers in the freezer away from the door where they will warm up slightly every time the door is opened.
- Place the freezer thermometer supplied by the milk bank in your freezer and adjust the controls to maintain as close to –20°C as possible.

Washing Your Pump Parts

- Rinse the parts of your pump that touch the milk in cold water, then wash thoroughly in hot, soapy water, rinsing them at least twice.
- Washing pump parts in a dishwasher is also an excellent way of cleaning your pump kits.
- Let pump parts dry on a clean paper towel.

Transporting Your Milk to the Milk Bank

- Bring your milk to the milk bank or arrange for a pick-up within 14 days of the previous milk pick-up or delivery of supplies. If delivering your milk, please call ahead to make sure that someone will be there to receive your milk.
- To transport your milk, place the milk in the shipping container supplied by the milk bank or a standard cooler. Wrap bottles in towels or plastic bubble wrap to help maintain frozen state if being transported short distances. If being shipped, follow the milk bank instructions for packing milk.

If You Have Questions

- Contact the milk bank.
- If you, your baby, or someone else in the house is sick, please contact the milk bank.
- If you take medications (including herbal preparations such as mother's milk tea) within 12 hours of pumping, do not save the milk for the milk bank.

- If you drink alcohol, do not pump for the milk bank for at least 12 hours.
- If you have a yeast infection on your nipples, your baby has thrush, or you have a fever blister, call the milk bank and do not donate milk until the infection is healed.
- If you are temporarily not saving your milk to donate, continue to pump. This keeps your milk supply even and your breasts comfortable. Your milk is fine for your baby.

Procedure 7.5.2
At the screening visit to the milk bank, the milk bank coordinator shall assess each donor's requirements for breastmilk collection bottles to cover a two-week period and determine the appropriate number to dispense to the donor. Resupply shall be determined based on the individual needs of the donor.

Procedure 7.5.3
Donors shall be provided with the following supplies:

- A shipping container
- Breastmilk collection bottles
- Preprinted labels with unique ID code on them
- One freezer thermometer

Policy 7.6

Milk collection procedures shall consist of the following:

Procedure 7.6.1
Mothers will wash their hands thoroughly with soap and water and dry with clean paper towels before beginning to express milk. Use of waterless hand cleaners is acceptable.

Procedure 7.6.2
If a mother chooses to use manual expression to obtain milk, milk should be expressed into a clean, wide-mouthed container and then poured into the containers provided by the milk bank. *Clean* is defined as having been washed in hot, soapy water, rinsed thoroughly and allowed to air dry or as having been washed in a dishwasher.

Note: Milk banks should provide a standard low-sudsing detergent for cleaning equipment and pump parts.

Note: Hypochlorite is not an appropriate cleaning solution.

Procedure 7.6.3
Clean kits or pumps will be used each time milk is pumped. *Clean* is defined as having been washed in hot, soapy water, rinsed thoroughly and allowed to air dry or as having been washed in a dishwasher. Kits/pumps need not be sterilized after each use.

Note: Milk banks should provide a standard low-sudsing detergent for cleaning equipment and pump parts.

Note: Hypochlorite is not an appropriate cleaning solution.

Procedure 7.6.4
If a mother is pumping her milk, collecting bottles supplied by the milk bank should be attached directly to the flange of the kit, avoiding the necessity of pouring the milk into a different container. If a mother wishes to express the milk in one breast while nursing on the contralateral breast, pump kits should be set up as single kits. Breast shells should not be used to passively collect milk from the breast that is not being actively nursed, as this milk is lower in fat content.

Procedure 7.6.5
Mothers should write the date and time of expression on the preprinted and coded collecting bottle label in indelible marker.

Procedure 7.6.6
Milk should be frozen immediately after expression.

Procedure 7.6.7
Layering of milk from several expressions in the same bottle should not be done.

Policy 7.7

Milk should be transported to the milk bank every 2 weeks at a minimum; more frequently if necessary.

Procedure 7.7.1
Upon pickup or delivery of a batch of milk, the donor signs a form verifying that she has followed the instructions for maintaining milk quality and safety (i.e., she has taken no drugs or medications, that the milk is undiluted and uncontaminated, and that the milk is hers).

Procedure 7.7.2
If the milk is picked up at the donor's residence, the donor should place the collecting bottles in the shipping container provided by the milk bank in the

presence of the employee/volunteer. Bottles are transported to the milk bank as expeditiously as possible.

Procedure 7.7.3
Any milk bank volunteer may pick up milk from a donor, or the donor may deliver the milk to the milk bank herself so that the chain of custody remains intact.

Procedure 7.7.4
Upon arrival at the milk bank, the number of ounces donated should be logged in the donor's file. Estimates of the number of ounces can be made by eyeballing the number of ounces of milk in the containers, or by weighing the containers and then subtracting the tare weight of the container itself (multiplied by the number of containers).

Procedure 7.7.5
Each bottle of donated milk is visually inspected. Bottles are rejected if they show any of the following:

Damage to the lid
Damage to the bottle
Breastmilk that has completely thawed and become liquid
Obvious impurities/debris in the milk

Procedure 7.7.6
All milk bank employees and staff shall wear gloves when handling bottles of milk and pasteurizing.

Policy 7.8

Freezers should meet evidence-based standards for human milk banks.

Procedure 7.8.1
Milk bank freezers should maintain –20°C or lower, have manual defrost, and provide convenient access. (Upright freezers may be easier to access.) Allowable latitude for milk bank freezers is –21° to –18°C.

Procedure 7.8.2
Freezers should be monitored by means of external recording thermometers and a temperature-sensitive alarm. Alarms that include automatic phone dialing devices are suggested.

Procedure 7.8.3
Freezers should be connected to an emergency power back-up system.

Procedure 7.8.4
Freezers should be installed so that the door closes automatically; e.g., they should be tipped slightly backward.

Procedure 7.8.5
Freezers used for donated milk should be in a secured area and must be locked during hours when the milk bank is not open.

Procedure 7.8.6
Access to keys to freezers should be restricted to a designated number of milk bank employees.

Procedure 7.8.7
Freezers should be calibrated monthly by milk bank staff to ensure that they maintain their ability to keep consistent low temperatures. Records of freezer temperatures should be logged and saved.

Procedure 7.8.8
Freezers used for milk storage should not be used for any other purpose.

Policy 7.9

Donated milk coming from out of state or a great distance should be shipped according to milk bank protocols.

Procedure 7.9.1
The donor will notify the milk bank that milk will be shipped on a specific date so that someone will be available to receive the milk in the milk bank.

Procedure 7.9.2
Donated milk should be shipped frozen, using containers and carriers provided by the milk bank.

Procedure 7.9.3
Donated milk should be shipped overnight by guaranteed shipping according to milk bank protocols.

Policy 7.10

Quality control: bacteriology.

Procedure 7.10.1
As milk is thawed for use, a sample of each donor's milk should be checked for bacteriological quality prior to pasteurization. Milk exceeding 10^5 CFU/ml shall be discarded and not used.

Procedure 7.10.2
Donors shall be notified if their milk exceeds bacteriological standards and reeducated with regard to proper collection techniques.

Procedure 7.10.3
A random sample of the batch postpasteurization shall be tested for bacteriological quality. Milk must show no bacterial growth to be acceptable for clinical distribution to recipients.

Procedure 7.10.4
Standard bacteriological testing shall be used.

Policy 7.11

Pasteurization

Procedure 7.11.1
All milk shall be pasteurized prior to being dispensed unless there is a medical need on the part of the recipient for raw (unpasteurized) milk.

Procedure 7.11.2
The method of pasteurization shall be an evidence-based method that causes the least amount of damage to the milk while at the same time assuring the maximum level of safety.

Procedure 7.11.3
Milk from several different donors shall be thawed and pooled to form a batch for pasteurization.

Procedure 7.11.4
When pasteurization is complete, a random sample of the batch will be taken for bacteriological analysis.

Procedure 7.11.5
A sample bottle from each batch will be analyzed for nutritional content.

Procedure 7.11.6
Labels for bottles in each batch shall be printed with:

- The milk bank name

- The unique batch number
- The time and date of pasteurization
- The nutritional content contained in each bottle in the batch

Procedure 7.11.7
Immediately after labeling, bottles shall be placed in the freezer in a section set aside for milk that is pasteurized but not ready for distribution.

Policy 7.12

Distribution of banked donor milk.

Procedure 7.12.1
Milk shall *only* be dispensed upon receipt of a prescription.

Procedure 7.12.2
Pasteurized milk shall *only* be dispensed once bacteriological testing has determined that there is no bacterial growth.

Procedure 7.12.3
Raw milk shall *only* be dispensed after both the physician and the recipient's guardian (or recipient himself, if an adult) sign consent forms acknowledging the risks of using raw milk.

Procedure 7.12.4
No recipient with a medical need for donor milk shall be refused access to donor milk for inability to pay the processing fee.

Procedure 7.12.5
Milk bank personnel shall work with the prescriber, the recipient, and the insurer to ensure reimbursement for banked donor milk.

STEP 8

Participate in a standardized quality assurance process and contribute data for system-wide research.

Policies 8.1–8.4

Title

Monitoring quality in the milk banking process.

Purpose

To ensure quality and safety of collection of donor milk and prevention of loss of components.

Supportive Data

Purchasers of care (insurers, employers), accreditation organizations such as The Joint Commission, government agencies involved with the healthcare system, consumers of health care (the public), and healthcare providers all want to be assured of the safety and efficacy of a healthcare service. This assurance comes only with internal and external quality monitoring. Individual milk banks are responsible for internal monitoring for compliance with policies, protocols, and procedures, and the governance of the milk banks is responsible for external oversight (Arnold, 2005; Carey, 2003). Quality control begins with the collection of data and statistics that demonstrate where system weaknesses occur and justify the existence of the service.

Rationale

Reluctance among physicians to prescribe donor milk is highly correlated with concerns about the safety and quality of donated milk. Current milk banking practices do not include self-audits for collecting, storing, processing, and distributing milk, nor is there an organization that provides quality assessment and monitoring for individual milk banks. This lack of quality control does not reassure the prescriber, causes perceptions of elevated risk to patients, and creates an environment of mistrust of donor milk (Arnold, 2005). Data collection is also important to justify the need for the organization to potential funders.

Scope

These policies apply to all DMB personnel including (but not limited to) the medical director, the milk bank coordinator, staff, and volunteers.

Policy 8.1

All community human milk banks will collect data in an ongoing manner. Data collections should include (but not be limited to):

- Number of donors (including number of donors who do not follow through)
- Number of recipients (with breakdown as to age category of recipient)
- Types of diagnoses for recipients

- Outcomes of recipients while on donor milk
- Number of ounces received
- Number of ounces distributed
- Number of ounces discarded and reasons for discarding
- Number of hospitals ordering

Procedure 8.1.1
Statistics will be reported on an annual basis and will become part of the public record.

Policy 8.2

The milk bank coordinator, in conjunction with the board of directors, shall conduct an annual audit of job performance of volunteers and employees.

Policy 8.3

The milk bank coordinator shall conduct an annual audit of policies and procedures and measure compliance with these policies and procedures by personnel.

Policy 8.4

The milk bank coordinator and medical director shall work with the local department of health and state regulatory commissions in the department of health to ensure that the donor milk bank is compliant with all state regulations for tissue banks.

STEP 9

Practice in an evidence-based manner compatible with ethical standards and avoid conflicts of interest.

Policies 9.1–9.3

Title

Sources of funding and supplies: evidence-based support.

Purpose

To create an environment in which donors and milk bank personnel are free of commercial pressures that may create a conflict of interest; and to promote, protect, and support breastfeeding through evidence-based practices that are consistent with donor criteria.

Supportive Data

Breastfeeding is more successful when there are fewer visible signs of commercial influence to undermine a mother's confidence. Funding and supplies for the milk bank's operations must come from grants and donations that are not connected with any industry that violates the International Code of Marketing of Breast-milk Substitutes, in order to remain free of commercial pressure to support the use of formula (see Armstrong & Sokol, 1994).

Use of non–evidence-based solutions to breastfeeding problems during counseling may negatively impact the health of the infant. Similarly, use of non–evidence-based methods to treat various conditions may introduce pathogens capable of compromising infant health. All milk bank personnel need to practice within their scope of practice to avoid legal complications (Arnold & Blair, 2007).

Rationale

In order to promote breastfeeding and help mothers gain confidence in their abilities to produce milk not only for their own infants, but for the infants of other women as well, it is important not to have materials that present conflicting messages and represent a conflict of interest when one is trying to promote human milk as the norm. It is also unethical for staff to be beholden to a commercial company, in particular one company to the exclusion of a competitor. Advertising for a commercial company is not within the job description of the staff of a milk bank. When dealing ethically with donors and recipients, lactation services must be provided in an evidence-based manner and confidentiality must be respected. Practicing evidence-based breastfeeding management also enhances the credibility of the staff of the milk bank and builds respect for the milk bank's work.

Scope

All DMB personnel including (but not limited to) the medical director, the milk bank coordinator, staff, and volunteers.

Policy 9.1

Grants and donations should not be accepted from businesses, commercial entities, or organizations that violate the International Code of Marketing of Breast-milk Substitutes. Examples of acceptable and unacceptable sources of funds are given below.

Acceptable funding sources include, but are not limited to:

- Private foundations that are not connected to the formula industry
- United Way and other community agencies
- Church groups
- Federal, state, county, and municipal agencies
- Private individuals
- Commercial entities that are independent of the formula industry
- Breast pump companies (provided all companies are solicited equally and favoritism for one brand is not shown)

Unacceptable funding sources include, but are not limited to:

- Formula companies
- Formula company research foundations
- Companies manufacturing and advertising feeding bottles and supplies

Policy 9.2

Solutions to breastfeeding problems that are compatible with clinical use of banked donor milk should be developed. Solutions that are incompatible with clinical use of banked donor milk (e.g., use of herbal preparations to increase milk supply) should not be used.

Policy 9.3

Milk bank staff should refer donors to their own healthcare providers if problems are outside the scope of practice of milk bank staff.

Procedure 9.3.1
Work with lactation and medical specialists in the community in a collegial manner, receiving and making referrals when appropriate.

STEP 10

Establish working relationships with all members of the community to support and maintain a community donor milk bank.

Policies 10.1–10.2

Title

Community representation and cooperation.

Purpose

To develop collegial working relationships with various members of the community and to develop a cadre of volunteers who will work with the milk bank staff.

Supportive Data

Group process is an important component of change and program development and implementation.

Rationale

Developing good working relationships with community groups and individuals ensures the acceptance of the milk bank in the community. Volunteers, be they board members or office volunteers, are the heart of the milk bank, and one volunteer's good experience leads to others volunteering to do more.

Scope

These policies apply to all DMB personnel including (but not limited to) the medical director, the milk bank coordinator, staff, and volunteers.

Policy 10.1

The board of directors of the milk bank should be interdisciplinary and composed of representatives from community agencies as well as consumer representatives, health professionals, and individuals with needed specific skills such as fund-raising, the law, and public relations.

Procedure 10.1.1
Include representation from community stakeholders on the board of directors of the milk bank.

Policy 10.2

The milk bank should develop a corps of volunteers who are willing to transport milk from collection sites to the milk bank, work in the office, deliver bottles to donors, raise funds, etc.

Procedure 10.2.1

Solicit and train volunteers from the community to do specific jobs for the milk bank, such as:

- Collecting milk from donors or collection sites
- Delivering donor supplies to donors as they need them
- Assisting in calculating milk donated (weighing, tallying number of bottles/ounces) and storing milk in milk bank freezers
- Making up and delivering donor publicity packets to other agencies, physicians' offices, etc., for distribution
- Doing routine office work, such as mailings, thank-you notes to past donors, collating statistics, helping with newsletters, and public relations events
- Assisting in fund-raising events

Procedure 10.2.2

All volunteers having contact with donors must respect donor confidentiality.

REFERENCES

American Academy of Pediatrics, Committee on Infectious Diseases (AAP). (2006). *2006 Red Book* (27th ed.). Elk Grove Village, IL: Author.

American Association of Blood Banks. (2006). *Standards for blood banks and transfusion services*. Arlington, VA: Author.

Arnold, L. D. W. (2003). *Policies and materials for use with nursing mothers*. East Sandwich, MA: The Center for Breastfeeding.

Arnold, L. D. W. (2005). *Donor human milk banking: Creating public health policy in the 21st century*. Doctoral dissertation, Union Institute and University.

Arnold, L. D. W., & Blair, A. C. (2007). *Ethical practice for lactation care providers*. (Unit 12, Lactation Consultant Series Two). Schaumburg, IL: La Leche League International.

Armstrong, H. C., & Sokol, E. (1994). *The international code of marketing of breast-milk substitutes: What it means for mothers and babies world-wide*. Raleigh, NC: International Lactation Consultant Association.

Carey, R. G. (2003). *Improving healthcare with control charts*. Milwaukee, WI: Quality Press.

Centers for Disease Control and Prevention (CDC). (1994). Guidelines for preventing transmission of human immunodeficiency virus through transplantation of human tissue and organs. *Morbidity Mortality Weekly Review*, *43*(RR-8), 1–17.

Department of Health and Human Services (DHHS). (2000a). *Healthy People 2010*. Washington, DC: Author.

Department of Health and Human Services, Office of Women's Health (DHHS). (2000b). *HHS blueprint for action on breastfeeding*. Washington, DC: Author.

Flatau, G., & Brady, S. (2006). *Starting a donor human milk bank: A practical guide*. Raleigh, NC: HMBANA.

Human Milk Banking Association of North America (HMBANA). (2008). *Guidelines for the establishment and operation of a donor human milk bank*. Raleigh, NC: Author.

Institute of Medicine (IOM). (1991). *Nutrition during lactation*. Washington DC: National Academy Press.

UNICEF/WHO. (1989). *Protecting, promoting and supporting breast-feeding: The special role of maternity services*. Geneva, Switzerland: Author.

United Kingdom Association of Milk Banks. (2003). *Guidelines for the establishment and operation of human milk banks in the UK*. London: Author.

United States Breastfeeding Committee (USBC). (2001). *Protecting, promoting, supporting breastfeeding in the United States: A national agenda*. Rockville, MD: U.S. Department of Health and Human Services, Health Resources and Services Administration, Maternal and Child Health Bureau.

World Health Organization (WHO). (1998). *Evidence for the ten steps to successful breastfeeding* (WHO/CHD/98.9). Geneva, Switzerland: Author.

Part V

The Ethics of Human Milk Use in the NICU

seventeen

chapter seventeen

Human Milk in the NICU and the Right to Ethical Care

HUMAN MILK AS A HUMAN RIGHT

The United Nations Conventions and Declarations

United Nations (UN) conventions and declarations have developed and disseminated those human rights that relate to the achievement of "the highest attainable standard of health" (UN, 1966, p. 4) and the right to adequate food (see Arnold, 2006b; Bar-Yam, 2003; Bar-Yam, 2004; Kent, 2004, 2006). These declarations and conventions include the *Universal Declaration of Human Rights* (UN, 1948), the *International Covenant on Economic, Social and Cultural Rights* (UN, 1966), the *Convention on the Elimination of All Forms of Discrimination Against Women* (UN, 1979), the *Convention on the Rights of the Child* (UN, 1989) and *The Right to Adequate Food* (UN, 1999). **Table 17-1** includes summaries of the pertinent sections and articles of these conventions and declarations.

Human rights, by definition, apply to all individuals, unless those rights specifically have been removed by the legal system, e.g., the rights of prisoners. These UN conventions have also delineated that special consideration and protection must be given to the rights of specific populations of individuals such as women and children. These groups have been targeted because of imbalances in power relationships. In many countries, women are considered inferior and have no rights of their own, including the right to own property, determine how their children are raised, or control their reproductive lives. Children, who cannot advocate for themselves, are dependent on

Table 17-1 United Nations Rights and Health Policy Statements Protecting the Right to Human Milk

Document	*Article*	*How It Supports Breastfeeding/ Expressed Breastmilk*	*How It Supports Banked Donor Human Milk*
Universal Declaration of Human Rights (adopted 1948)	25: "Everyone has the right to a standard of living adequate for the health and well-being of himself and of his family, including food . . ." Mothers and children are entitled to special protection, care, and assistance.	Human milk (at breast or expressed) provides health and well-being for all individuals from birth through the first several years of life. Impacts adult health as well.	In the absence of mother's own milk, donor milk provides the same protection and promotion of optimal health, both short- and long-term, for populations at risk.
International Covenant on Economic, Social and Cultural Rights (adopted 1966)	11: Recognizes the "fundamental right of everyone to be free from hunger . . ." 12: *All* individuals have the right to "the highest attainable standard of physical and mental health." Countries should take steps to lower infant mortality rates and increase "healthy development of the child . . ." including assurance of adequate medical services.	A direct relationship between breastfeeding and lower infant mortality rates makes it an integral component in achieving the right to optimal health; e.g., preemies deserve protection from NEC and consequences of NEC.	In the absence of mother's own milk, donor milk can provide definite improvements in health and long-term outcomes.
Convention on the Elimination of All Forms of Discrimination Against Women (adopted 1979)	5: Certain groups require special protection. The ". . . interest of the children is the primordial consideration in all cases."	Optimal nutrition should be a priority through protection, promotion, and support of breast-feeding and use of human milk.	Donor milk becomes an element that needs special protection as part of the child's best interests.

Table 17-1 United Nations Rights and Health Policy Statements Protecting the Right to Human Milk (continued)

Document	*Article*	*How It Supports Breastfeeding/ Expressed Breastmilk*	*How It Supports Banked Donor Human Milk*
Convention on the Rights of the Child (CRC) (adopted 1989)	3: Best interests of the child are primary. 18: Institutions and legislatures should provide assistance in protection of these rights. 24: Recognizes the "right of the child to the enjoyment of the highest attainable standard of health . . ." States will combat malnutrition problems and decrease infant mortality. States specifically that breastfeeding is an activity for the entire society.	Recognizes rights of all children, not just healthy ones. In order for all children to reach the highest attainable standard of health, parents must remedy the situation through breastfeeding to improve outcomes.	Use of banked donor human milk as a remedy; takes on greater significance for sick and premature infants.
The Right to Adequate Food (general comment No. 12) (1999)	Defines what constitutes "adequate food."		

Source: Arnold 2006; Bar-Yam 2003, 2004; Kent 2004, 2006.

parents to advocate for them and care for them in a manner that is in the best interests of the children.

The Right to the Highest Attainable Standard of Health

When applied to premature infants, the right to achieve the highest attainable standard of health means that they should be cared for in a manner that promotes their optimal development, both physical and mental. Optimal development leads to improved health and puts the preterm infant on a level playing field with his born-at-term counterparts. Breastfeeding/provision of breastmilk and other hospital and NICU policies and practices that foster optimal milk supplies are therefore essential to the achievement of each individual preterm infant's highest attainable standard of health. I have provided evidence throughout this book showing that human milk, either mother's own or banked donor milk, achieves better outcomes than formulas when given to preterm infants. Improved outcomes are both short term and long term; in the short term reducing morbidity and mortality especially related to the prevention of NEC and its consequences, and in the long term providing better developmental outcomes for extremely low birth weight babies at 18 months and 30 months of age (Vohr, Poindexter, Dusick, McKinley, Higgins, Langer, et al., 2008; Vohr, Poindexter, Dusick, McKinley, Wright, Langer, et al., 2006). The provision of human milk and an environment supportive of the mother providing her own milk fulfills the obligations of these human rights documents. I have argued elsewhere (2006b) that the use of donor milk will fulfill the obligation of providing for optimal health. A NICU, therefore, that does not provide this environment and give the mother the education and support she needs to succeed in establishing a milk supply and then transitioning to breastfeeding is in violation of the intent of these human rights documents. A NICU that does not have banked donor milk available is also in violation of these rights.

The Right to Adequate Food

The International Covenant on Economic, Social and Cultural Rights (UN, 1999) states that individuals have the "fundamental right to freedom from hunger and malnutrition" (Article 11).

The Merriam-Webster dictionary (1998) gives several definitions of *hunger*. One is the ". . . urgent need for food or a specific nutrient"; another is "a weakened condition brought about by prolonged lack of food" (p. 565). In 1999, the Committee on Economic Social and Cultural Rights of the

UN Economic and Social Council defined what is meant by *adequate food that would prevent hunger and malnutrition* (UN, 1999). The committee stated unequivocally that this right applied to *everyone*. Furthermore it stated that adequate food was "indispensible for the fulfillment of other human rights" and was "inseparable from social justice" (¶ 4). It also pointed out that hunger and malnutrition are not just problems of developing countries, but they are also problems in some of the most economically advantaged countries. The problem arises in *lack of access* to enough nutritious food that will prevent hunger and malnutrition. The clarification statement goes on to say that the right to adequate food should "not be interpreted in a narrow or restrictive sense which equates it with a minimum package of calories, proteins and other specific nutrients" (¶ 6). In order to ensure that food resources are adequate, they must also be sustainable and secure, meaning that they will be available for the long term and accessible, both physically and economically, and that they will be safe.

Consider the case of the preterm infant in this regard. While formula may be considered adequate nutritionally, is it safe and of sufficient quality? Is it free from adverse substances? *Not* if we are concerned about contamination with enterobacteria. *Not* if formula companies have recalls because of missing elements, too much of a specific ingredient, or misleading or inaccurate labeling information. Is it accessible? *Not* if the mother cannot afford enough formula to ensure her infant's optimal nutrition once he is discharged from the hospital.

What about breastfeeding and human milk for the preterm infant in regard to freedom from hunger? Human milk is the ideal food. It is sustainable in that as demand increases, so do most mothers' milk supplies. It is the ultimate in renewable resources and is available economically and physically, as long as the mother is in close proximity. It is also locally produced and in most cases safe for the baby to consume. We have no concerns related to the healthy, term baby getting enough or too much because feeding at the breast is baby led and the baby determines when and how much he will ingest. He determines, for example, how much fat he gets over the course of the day. However, it is different with a preterm infant. When we restrict volume of feedings artificially and feed on a formula-feeding schedule, we are depriving the infant of adequate food. Discussion in the literature of feeding preterm infants more aggressively from the moment of birth provides ammunition for the argument that preterm infants being fed expressed human milk are not being protected adequately from hunger and malnutrition because they are not being fed *enough* human milk.

Conflicting Rights

Kent (2006) asks the question, what happens when the mother's rights conflict with the baby's rights? Most of us agree that mothers have the right to breastfeed. But do babies have the right to be breastfed? Most of us would also agree that mothers should not be forced into breastfeeding when they truly do not want to and some would argue, based on the *Convention on the Rights of the Child* statement that all actions regarding children should be in the "best interests of the child" (UN, 1989, p. 2, Article 3.1) that babies have the right to be breastfed. However, babies are not in positions of power to force an unwilling mother to breastfeed. Kent argues for considering that both mothers and babies should be protected from outside interference in the mother–child relationship. "Outsiders are obligated to refrain from doing anything that might interfere with a mother's freely made and informed decision" (Kent, 2006, p 16). Mothers make their decisions based on the information they have and usually act in what they believe to be the best interests of the child. If they lack information, they act on personal beliefs and feelings rather than hard facts. If they have an abundance of conflicting and nonobjective information, then it is difficult for mothers to make fully informed decisions. If the major source of information is commercially produced information that is biased or inaccurate, women similarly are deprived of enough evidence with which to make an informed decision. Education about the importance of breastfeeding and human milk is therefore critical to the acquisition of adequate food and the prevention of hunger and malnutrition, and mothers in the NICU need to be protected from interference in the flow of evidence-based information.

Who Is Responsible?

In the UN documents, it is "States" (meaning nations) that are mentioned as being responsible for the fulfillment of these rights, since they are the entities that will be enacting legislation, implementing it, and monitoring compliance. However, this does not mean that all others are exempt from participating. Article 20 of the general comments on the right to adequate food states:

> . . . all members of society—individuals, families, local communities, non-governmental organizations, civil society organizations, as well as the private business sector—have responsibilities in the realization of the right to adequate food. The State should provide an environment that facilitates implementation of these responsibilities.

In another section, the document notes that violations of the right to food can occur when other entities are insufficiently regulated by states. In the case of the preterm infant in the hospital setting, it is the obligation of hospital staff to provide evidence-based information to the mother in a manner that she can understand so that she can make an informed decision about whether to supply her milk or not and whether to continue by transitioning to breastfeeding when the infant is ready. It is also the obligation of the individuals controlling the feeding not to violate the right to food and to feed the infant adequate amounts of appropriate nutrition. Since hospital staff make the determination of how much and how often the preterm infant is fed, it is their obligation also not to violate the right to adequate food by feeding human milk on a formula-feeding schedule and in restricted volumes. The right to food and a safe, sustainable, and accessible source of nutrition helps achieve the right to the highest attainable standard of health. The healthcare system in its protection, promotion, and support of breastfeeding plays an integral part in assuring that the highest attainable standard of health is achieved by every individual, beginning prenatally. In the NICU, this ensures the best possible health outcomes for preterm infants.

WHO/UNICEF POLICIES

WHO and UNICEF, both independently and jointly, have developed a number of policy documents that help ensure the right of children to the highest attainable standard of health and the right of women to receive full and unbiased information and adequate health care so that they can make choices in the best interests of themselves and their children. There are several WHO/UNICEF policy statements that are applicable to the achievement of the highest attainable standard of health. Their contribution lies in the application of adequate food for children. Only through adequate nutrition can children develop physically and mentally, learn in school, and become contributing members of society as they grow into adults. The *Global Strategy for Infant and Young Child Feeding* (WHO/UNICEF, 2002) describes it best: "The life-long impact [of inadequate quality nutrition] includes poor school performance, reduced productivity, and impaired intellectual and social development" (p. v). The foundation for good development and health lies in breastfeeding. Although these international resolutions and declarations that protect, promote, and support breastfeeding are nonbinding, they have contributed substantially to national health policies. These are the

GOBI Initiative, the Hierarchy of Infant Feeding Choices, the International Code of Marketing of Breast-milk Substitutes (1981), the Baby-Friendly Hospital Initiative (WHO/UNICEF, 1989), and the *Global Strategy for Infant and Young Child Feeding* (WHO/UNICEF, 2002). Several of these resolutions and declarations were discussed in Chapter 15 as they relate to donor human milk banking. Kent (2006) also includes the *Innocenti Declaration on the Protection, Promotion and Support of Breastfeeding* of 1990 (principles reaffirmed in 2005) and the *Maternity Protection Convention 103* from the International Labour Organization (revised in 2000 as *ILO Convention 183*) as having roles in assuring optimal health and adequate food, the latter by protecting maternity and breastfeeding rights for working women.

The Baby-Friendly Hospital Initiative has been adapted in this book to present a 10-step model that promotes, protects, and supports breastfeeding optimally in the NICU. Two of these steps (step 6 and step 9) pertain directly to implementation of the International Code of Marketing of Breast-milk Substitutes and protect the mother from direct contact with marketing materials printed by formula companies. These steps also ensure that her baby receives only human milk unless there is a medical need for formula. Additionally, formula, fortifiers made out of bovine products, and all feeding supplies such as bottles and teats should be purchased at fair market value to avoid conflict of interest from free samples and gifts. In Chapters 13–16, banked donor human milk was discussed as an alternative to formula when a mother's own supply of milk is inadequate.

The *Global Strategy* (WHO/UNICEF, 2002) presents a plan of action in fulfilling the child's right to adequate food—access to safe and nutritious food—and thus the right to the "enjoyment of the highest attainable standard of health" as delineated in the *Convention on the Rights of the Child* (UN, 1989, p. 7, Article 24). Breastfeeding is the foundation of good health in this document. The *Global Strategy* addresses the needs of low-birth-weight infants by saying, "Breast milk is particularly important for preterm infants and the small proportion of term infants with very low birth weight; they are at increased risk of infection, long-term ill-health, and death" (WHO/UNICEF, 2002, p. 11) even in a developed country. Mothers and babies should be provided with accurate information and support from all sectors of the healthcare system. This should include skilled practical help from peer counselors and trained health workers, including lactation care providers. Specifically, support from the healthcare system as it applies to the preterm infant and the NICU optimally includes:

- Skilled counseling and help with infant and young child feeding
- Hospital routines that support the initiation and establishment of breastfeeding along the lines of the Ten Steps
- Support for continued breastfeeding
- Support for adequate intake of safe and sustainable food
- Effective therapeutic feeding of sick and malnourished infants and children (to include banked donor milk)
- Training for healthcare workers in skills necessary to assist mothers with regard to ongoing breastfeeding and milk expression

In this way, hospitals and healthcare systems, and NICUs in particular, can ensure that the basic human right of adequate food and the best health attainable for preterm infants is provided through the use of human milk and the transition to full breastfeeding.

U.S. HEALTH POLICIES

I have previously described (2008) the U.S. health policies that impact breastfeeding and have shown where they can be applied to donor human milk banking. Perhaps the most important of these health policies are those from health professional associations that set a standard of practice with their policies. The American Academy of Pediatrics (AAP) has stressed the importance of breastfeeding in the nutritional management of preterm infants (AAP, 2005). AAP states that:

> Hospitals and physicians should recommend human milk for premature and other high-risk infants either by direct breastfeeding and/or using the mother's own expressed milk. Maternal support and education on breastfeeding and milk expression should be provided from the earliest possible time. Mother–infant skin-to-skin contact and direct breastfeeding should be encouraged as early as feasible. Fortification of expressed human milk is indicated for many very low birth weight infants. Banked human milk may be a suitable feeding alternative for infants whose mothers are unable or unwilling to provide their own milk. (p. 500)

A standard of NICU care has thus been established that includes education and support for mothers. The American Breastfeeding Institute's Ten Steps model for the NICU that has been developed in this book provides a guide for NICUs to develop practice that supports this standard of care.

ETHICAL CARE IN THE NICU

I believe that most healthcare providers want to practice in an ethical manner and would be horrified if they discovered they were not doing so. Ethical practice, however, is evidence-based practice. Therefore, ethics should be questioned in situations where outdated, non–evidence-based policies and procedures are in practice. In spite of an ever-growing body of research about the care and nutrition of preterm infants, there are also many questions that remain unanswered, particularly in relation to infants who are really small and of very early gestation. Evidence from term infants or even larger and gestationally older preterm infants does not always apply. There are still ways to provide evidence-based ethical care that do not deprive infants of their basic human rights to quality nutrition and nurturant care and do not deprive mothers of their rights to breastfeed and care for the baby in every way they can. Evidence tells us we should be caring for these mothers and babies in a different way from the example given in Chapter 1.

How Ethical Principles Apply to Bonnie's Case

There are seven principles of biomedical ethics—autonomy, veracity, beneficence, nonmaleficence, confidentiality, justice, and role fidelity. **Table 17-2** gives a brief description of each principle and what it entails. What is presented next is an analysis of Bonnie's case (presented in Chapter 1) in light of each of these ethical principles; how principles were honored and how they were violated by the behavior of those providing the care for Bonnie and her son.

Autonomy

Violations of Bonnie's autonomy began in the first hospital. The clearest example of this is her inability to access a breast pump in the hospital with staff who obstructed her desires and failed to respond to her requests for help in securing a breast pump, learning how to use the pump, and finding one in the community that she could continue to use to express her milk once she was discharged. Bonnie actually had more knowledge than the postpartum staff did about breast pumps and when she should begin pumping. The lack of staff knowledge and skills prevented her from following through on her decision to express milk. Another example of violation of autonomy lies in the misinformation she was given about pumping by hospital staff. Rest and wearing a good supportive bra are irrelevant to establishing and maintaining a milk supply.

Table 17-2 Principles of Biomedical Ethics

Autonomy	The ability of a patient to make an informed decision about his/her health care. This decision is predicated on having enough information with which to make a decision and is the basis of informed consent. Autonomy means self-governance. Coercion, deceit, constraint, and duress must be absent in order for autonomy to function. Patients must also be able to understand and be competent to make a decision, and they must have the power to make the choice. In the case of children, the parents have this decision-making power. Intentionally limiting information to prejudice the patient's decision (paternalism, benevolent deception) also interferes with autonomy.
Veracity	Truthfulness. In a two-party interaction such as doctor and patient, both parties must be truthful, otherwise the patient could get inappropriate care. Withholding information or giving a false piece of information can actually cause harm or maleficence.
Beneficence	This is the obligation to promote health and well-being of a patient. If the surgery that someone has removes the bone cancer but causes paralysis, then the promotion of health and well-being was not achieved because the patient may be worse off. Quality of life decisions involve beneficence.
Nonmaleficence	This is the active avoidance of inflicting harm on a patient. It is somewhat different from beneficence in that care providers should not do something that knowingly causes harm. The physician who continually writes prescriptions for pain killers knowing that the individual really needs to go to rehab is violating nonmaleficence. He is causing harm by furthering an addiction.
Confidentiality	Patients have a right to privacy, and patient information should not be shared without consent.
Justice	In health care, this is primarily about distribution of services and scarce resources. Who receives them and who determines the distribution? Organ transplants, where there are more recipients in need of organs than available organs, are examples of a system that has been set up to determine who should get the service. It is based on need and potential benefit to the individual.
Role fidelity	Sometimes referred to as simply fidelity, this means that one practices within one's scope of practice. If someone is not licensed to perform surgery, it is out of his or her scope of practice to amputate someone's leg.

Staff of the second hospital also violated Bonnie and her son's autonomy. Bonnie's decision to express her milk was consistently disregarded by NICU staff who gave her no help and scant education. Support was provided by the baby's grandmother and the grandmother's professional colleagues. For autonomy to work in the healthcare system, mothers must be given information by staff with which to make an informed decision and staff must have the competency (knowledge and skills) to help her achieve her goals. We see this lack of competency several times as Bonnie abandons her goals when no staff member can help her. She was forced to agree to the use of bovine-based fortifiers for her milk when she realized that, even though her milk could be fortified in other ways, the staff lacked competency to do it any other way. Nurses who observed Bonnie's unsuccessful attempts to breastfeed offered no help; even after suggesting a nipple shield might help, they were unable to offer competent assistance or instruction on how to use one. Bonnie became so discouraged by the lack of help she decided to wait until her son was discharged to learn how to breastfeed at home.

Autonomy is not served when coercion or threats are implied/inferred. Coercion and threats were made in Bonnie's case when the nurse manager suggested that Bonnie was having difficulty becoming a mother and said that she had made an appointment for a counselor to interview her. The implied threat was that the baby would be taken away from her; she demanded what was best for her baby as she understood it and with the help of many support people who were experts in the fields of lactation and neonatology, but in doing so made enemies among the nursing staff who retaliated with threats. Resolution was not satisfactory because the patient advocate and the nurse manager were one and the same.

The baby's autonomous choice also was denied in that he was denied physiological stability from his mother's body through STS contact. When given a choice, babies choose STS contact/KMC and their own mother's milk.

Veracity

In the first hospital when Bonnie reports to the obstetrician and nurses that she does not use drugs her truth is ignored and dismissed. Veracity is not only telling the truth but also accepting what someone tells you as the truth until proven otherwise. In both cases, staff were very disrespectful of the truth of Bonnie's statements. When the baby speaks the truth by crying, disbelief is also seen. Veracity is again violated when Bonnie is told untruths, such as "wear a good supportive bra" and rest is more important than pumping. These statements are patently untrue.

In the second hospital, other untruths were told to Bonnie: if she drank too much milk while pumping she would make her son lactose intolerant; breastfeeding was more stressful than bottle-feeding; babies have to learn to bottle-feed before they can learn to breastfeed; breastfeeding pillows are the solutions to all breastfeeding problems; STS care/KMC was too stressful and would cause her son to get cold; babies' bones hurt if they are held too much; babies over 4 pounds are too big for STS care/KMC. These untruths come from a paucity of evidence-based information on the part of staff and indicate lack of education and competency in very basic skills sets that should be standard of care in all level 3 NICUS. Of greater concern, however, is the false reporting of the nurses when they tried to avoid responsibility for their actions and blamed others for things that had happened during their care of the baby. For example:

- No promised discussion of fortifiers occurred before they were fed to her son.
- Nurses interpreted physicians' orders for STS care/KMC as being implemented at the discretion of the nurse.
- The baby was unswaddled in the isolette because the nurse had been checking the baby's leads in one version of the story, which then changed to blaming Bonnie or a physician for taking his clothes off and leaving him uncovered.
- The nurse gave morphine instead of weaning the baby off the ventilator after LASIK surgery and said that the doctor had told her to administer morphine.
- The head circumference was misreported after placement of the cerebral reservoir.

Equally disturbing is the chaos of communication between doctors and nurses in this NICU and the blaming that went on. It would appear that the blame game then fostered an atmosphere of distrust where no one believed anybody and it was impossible to come to agreement about the development of policies such as the use of STS care/KMC. Veracity was not well served in this unit in day-to-day operations.

Beneficence

When Bonnie complained of nipple pain from pump flanges that were too small, the lactation consultant (LC) dismissed her concerns, most likely due to lack of competency on the LC's part. This did not promote Bonnie's well-being. It caused maleficence or harm because Bonnie's nipples continued to be damaged by the design and size of the pump flanges. The LC was not inflicting the harm, but by failure to remove the source of harm she was violating beneficence.

The tapping of the baby's cerebral reservoir would have been a procedure that is beneficent because it relieves fluid pressure on the brain that could cause brain damage. However, if done unnecessarily because nurses reported the head circumference incorrectly, the increased risk of infection might have outweighed the benefits.

Nonmaleficence

Active prevention of harm was not evident in the emergency room in the first hospital. The internal ultrasound most likely precipitated a speedier delivery. Maleficence is also evident when the baby was allowed to lie on the bed for minutes in the amniotic sac, and again when staff were unable to intubate the baby or care for the critically ill baby in the newborn nursery. They could not stabilize him for transport or intubate him and had to wait several hours for the tertiary transport team to arrive, stabilize the baby, and transport him. Weather conspired to make the delay even longer as helicopter transport could not be used and the ambulance had to travel several hours through driving sleet and snow to get to the first hospital and then return to the tertiary care center.

In both hospitals, emotional maleficence was precipitated by attitudes and comments from nurses and doctors. Inflicting emotional harm may be just as much a violation of nonmaleficence as inflicting physical harm: Bonnie was told that they would find out soon enough if she was a drug user. It was inflicted again when nurses referred to her carefully expressed milk as formula and when they belittled the amount of milk she got after one pumping session. Not using her colostrum was another blow, as was watching her milk being poured down the sink after too much had been thawed. Emotional harm was also inflicted when she was told that no one would help her monitor her milk supply in the NICU freezers when she couldn't visit because of weather or her job. Unfounded staff threats of involvement of child protective services also constituted maleficence.

Confidentiality

It is hard to say whether confidentiality was, in fact, violated in this case because in the NICU setting, nurses and physicians need to be talking to each other to ensure continuity of care from one shift to another. In a NICU setting, it is also common to have social services, respiratory therapists, dietitians, pharmacists, lactation consultants, and others all involved in a case. Besides the regular staff of the NICU, Bonnie's son was also being seen by specialists because of his grade IV bleed. However, the manner in which information about the case was conveyed is of concern, and although Bonnie does not say it, I think there was a great deal of behind-the-scenes negative and derogatory discussion about Bonnie and her actions going on among some staff, which then poisoned other staff attitudes about Bonnie as a person and mother. This is disrespectful and decreases the quality of care to the point that maleficence can be caused. In one phone communication to me, Bonnie reported that she had angered the nurse and she felt the nurse took it out on her son, purposely handling him very roughly while she was dressing him in Bonnie's presence. In any case, there was a prevailing attitude in this NICU that was detrimental to quality care.

Justice

Justice is about the distribution of services, and in Bonnie's case, what prevented justice from being fulfilled was lack of knowledge, skills, and competency on the part of nurses, who could help her achieve her breastfeeding goals over the long term. Bonnie received few of the services to which she should have been entitled, such as frequent lactation support and assistance.

Role Fidelity

At the first hospital, several individuals seemed to violate the principles of role fidelity and scope of practice. The ultrasound technician did an internal ultrasound despite the fact that Bonnie was showing evidence of cramping and bleeding. The diagnosis of pregnancy had already been determined. This internal exam should not have been done without the consent of the physician. Making the decision to go ahead on his/her own exceeded the scope of practice of this technician. Furthermore, no one examined Bonnie again to see if the internal ultrasound had caused her to dilate.

In the first hospital, failure to answer calls to the nurses' station for assistance verges on dereliction of duty, a different form of role fidelity violation than exceeding one's scope of practice. In this case, it is the role of the nurse to respond to the phone and to respond to requests for assistance. Ignoring these requests is abrogating the responsibilities of one's role and violating role fidelity.

In the second hospital, the biggest role fidelity violation is seen in the conflict of interest between the nurse manager's role as an advocate for her nurses and her role as a patient advocate. These two roles clashed when Bonnie and the nurses became adversaries, and the nurse manager, in supporting her nurses, could not fairly be an ombudsman for Bonnie's concerns about her treatment. Another violation of role fidelity came when the nurse gave morphine in contradiction to the physician's desire to wean the baby off the ventilator after eye surgery.

CONCLUSIONS

This chapter has dealt with the ethical and human rights violations that Bonnie and many other parents of infants in the NICU experience routinely as part of their infants' care. Although I have focused on a single case here, similar stories have been told to me over the years of my work in this field. Many of them are too painful to put in writing even years later. What makes Bonnie's case unique is that she was able to put it in writing and actually sent a letter describing her experiences to the CEO of the hospital where the level 3 NICU was located. Reaction from administration was immediate and positive on her behalf, and while the hospital cannot rectify the wrongs done to Bonnie and her son, they are trying to ensure that practices and policies change so that other mothers will not go through similar experiences. This means changing an entire climate—changing attitudes and beliefs and changing policies and practices. "The way we've always done it" is no longer adequate or ethical and violates basic human rights.

This entire book is intended to provide hospital staff with model breastfeeding policies that can be adapted for a NICU/SCN. By having evidence-based policies and procedures in place, NICUs may be able to prevent ethical and human rights violations from occurring. Practicing in an evidence-based manner also can prevent litigation. Policies need to be supportive of the use of human milk and transitioning to breastfeeding (Chapter 3, step 1). Once policies and procedures are in place, staff should be adequately trained in implementing the policies. Beyond just knowing the literature and principles behind the policies, they also need to have the competency skills that will enable them to support mothers in expressing their milk, practicing STS contact/KMC, and transitioning to breastfeeding so that the mother gains confidence and competence in her ability to mother the infant (Chapter 4, step 2). Benefits of human milk for preterm infants needs to be discussed in a proactive manner by all staff, with the neonatologist taking the lead in expressing how important a mother's milk is for her infant (Chapter 5, step 3). Helping mothers to become mothers by decreasing separation and allowing them to have more of a role in caring for their infants will decrease emotional stress and depression and help mothers succeed at milk expression. Strategies for improving bonding such as the use of touch are seen as improving the mother's psychological frame of mind and the way she interacts with her infant, and also improving infant outcomes (Chapter 6, step 4). Chapter 7 (step 5) assists staff in understanding the principles of establishing and maintaining a milk supply through mechanical or manual expression. Daily encouragement and praise are needed to make it possible for many mothers to continue this effort over a long period of time. Storage and handling of milk also requires separate policies and procedures, and recommendations for collection, storage, and handling of human milk in the NICU are provided. Giving preterm infants only human milk unless formula is medically indicated is the goal for a standard of care (Chapter 8, step 6). Staff should understand the implications of a formula-feeding model and how this impacts achievement of the goal. NICU staff also need to be able to talk to mothers about the use of banked donor human milk as an alternative to formula (see also Chapters 13–16) and teach them how to safely prepare formula and store it if they choose to formula feed. These are part of the skill set and competencies that every nurse should have in the NICU (Chapter 8, step 6). Skill sets for facilitating skin-to-skin care for mothers and preterm infants are vital to the health and well-being of both the mother and the infant, and continuous STS care/KMC should be firmly established as a standard operating procedure for most preterm infants, whether or not they are breastfed (Chapter 9, step 7). Knowing that infants can learn how to breastfeed and transfer milk at the breast at much earlier ages than previously thought, policies that begin to transition preterm infants to the breast early should be in place. This requires skills and technical knowledge on the part of nurses so that they can assist the mother effectively and provide encouragement along the way as the infant begins to develop these skills (Chapter 10, step 8). There should be policies and procedures that clearly outline for staff behaviors that are considered conflicts of interest with commercial entities. When staff are obligated to a commercial company through a gift arrangement, breastfeeding support cannot be effective (Chapter 11, step 9). Finally, to effectively increase use of human milk/breastfeeding initiation and duration rates, support for breastfeeding needs to be provided effectively through peers and professionals in a peripartum setting, in the NICU and postdischarge (Chapter 12, step 10).

Cadwell and Turner-Maffei (2009) cite a study by Raisler (2000) in which low-income mothers were interviewed about their experiences being helped to breastfeed. **Table 17-3** summarizes what was helpful and what was not helpful. Most of the unhelpful strategies could be seen in play in Bonnie's situation. Key elements to breastfeeding success for women with healthy, term infants are freedom to decide whether or not to breastfeed based on accurate information; psychosocial support during labor; consistency of information across the postpartum stay; individualized feeding assessment and hands-off teaching when problems arise; and adequate support both emotionally and physically that is also unhurried and indicative

Table 17-3 Help with Breastfeeding: What Works; What Doesn't

Care providers were *helpful* when they:	Care providers were *unhelpful* when they:
• Knew correct information	• Missed opportunities to discuss breastfeeding
• Established supportive personal relationships	• Gave misinformation
• Referred women to a breastfeeding specialist for problems	• Encouraged formula supplementation
• Showed enthusiasm for breastfeeding	• Provided perfunctory or routine breastfeeding care
• Facilitated breastfeeding through concrete interaction during the childbearing period	• Were hard to contact when problems arose

Source: Cadwell & Turner-Maffei, 2009, p. 142. Used with permission.

that the person supporting the mother really cares. Having these elements present in the NICU would have also helped Bonnie to achieve her goals of exclusive breastmilk and a transition to breastfeeding. Had these elements been in place, along with policies and practices supportive of breastfeeding success similar to those in this book, continuity of care would have been achieved, and Bonnie's rights to ethical and humane care would have been realized.

REFERENCES

American Academy of Pediatrics, Section on Breastfeeding (AAP). (2005). Breastfeeding and the use of human milk. *Pediatrics, 115*(2), 496–506.

Arnold, L. D. W. (2006a). The ethics of donor human milk banking. *Breastfeeding Medicine, 1*(1), 3–13.

Arnold, L. D. W. (2006b). Global health policies that support the use of banked donor human milk: A human rights issue. *International Breastfeeding Journal, 1*, 26.

Arnold, L. D. W. (2008). U.S. health policy and access to banked donor human milk. *Breastfeeding Medicine, 3*(4), 221–229.

Bar-Yam, N. (2003). Breastfeeding and human rights: Is there a right to breastfeed? Is there a right to be breastfed? *Journal of Human Lactation, 19*(4), 357–361.

Bar-Yam, N. (2004). Author's response to "Response to breastfeeding and human rights" [Letter to the editor]. *Journal of Human Lactation, 20*(2), 148.

Cadwell, K., & Turner-Maffei, C. (2009). *Continuity of care in breastfeeding: Best practices in the maternity setting*. Sudbury, MA: Jones and Bartlett.

Kent, G. (2004). Response to "breastfeeding and human rights." [Letter to the editor]. *Journal of Human Lactation, 20*(2), 146–147.

Kent, G. (2006). Child feeding and human rights. *International Breastfeeding Journal, 1*(27), 1–27.

Merriam-Webster's collegiate dictionary (10th ed.). (1998). Springfield, MA: Merriam-Webster, Inc.

Raisler, J. (2000). Against the odds: Breastfeeding experiences of low income mothers. *Journal of Midwifery and Women's Health, 45*(3), 253–263.

United Nations (UN). (1948). *Universal declaration of human rights.* Retrieved May 12, 2009, from http://www.un.org/en/documents/udhr/index.shtml

United Nations (UN). (1966). *International covenant on economic, social and cultural rights.* Retrieved May 12, 2009, from http://www2.ohchr.org/english/law/pdf/cescr.pdf

United Nations (UN). (1979). *Convention on the elimination of all forms of discrimination against women.* Retrieved May 12, 2009, from http://www2.ohchr.org/english/law/cedaw.pdf

United Nations (UN). (1989). *Convention on the rights of the child.* Retrieved May 12, 2009, from http://www2.ohchr.org/english/law/pdf/crc.pdf

United Nations (UN). (1999). *The right to adequate food. Substantive issues arising in the implementation of the international covenant on economic, social and cultural rights: General comment 12.* Retrieved May 12, 2009, from http://www.unhchr.ch/tbs/doc.nsf/MasterFrameView/3d02758c707031d58025677f003b73b9?Opendocument

Vohr, B., Poindexter, B., Dusick, A., McKinley, L., Higgins, R., Langer, J., et al. (2008). Persistent beneficial effects of breast milk ingested in the neonatal intensive care unit on outcomes of extremely low birth weight infants at 30 months of age. *Pediatrics, 120*(4), e953–e959.

Vohr, B., Poindexter, B., Dusick, A., McKinley, L., Wright, L., Langer, J., et al. (2006). Beneficial effects of breast milk in the neonatal intensive care unit on the developmental outcome of extremely low birth weight infants at 18 months of age. *Pediatrics, 118*(1), e115–e123.

World Health Organization/UNICEF (WHO). (1989). *Protecting, promoting and supporting breast-feeding: The special role of maternity services*. Geneva, Switzerland: Author.

World Health Organization/UNICEF (WHO). (2002). *Global strategy for infant and young child feeding*. Geneva, Switzerland: Author.

Index

Boxes, figures, and tables are indicated by b, f, and t following the page number.

C

D

I

Q

R

T

U

Z